Clinical Advances in Arthroplasty

Clinical Advances in Arthroplasty

Editor: Matthew Glenn

AMERICAN
MEDICAL PUBLISHERS
www.americanmedicalpublishers.com

AMERICAN
MEDICAL PUBLISHERS
www.americanmedicalpublishers.com

Cataloging-in-Publication Data

Clinical advances in arthroplasty / edited by Matthew Glenn.
p. cm.
Includes bibliographical references and index.
ISBN 978-1-63927-391-1
1. Arthroplasty. 2. Orthopedic surgery. 3. Joints--Surgery. 4. Surgery, Plastic. I. Glenn, Matthew.
RD686 .A78 2022
617.472 059 7--dc23

American Medical Publishers,
41 Flatbush Avenue,
1st Floor, New York,
NY 11217, USA

ISBN 978-1-63927-391-1 (Hardback)

Contents

Preface

Every book is initially just a concept; it takes months of research and hard work to give it the final shape in which the readers receive it. In its early stages, this book also went through rigorous reviewing. The notable contributions made by experts from across the globe were first molded into patterned chapters and then arranged in a sensibly sequential manner to bring out the best results.

Arthroplasty is a surgical procedure within the domain of orthopedics. In this procedure, the articular surface of a musculoskeletal joint is replaced, remodeled or realigned by osteotomy. The aim of arthroplasty is to relieve pain and restore function to the joint after damage by arthritis or some other type of trauma. The most successful and common form of arthroplasty is the joint replacement arthroplasty. Other types of arthroplasty include interpositional arthroplasty, excisional arthroplasty, resurfacing arthroplasty, mold arthroplasty, etc. However, arthroplasty can cause various complications, such as deep vein thrombosis, infection, bleeding and periprosthetic fracture. The prosthesis selected in arthroplasty must be non-toxic yet resistant, compatible and durable. The technology has been improved in the recent years with a porous-coated prosthesis which helps in bonding to the body. This book strives to provide a fair idea about this discipline and to help develop a better understanding of the latest advances within this field. It consists of contributions made by international experts. This book is a vital tool for all researching or studying arthroplasty as it gives incredible insights into emerging trends and concepts.

It has been my immense pleasure to be a part of this project and to contribute my years of learning in such a meaningful form. I would like to take this opportunity to thank all the people who have been associated with the completion of this book at any step.

Editor

1

Tranexamic acid in total shoulder arthroplasty and reverse shoulder arthroplasty

Liang-Tseng Kuo[1,2,3], Wei-Hsiu Hsu[1,4], Ching-Chi Chi[2,4,5*†] and Jae Chul Yoo[6*†]

Abstract

Background: The effects of tranexamic acid (TXA) in the setting of shoulder arthroplasty are unclear. The objective of this study was to examine the effects of TXA in reducing the need for blood transfusions and blood loss in patients undergoing primary total shoulder arthroplasty (TSA) and reverse total shoulder arthroplasty (RTSA).

Methods: We conducted a systematic review and meta-analysis of randomized controlled trials (RCTs) and retrospective cohort studies (RCS) that compared outcomes of patients who did and did not receive TXA during TSA or RTSA. We searched Cochrane Central Register of Controlled Trials, EMBASE, and MEDLINE for relevant studies. We assessed the risk of bias of the included studies and calculated pooled risk estimates. The primary outcome was transfusion rate, and secondary outcomes were changes in hemoglobin, estimated total blood loss (ETBL), blood loss via drainage, operative time, hospital stay, overall complications, and thromboembolic events.

Results: We identified 3 RCTs and 3 RCS including 677 patients with 680 shoulders (343 TXA and 337 non-TXA). The random-effects model meta-analysis showed that TXA group had a lower transfusion rate (risk ratio (RR) 0.34, 95% CI 0.14 to 0.79), less change in hemoglobin (mean difference (MD) -0.64 g/dl, 95% CI -0.81 to − 0.46), and reduced ETBL (MD -249.24 ml, 95% CI -338.74 to − 159.74). In patients with RTSA, the TXA group had a lower transfusion rate (RR 0.28, 95% CI 0.14 to 0.79), less ETBL (MD -249.15 ml, 95% CI -426.60 to − 71.70), less change in hemoglobin (MD − 0.64 g/dl, 95% CI -0.86 to − 0.42), and less blood loss via drainage (MD − 84.56 ml, 95% CI -145.72.14 to − 23.39) than non-TXA group.

Conclusions: The use of TXA in primary shoulder arthroplasty appears safe, and can reduce transfusion rate, changes in hemoglobin, and perioperative total blood loss, especially in patients with RTSA.
Level of Evidence: Systematic Review and meta-analysis, III.

Keywords: Total shoulder arthroplasty, Reverse total shoulder arthroplasty, Tranexamic acid, Blood loss, Transfusion

* Correspondence: chingchi@cgmh.org.tw; chingchichi@gmail.com; shoulderyoo@gmail.com
†Equal contributors
[2]Centre for Evidence-Based Medicine, Chang Gung Memorial Hospital, Chiayi, Taiwan
[6]Department of Orthopedic Surgery, College of Medicine, Samsung Medical Center, Sungkyunkwan University School of Medicine, 81 Irwon-ro, Gangnam-gu, Seoul 135-710, Republic of Korea
Full list of author information is available at the end of the article

Background

With improvements in implant design and surgical techniques, total shoulder arthroplasty (TSA) and reverse total shoulder arthroplasty (RTSA) are gaining popularity and are widely indicated for various shoulder conditions including end-stage shoulder arthropathy, cuff tear arthropathy, traumatic shoulder injuries, tumors, and failure of prior arthroplasty. However, shoulder arthroplasty, including both TSA and RTSA, is associated with a considerable risk of perioperative blood loss, and a reported allogeneic blood transfusion rate ranging from 4.3% to 43% [1–7]. The risk factors for requiring a transfusion after shoulder arthroplasty include old age, female sex, preoperative anemia, ischemic heart disease, and reverse shoulder replacement [2–4, 6–8].

The complications of blood transfusions include allergic reactions, immunosuppression, infection, and transfusion-related cardiopulmonary injury [9, 10]. A previous study of a healthcare database reported that patients who received a perioperative blood transfusion had a higher risk of medical complications including myocardial infarction, pneumonia, sepsis, and cerebrovascular accidents, as well as venous thromboembolic events and surgical complications including periprosthetic infections, periprosthetic fractures, and mechanical complications [11]. Though sicker patients that are more likely to require transfusions are also more likely to have complications mentioned above such as MI, pneumonia, stroke, etc. It is not likely the transfusion itself that causes these complications.

Many methods are available to reduce perioperative blood loss, including hypotensive anesthesia, hemodilution, autologous blood transfusion, reinfusion drainage, and the use of intravenous or topical tranexamic acid (TXA) [12, 13]. TXA interferes with the process of fibrinolysis and thereby reduces perioperative blood loss and the need for a transfusion [14]. Previous systematic reviews and meta-analyses have shown that the use of TXA in total knee arthroplasty and total hip arthroplasty can reduce blood loss and blood transfusion rates without increasing venous thromboembolism or other complications [15–18]. However, even though a few studies have investigated the use of TXA in shoulder arthroplasty, its effectiveness remains unclear [19, 20]. To date, few meta-analysis of randomized controlled trials (RCTs) and retrospective cohort studies (RCS) has investigated the effects of TXA in TSA [21, 22]. Even though more current studies on this issue have been published recently [23, 24], systematic evaluations of the latest evidence on the use of TXA in shoulder arthroplasty, and especially in RTSA, are lacking. Therefore, to comprehensively examine the effects of TXA in shoulder arthroplasty, we conducted this systematic review and meta-analysis to evaluate outcomes including transfusion rate, total blood loss, changes in postoperative hemoglobin (Hb), operative time, hospital stay and thromboembolic events. Our hypothesis is that TXA can reduce allogenic blood transfusion rate and blood loss effectively in patients with shoulder arthroplasty.

Methods

Data source and search strategy

We searched the Cochrane Central Register of Controlled Trials (CENTRAL), EMBASE, and MEDLINE from inception to August 15th, 2017 for RCTs and RCS that compared surgical outcomes in patients who did and did not receive TXA during TSA or RTSA. We also checked the references of the included studies for potentially relevant studies. There were no language restrictions.

The key words used in the search included "tranexamic acid", "total shoulder arthroplasty", and "reverse total shoulder arthroplasty". Search details are shown in the supplementary document (see Additional file 1: Appendix 1). We also searched the U.S. National Institutes of Health trials registry (http://clinicaltrials.gov). In addition, we contacted experts in this field for relevant ongoing trials or unpublished studies.

Selection criteria

Studies were included if they met the following criteria: (1) they were designed as a RCT or RCS; and (2) they compared the outcomes in patients who did and did not receive TXA during TSA or RTSA. There were no restrictions on the route of TXA administration. Two authors (LTK and CCC) independently checked the citations identified from the searches against the inclusion criteria.

Data extraction and risk of bias assessment

Two authors (LTK and WHH) independently extracted the data from the included trials using a formal data extraction sheet. The items were as follows: first author, year of publication, diagnosis, study design, sample size, participant characteristics (e.g., age and sex), the regimen of TXA (dose and route), and the operative details such as the prosthesis type and surgical approach. Outcome data including operative time (minutes), hospital stay (days), blood loss through an intra-articular drain (ml), estimated blood loss (ml), changes in postoperative Hb (g/dl), transfusion rate and complications including overall and thromboembolic events were also extracted. The third author (CCC) arbitrated in cases where LTK and WHH could not agree.

LTK and WHH independently assessed the risk of bias of the included studies, and CCC resolved differences in opinions. The Cochrane Collaboration's tool was used to evaluate the risk of bias of the included

RCTs. The Cochrane risk of bias tool included the following domains on biased estimates of intervention effects: randomization sequence, allocation concealment, performance bias (blinding of patients and personnel), detection bias (blinding of outcome assessors), attrition bias (incomplete outcome data), selective reporting, and other biases [25, 26]. For each domain, a high, low, or unclear risk of bias was judged per the quality of the RCT [25]. The Newcastle-Ottawa Scale was applied to assess the bias of the included RCS [27].

The primary outcome was blood transfusion rate. The secondary outcomes included estimated total blood loss, changes in postoperative Hb (g/dl), blood loss via the drain (ml), operative time (minutes), hospital stay (days), and thromboembolic and overall complications.

Statistical analysis

Quantitative analysis was performed for blood loss via drainage, estimated total blood loss, changes in postoperative Hb, operative time, and hospital stay, for which continuous data were presented as mean difference (MD) with a 95% confidence interval (CI). Dichotomous data including transfusion rate, overall complications, and thrombotic complications were reported as risk ratio (RR) with a 95% CI. We examined between-study variance using the tau-square (τ 2) statistic [26]. χ^2 and I^2 statistics were used for statistical heterogeneity, and significance was set at $P <$ 0.10. I^2 values of 0–24.9%, 25–49.9%, 50–74.9%, and 75–100% were assigned as none, low, moderate, and high heterogeneity, respectively [28, 29]. We performed a random-effects model meta-analysis for all outcomes, because we expected clinical heterogeneity across the included RCTs and RCS [30]. For continuous data, if the standard deviation (SD) was not reported, we estimated the mean and variance from the reported median, range, and sample size as previously reported [31]. When the SD and range were not available, variance was estimated from the P value in the t test [26]. A forest plot was used to summarize the results. Review Manager 5.3 (The Nordic Cochrane Centre, The Cochrane Collaboration, 2014) was used for meta-analysis.

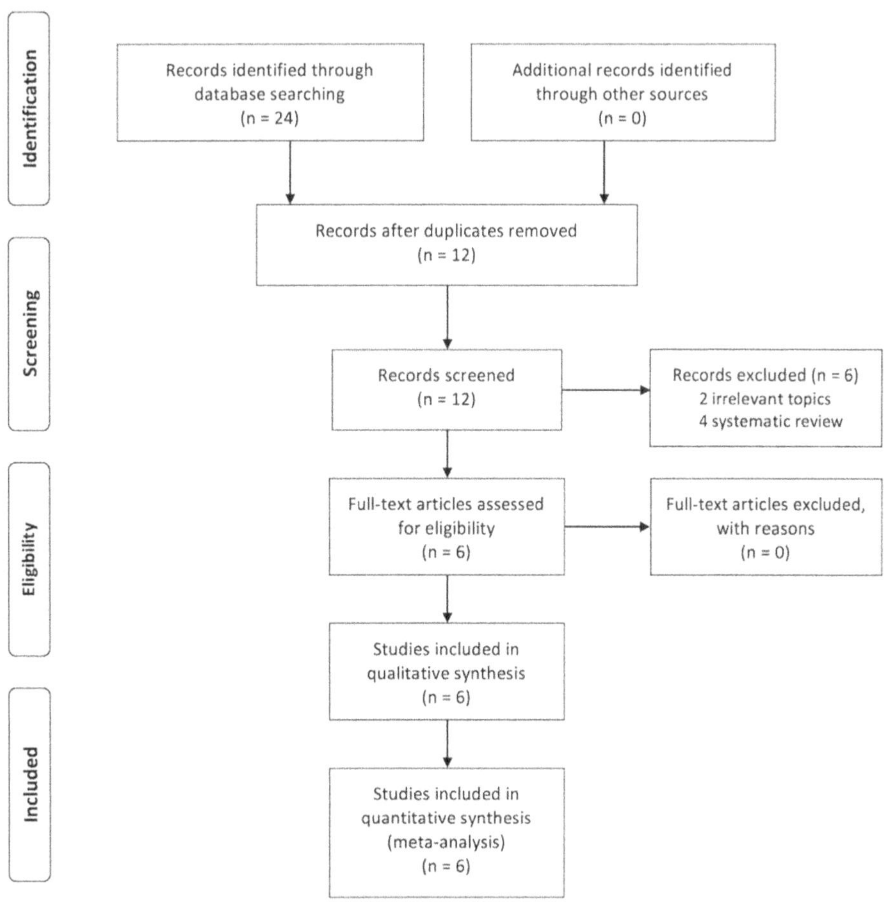

Fig. 1 PRISMA 2009 (Preferred Reporting Items for Systematic Reviews and Meta-Analyses) flow diagram of the study

Table 1 Characteristics of the included studies

Author	Year	Patients' diagnosis	Surgery	Study design	Enrolled sample number (M/F)	Average age, years	Outcome measurement	Quality assessment
Gillespie [20]	2015	OA	TSA 44 RTSA 67	Randomized controlled trial	TXA 56 (27/29) Placebo 55 (22/33)	TXA: 67.59 Placebo:66.45	Blood loss via drainage, Hb change, ETBL, transfusions, complications	Detail shown in Fig. 2
Pauzenberger [20]	2017	Not mentioned	TSA 26 RTSA 28	Randomized controlled trial	TXA 27(20/7) Placebo 27(18/9)	TXA: 70.3 ± 9.3 Placebo:71.3 ± 7.9	Blood loss via drainage, Hb/Hct change, ETBL, haematoma, complications	Detail shown in Fig. 2
Vara [34]	2017	Massive rotator cuff deficiency ± glenohumeral arthrosis	RTSA 102	Randomized controlled trial	TXA 53(20/33) Placebo 49(22/27)	TXA: 67 ± 9 Placebo:66 ± 9	Blood loss via drainage, Hb change, ETBL, operation time, hospital stay, transfusions, complications	Detail shown in Fig. 2
Abildgaard [33]	2016	TSA:1 ON and 7 OA RTSA:45 CTA, 34 massive cuff tear, 1 ON, 1RA, 11OA, and 2 fractures	TSA 77 RTSA 94	Retrospective cohort study	TXA 77 (49/28) Placebo 94 (51/43)	TSA: TXA: 70 (53–87) Placebo:71 (58–87) RTSA TXA: 74 (54–90) Placebo: 76(54–89)	Blood loss via drainage, Hb/Hct change, ETBL, transfusions, complications	9[a]
Friedman [19]	2016	Not mentioned	TSA 97 RTSA 97	Retrospective cohort study	TXA 106 (46/60) Placebo 88 (33/55)	not mentioned	Hb/Hct, recover room time, operation time, hospital stay, transfusions, complications	8[a]
Kim [24]	2017	CTA	RTSA 48	Retrospective cohort study	TXA 24 (3/21) Placebo 24 (6/18)	TXA: 73.2 ± 4.4 Placebo: 74.2 ± 4.4	Hb/Hct change, operation time, blood loss via drainage	8[a]

CTA Cuff tear arthropathy; *ETBL* Estimated total blood loss; *F* Female; *Hb* Hemoglobin; *Hct* Hematocrit; *M* Male; *OA* Osteoarthritis; *ON* Osteonecrosis; *RA* Rheumatoid arthritis; *RTSA* Reverse total shoulder arthroplasty; *TSA* Total shoulder arthroplasty; *TXA* Tranexamic acid

[a]Quality scores derived from the Newcastle-Ottawa Scale

Subgroup analysis

If data were available, we planned to perform subgroups analysis including:

(1) RCTs alone;
(2) Different routes of TXA administration: intravenous (IV) versus topical;
(3) RTSA or TSA only.

Results

The details of the study selection process are presented in Fig. 1 [32]. Our search of the MEDLINE, EMBASE, and CENTRAL databases returned 24 published studies. No additional studies were identified from the references of the included studies. After excluding 12 duplicates and 6 studies (two irrelevant topics and four systematic reviews), we finally included the following six studies in this meta-analysis: Abildgaard et al. [33], Friedman et al. [19], Gillespie et al. [20], Kim et al. [24], Pauzenberger et al. [23], and Vara et al. [34].

Study characteristics and patient populations

The included trials were published between 2015 and 2017 (Table 1). The sample sizes ranged from 48 to 194, with a total 677 patients (680 shoulders, 343 in the TXA group and 337 in the non-TXA group). Three included studies [20, 23, 34] were RCTs that prospectively compared outcomes, and the other three RCS [19, 24, 33] compared results using retrospective analysis (Table 1). Further perioperative characteristics of the included studies are described in Table 2.

Risk of bias of the included studies

Data on the risk of bias of the six studies included in the meta-analysis are summarized in Table 1 and Fig. 2. The three RCS [19, 24, 33] were of high quality (Newcastle-Ottawa Scale score > 7). For the risk of bias of the RCTs, random sequence generation and allocation concealment were not described in two trials [20, 34], and therefore the risk of bias was rated as being unclear. Blinding of the surgeon was not explicitly mentioned in one trial [23], which was therefore also rated as having an unclear risk of bias. Other items with regards to the risk of bias were rated as low risk when appraised using the Cochrane Collaboration's tool.

Outcomes

Summaries of the findings and subgroup analysis are shown in Table 3.

Table 2 Perioperative details of the included studies

Author	Year	Intervention	Prosthesis properties	Approach	Transfusion protocol	Thromboprophylaxis
Gillespie [20]	2015	TXA: 2 g in 100 ml NS for 5 min Placebo: 100 ml NS for 5 min	N/S	DP	1) Hb < 7.0 g/dl 2) 7.1 g/dl < Hb < 9.0 g/dl + symptoms	N/S
Pauzenberger [23]	2017	TXA: 1 g TXA intravenously in 100 ml NS, 2 doses Placebo: 100 ml NS, 2 doses	TSA (Eclipse; Arthrex Inc., Naples, Florida) RTSA (Delta Xtend; DePuy Synthes, Warsaw, Indiana)	DP	1) Hb < 8 g/dl 2) 8 g/dl < Hb < 10 g/dl + symptoms	Chemical prophylaxis (subcutaneous 40 mg of enoxaparin sodium + aspirin)
Vara [34]	2017	TXA: 10 mg/kg IV, 1st dose within 60 mins before surgery, 2nd dose at wound closure Placebo: NS	102 Non-cemented RTSA (79 Zimmer; 11 DePuy; 4 Biomet; 2 Encore,)	DP	1) Hb < 7 g/dl 2) 7 g/dl < Hb < 9 g/dl + symptoms	Chemical prophylaxis (subcutaneous heparin + oral aspirin) Mechanical prophylaxis (compression stockings)
Abildgaard [33]	2016	TXA: 1 g IV at skin preparation Placebo: no TXA	TSA (Bigliani/ Flatow Anatomical Total Shoulder; Zimmer, Warsaw, IN, USA) RTSA (Trabecular Metal Inverse/Reverse Total Shoulder, Zimmer)	DP	1) Hb < 7 g/dl 2) 7 g/dl < Hb < 9 g/dl + symptoms	Chemical prophylaxis was not routinely used postoperatively
Friedman [19]	2016	TXA: 20 mg/kg IV at skin preparation Placebo: no TXA	RTSA: cemented; brand N/S TSA: 90% non-cemented;	N/S	N/S	N/S
Kim [24]	2017	TXA: 500 mg IV	25 DJO Reverse Shoulder Prosthesis; 16 Tornier reverse shoulder prosthesis; 7 Biomet Comprehensive Reverse Total Shoulder Replacement	DP	No absolute guideline	N/S

DP Deltopectoral approach; *Hb* Hemoglobin; *IV* Intravenous; *NS* Normal saline; *N/S* Not shown; *RTSA* Reverse total shoulder arthroplasty; *TSA* Total shoulder arthroplasty; *TXA* Tranexamic acid

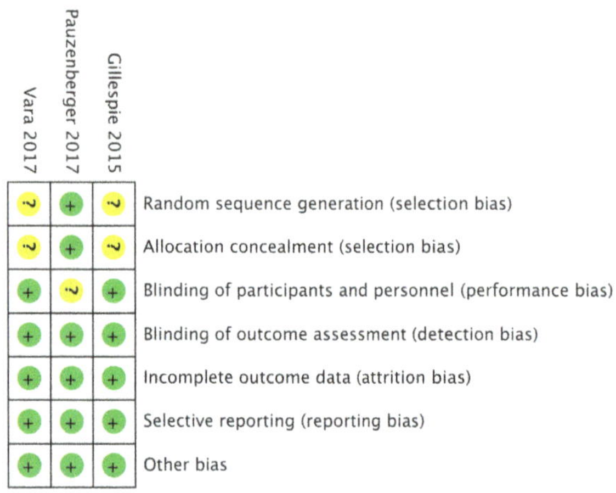

Fig. 2 Risk of bias summary. Authors' judgments about the risk of each bias item for each included study. "+" represents low risk of bias; "?" represents unclear risk of bias; "–" represents high risk of bias

Allogenic blood transfusion rate

Five included studies [19, 20, 23, 33, 34] reported the blood transfusion rate in the TXA and non-TXA groups. The risk of the need for a blood transfusion was lower in the TXA group compared to the non-TXA group (7/319 vs. 20/313, RR 0.34, 95% CI 0.14–0.79; $P = 0.01$; $I^2 = 0\%$; Fig. 3a).

Estimated total blood loss

Of the included studies, three compared estimated blood loss in the two groups (157 patients in the TXA group vs. 170 patients in the non-TXA group) [23, 33, 34]. The pooled MD for estimated blood loss was − 249.24 ml (95% CI -338.74 to − 159.74 ml; $P < 0.00001$; $I^2 = 20\%$; Fig. 4a), indicating that the post-operative estimated blood loss was 249.24 ml lower in the TXA group compared to the non-TXA group.

Table 3 Summary of findings of shoulder arthroplasty

Outcomes	N	Patients (TXA/non-TXA)	Overall effect		Heterogeneity	
			RR or MD (95% CI)	*P*	I^2	*P*
Rate of blood transfusion						
All included studies	5	319/313	0.34 [0.14, 0.79]	0.02	0%	0.42
Randomized controlled trials	3	136/131	0.23 [0.07, 0.77]	0.01	NA	NA
RTSA	4	141/150	0.28 [0.10, 0.83]	0.02	0%	0.47
Estimated total blood loss (ml)						
All included studies	3	157/170	-249.24 [−338.74, −159.74]	< 0.00001	20%	0.29
Randomized controlled trials	2	80/76	− 357.92 [− 504.25, −211.59]	< 0.00001	0%	0.87
RTSA	2	95/101	−249.15 [−426.60, −71.70]	0.006	64%	0.10
Hb change within 48 h after surgery (g/dl)[a]						
All included studies	5	316/310	−0.64 [− 0.81, − 0.46]	0.009	0%	0.72
Randomized controlled trials	2	109/104	−0.65 [− 1.14, − 0.16]	< 0.00001	42%	0.19
RTSA	4	153/158	−0.64 [− 0.86, − 0.42]	< 0.0001	0%	0.66
IV TXA	5	260/255	−0.60 [− 0.79, − 0.41]	< 0.0001	0%	0.79
Topical TXA	1	56/55	−0.90 [− 1.42, − 0.38]	0.0007	NA	NA
Blood loss via drainage within 48 h after surgery (ml)[a]						
All included studies	4	160/155	−95.41 [−139.86, − 50.96]	< 0.001	65%	0.04
Randomized controlled trials	3	136/131	−105.78 [− 159.88, −51.68]	0.001	71%	0.03
RTSA	3	111/106	−84.56 [−145.72, −23.39]	0.007	80%	0.007
IV TXA	3	104/100	−110.04 [− 159.03, −61.06]	< 0.0001	65%	0.04
Topical TXA	1	56/55	−60.00 [−103.29, − 16.71]	0.007	NA	NA
Operation time (min)	3	183/161	−1.08 [−4.91, 2.74]	0.58	0%	0.42
Hospital stay (day)	2	159/137	− 0.04 [− 0.45, 0.37]	0.84	75%	0.05
Overall complications	6	343/337	0.44 [0.07, 2.96]	0.40	0%	0.95
Thromboembolic events	6	343/337	0.31 [0.01, 7.40]	0.47	NA	NA

CI Confidence interval; *Hb* Hemoglobin; *MD* Mean difference; *N* Number of studies; *NA* Not applicable; *RTSA* Reverse total shoulder arthroplasty; *TXA* Tranexamic acid

[a]Data from Gillespie 2015 and Friedman 2017 were estimated from median and range

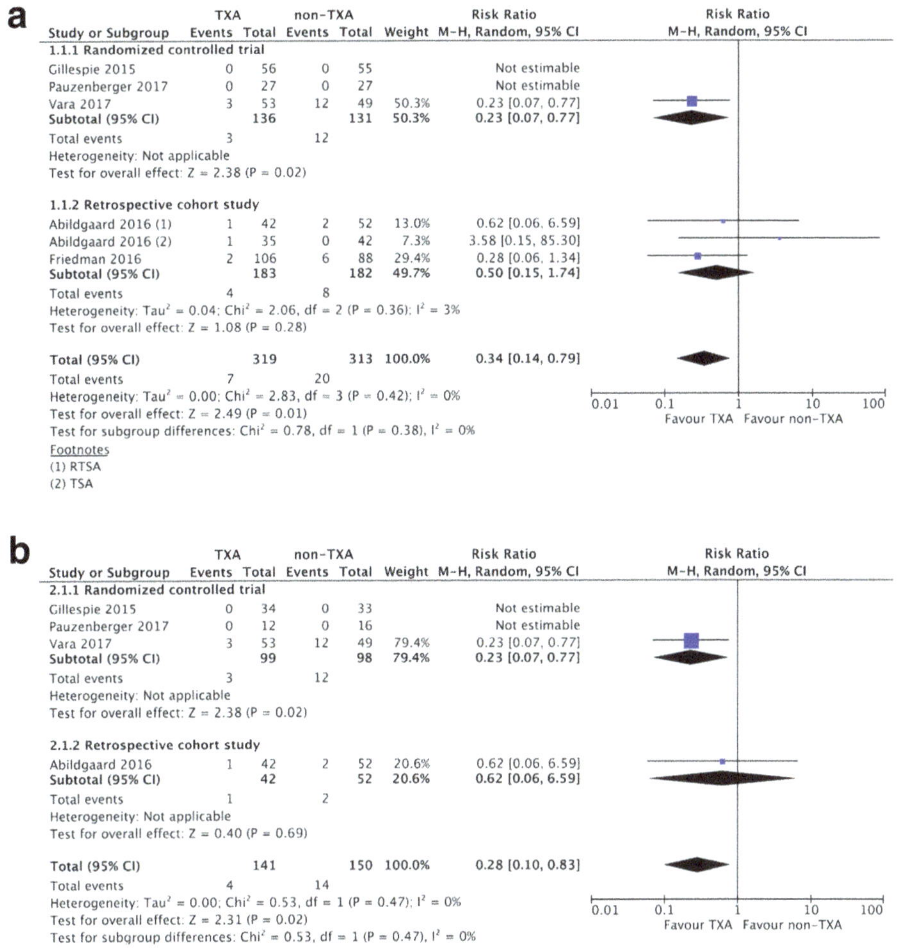

Fig. 3 Forest plot and meta-analysis of the rate of blood transfusion. **a** All included studies (**b**) RTSA group

Changes in Hb (within 48 h after surgery)

Five studies reported changes in Hb within 48 h after surgery [19, 20, 24, 33, 34], with a pooled MD of – 0.64 g/dl (95% CI -0.81 to – 0.46 g/dl; $P <$ 0.00001; $I^2 = 0\%$; Fig. 5a). This indicated that the postoperative decrease in Hb was 0.64 g/dl lower in the TXA group compared to the non-TXA group.

Blood loss via drainage (within 48 h after surgery)

Three RCTs [20, 23, 34] and one RCS [24] compared blood loss in drainage in the TXA and the non-TXA groups, which consisted of 160 and 155 patients, respectively. The pooled MD of blood loss via drainage was – 95.41 ml (95% CI -139.86 to – 50.96 ml; $P = 0.04$; $I^2 = 65\%$; Fig. 6a), indicating that postoperative blood loss via drainage was 95.41 ml lower in the TXA group within 48 h after surgery.

Operative time and hospital stay

Of the included studies, three compared operative time between the two groups [19, 24, 34]. The pooled data showed that there was no significant difference between the two groups (MD – 1.08 min, 95% CI -4.91 to 2.74 min; $P = 0.58$; $I^2 = 0\%$; Fig. 7). Two studies compared the hospital stay between the two groups [19, 34], and the pooled data indicated that there was no significant difference regarding hospital stay between the two groups (MD – 0.04 days, 95% CI -0.45 to 0.37 days; $P = 0.84$; $I^2 = 75\%$; Fig. 8).

Overall complications and thromboembolic events

All six included studies reported data on the proportion of patients who developed complications and thromboembolic events during the study period. There were no significant differences in overall complications or thromboembolic events between the TXA and the non-TXA groups (overall complications: 1/343 vs. 3/337, RR 0.44, 95% CI 0.07 to 2.96; $P = 0.95$.; $I^2 = 0\%$; Fig. 9a; thromboembolic events: 0/343 vs. 1/337, RR 0.31, 95% CI 0.01 to 7.40; $P = 0.47$; Fig. 9b).

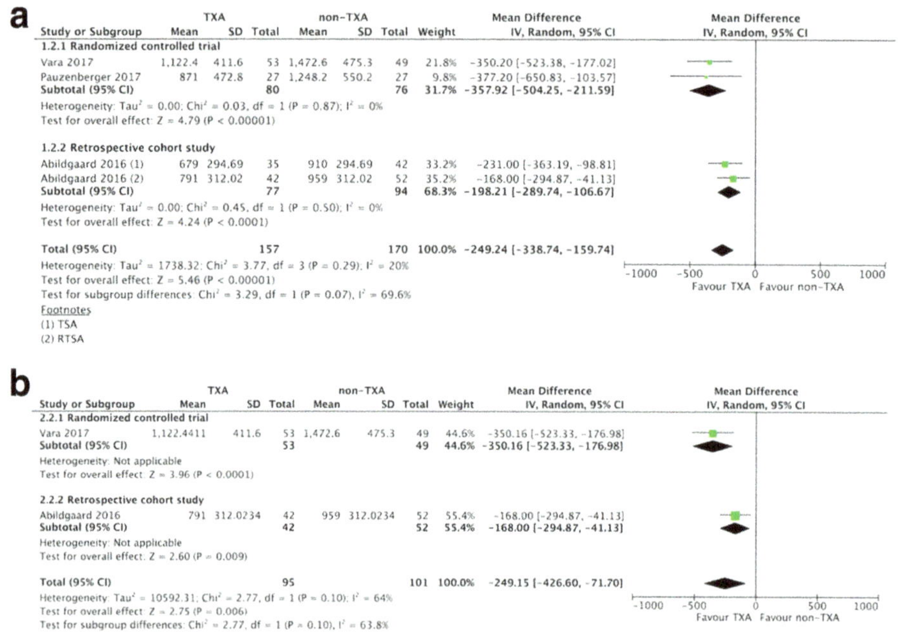

Fig. 4 Forest plot and meta-analysis of estimated total blood loss. **a** All included studies (**b**) RTSA group

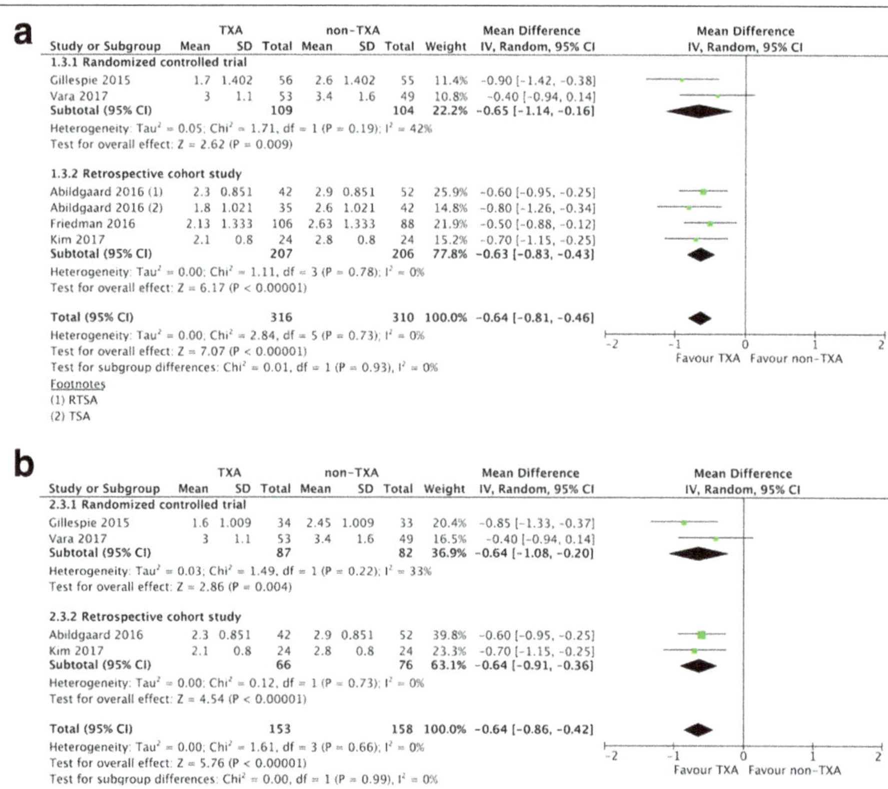

Fig. 5 Forest plot and meta-analysis of Hb change. **a** All included studies (**b**) RTSA group (data from Gillespie 2015 were estimated from median and range)

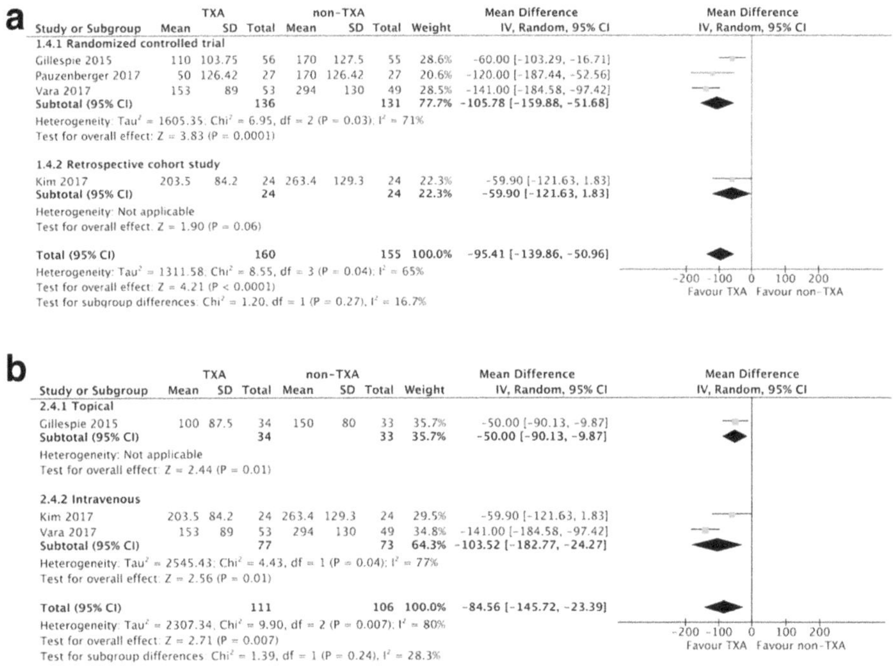

Fig. 6 Forest plot and meta-analysis of blood loss via drainage. **a** All included studies (**b**) RTSA group (data from Gillespie 2015 and Friedman 2017 were estimated from median and range)

Subgroup analysis

Subgroup analysis only including the three RCTs [20, 23, 34] did not affect the direction of effects of any of the outcomes including allogeneic blood transfusion rate, estimated total blood loss, change in postoperative Hb, and overall complications (Table 3). For data limited to RTSA, the TXA group had a lower allogenic blood transfusion rate, less estimated total blood loss, less change in Hb, and less blood loss via drainage compared with the non-TXA group (Table 3, Fig. 3-6b).

Considering the route of TXA administration, one study examined the topical use of TXA [20], and the other four studies examined the IV administration of TXA [19, 23, 24, 33, 34]. Regardless of whether topical or IV administration was used, the TXA group had less change in Hb than the non-TXA group, and there was no difference between the two routes of administration (subgroup difference, $P = 0.27$; Table 3, see Additional file 2: Figure S1). Four studies reported blood loss via drainage [20, 23, 24, 34]. The TXA group had less blood loss compared with the non-TXA group in both topical and IV subgroups (MD − 60.00 ml, 95% CI -103.29 to − 16.71 ml, $P = 0.007$; MD -110.04 ml, 95% CI -159.03 to − 61.06 ml, $P < 0.0001$, respectively; Table 3, see Additional file 3: Figure S2). Comparing these two subgroups, IV TXA was as effective as topical TXA in reducing blood loss via drainage (subgroup difference, $P = 0.13$, Table 3, see Additional file 3: Figure S2).

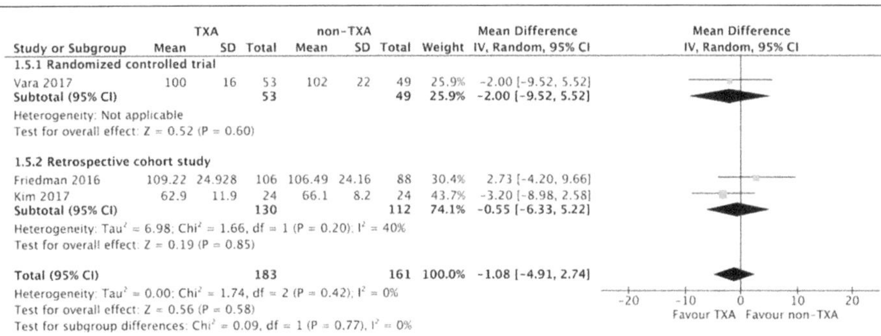

Fig. 7 Forest plot of and meta-analysis of operative time

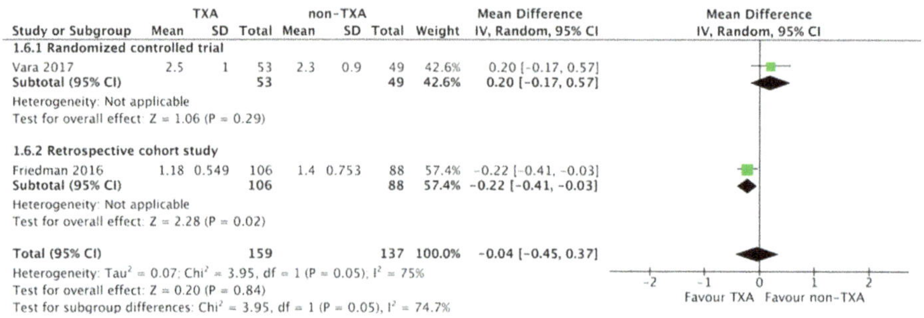

Fig. 8 Forest plot of and meta-analysis of hospital stay

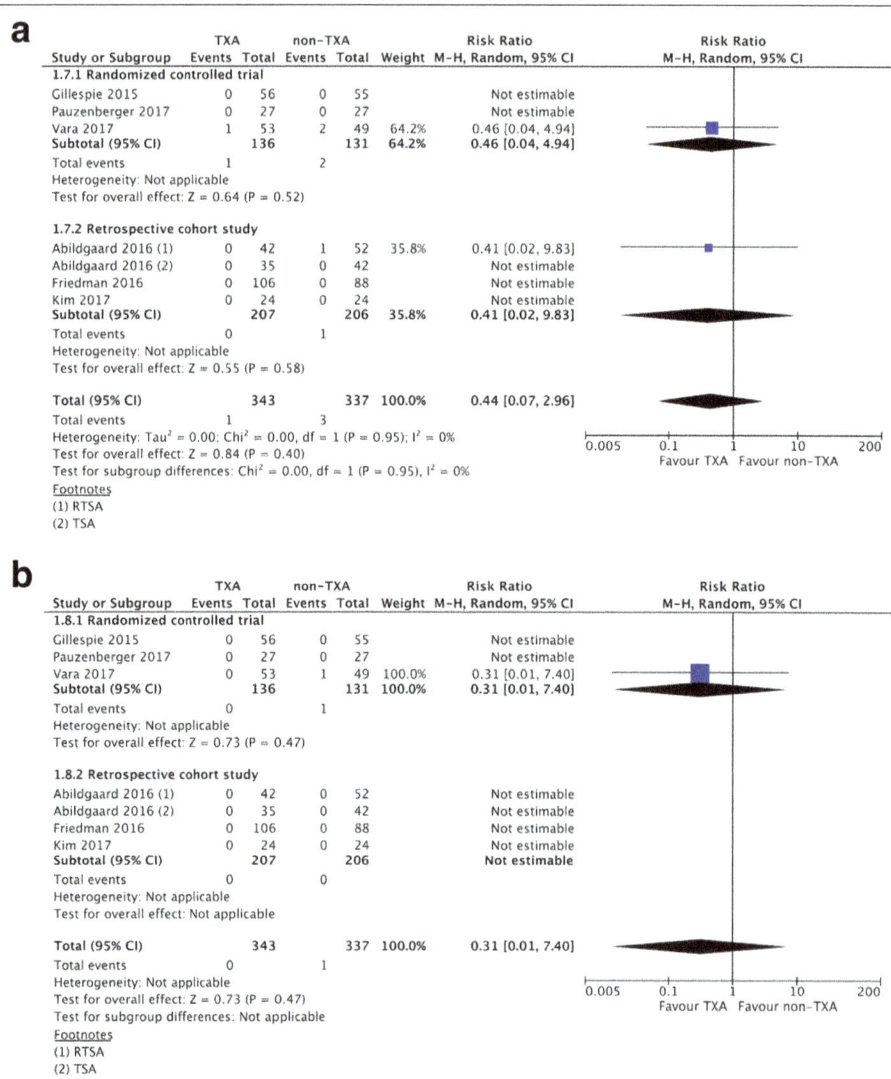

Fig. 9 **a** Forest plot and meta-analysis of overall complications. **b** Forest plot and meta-analysis of thromboembolic complications

Discussion

The main findings of this study are that the use of TXA in shoulder arthroplasty can reduce blood loss parameters including allogeneic blood transfusion rate, estimated total blood loss, change in Hb level, and blood loss via drainage without increasing the operative time, hospital stay, or the incidence of perioperative complications.

RTSA has been reported to be an independent predictor of the need for a blood transfusion after shoulder arthroplasty [2], which implied that patients undergoing RTSA bled more than TSA. Both the reverse design of implant geometry and the lack of intact cuff contribute to greater potential dead space in RTSA, resulting in more bleeding [24]. Our study shows that TXA reduces blood loss and the need for blood transfusion, suggesting that it could be applied to patients undergoing RTSA.

TXA has been shown to reverse the effect of plasminogen, thereby reducing blood loss and requirement for an allogeneic blood transfusion [35]. However, the most appropriate route of TXA administration is still under debate. One meta-analysis comparing the effectiveness and safety of IV versus topical administration of TXA in patients undergoing total knee arthroplasty showed that both IV and topical TXA had comparable efficacy in reducing blood loss and blood transfusion rates [36]. Another meta-analysis on total hip and knee arthroplasty also demonstrated similar results [37]. In the present study, both the IV and topical administration of TXA were effective in reducing blood loss and transfusion rates. For patients with a history of pulmonary embolism (PE) or deep vein thrombosis (DVT), the topical administration of TXA may be preferable.

Theoretically, TXA has a potential risk of thrombosis [14]. However, previous studies on total knee or total hip arthroplasty have not found an increased risk of thromboembolic events [16, 36–38]. Our findings suggest that TXA may not increase the risk of venous thromboembolic complications including PE and DVT in shoulder arthroplasty. This may be due to the use of allogeneic blood transfusion protocols with thromboprophylaxis including heparin, aspirin and mechanical prophylaxis in most of the included studies [23, 33, 34]. The low incidence of thromboembolic events may also be due to the routine use of chemical prophylaxis or the careful selection of patients with a higher risk of thromboembolism or the different nature between upper limb and lower limb surgery. In one study investigating the use of TXA in patients undergoing total hip arthroplasty without chemical prophylaxis for DVT, TXA was found to significantly increase the incidence of total DVT compared with the control group [39]. Since we found that both IV TXA and topical TXA were effective in reducing blood loss and transfusion rates, the topical administration of TXA may be preferable for patients with a history of PE or DVT.

To the best of our knowledge, this study is the most up-to-date systematic review and meta-analysis focusing on the use of TXA in shoulder arthroplasty. Compared to the previous systematic review, this study provides additional information about the efficacy of TXA with regards to the different types of shoulder arthroplasty and different routes of administration. This study also provides evidence supporting that TXA is a safe and efficient agent in reducing perioperative blood loss and transfusion rates without increasing complications, and that it can be applied in shoulder arthroplasty, especially for those at risk of requiring a blood transfusion.

This study has several important limitations. First, of the six studies, three were observational, with bias leading to inherent heterogeneity, even with high-quality scores. However, the subgroup analysis only including RCTs did not affect the direction of effects of any of the outcomes. In addition, we identified two ongoing trials from trial registries (NCT02569658, NCT01937559), and the findings of the present study may be different after including the results of these two trials. Second, the current study provides information on the route of TXA administration. However, this study can only provide indirect evidence about the comparison between the efficacy of IV TXA and topical TXA. Further trials with direct comparisons between IV TXA and topical TXA are needed to validate this finding. Finally, this study cannot make any conclusions on the optimal dose of TXA. Further head-to-head trials comparing different doses of TXA in shoulder arthroplasty are required to determine the optimal dose. Other limitations included non-standardized doses of TXA, variable postoperative chemoprophylaxis, and heterogeneous transfusion protocols which may have a significant effect on one of the main study endpoints.

Conclusions

When used in shoulder arthroplasty, TXA is safe and effective in reducing perioperative blood loss and the need for a blood transfusion without increasing complications including thromboembolic events. TXA can be included as part of a comprehensive strategy for shoulder arthroplasty, especially for patients at a high risk of requiring a blood transfusion.

Additional files

Additional file 1: Appendix 1. Database search strategy.

Additional file 2: Figure S1. Forest plot and meta-analysis of Hb change. The TXA group had a lower change in Hb than the non-TXA group in both the topical TXA and IV TXA subgroups. There was no significant subgroup difference. (data from Gillespie 2015 and Friedman 2017 were estimated from median and range).

Additional file 3: Figure S2. Forest plot and meta-analysis of blood loss via drainage. The TXA group had less blood loss via drainage than the non-TXA group in both topical TXA and IV TXA subgroups. There was no significant subgroup difference. (data from Gillespie 2015 and Friedman 2017 were estimated from median and range).

Abbreviations
CI: Confidence interval; CTA: Cuff tear arthropathy; DP: Deltopectoral approach; ETBL: Estimated total blood loss; F: Female; Hb: Hemoglobin; Hct: Hematocrit; IV: Intravenous; M: Male; MD: Mean difference; N: Number of studies; N/S: Not shown; NA: Not applicable; NS: Normal saline; OA: Osteoarthritis; ON: Osteonecrosis; RA: Rheumatoid arthritis; RTSA: Reverse total shoulder arthroplasty; TSA: Total shoulder arthroplasty; TXA: Tranexamic acid

Acknowledgements
We thank Ms. Yu-Shiun Tsai for help in the searching the databases and obtaining the full-text of the articles.

Funding
No funding was obtained for this study.

Authors' contributions
LTK was responsible for the study concept and design and drafting of the manuscript. LTK and WHH were responsible for the trial selection and appraisal of methodological quality. LTK and CCC participated in acquisition, analysis, and interpretation of data. CCC provided consultation for statistics and methodology. CCC and JCY were in charge of the study concept and design, supervised the study and critically revised the manuscript for important intellectual content. All authors read and approved the final manuscript.

Consent for publication
Not applicable

Competing interests
The authors declare that they have no competing interests.

Author details
[1]Division of Sports Medicine, Department of Orthopedic Surgery, Chang Gung Memorial Hospital, Chiayi, Taiwan. [2]Centre for Evidence-Based Medicine, Chang Gung Memorial Hospital, Chiayi, Taiwan. [3]Chang Gung University of Science and Technology, Chiayi, Taiwan. [4]College of Medicine, Chang Gung University, Taoyuan, Taiwan. [5]Department of Dermatology, Chang Gung Memorial Hospital, Linkou, 5, Fuxing St, Guishan Dist, Taoyuan 33305, Taiwan. [6]Department of Orthopedic Surgery, College of Medicine, Samsung Medical Center, Sungkyunkwan University School of Medicine, 81 Irwon-ro, Gangnam-gu, Seoul 135-710, Republic of Korea.

References
1. Ahmadi S, Lawrence TM, Sahota S, Schleck CD, Harmsen WS, Cofield RH, et al. The incidence and risk factors for blood transfusion in revision shoulder arthroplasty: our institution's experience and review of the literature. J Shoulder Elb Surg. 2014;23:43–8.
2. Gruson KI, Accousti KJ, Parsons BO, Pillai G, Flatow EL. Transfusion after shoulder arthroplasty: an analysis of rates and risk factors. J Shoulder Elb Surg. 2009;18:225–30.
3. Hardy JC, Hung M, Snow BJ, Martin CL, Tashjian RZ, Burks RT, et al. Blood transfusion associated with shoulder arthroplasty. J Shoulder Elb Surg. 2013; 22:233–9.
4. Millett PJ, Porramatikul M, Chen N, Zurakowski D, Warner JJ. Analysis of transfusion predictors in shoulder arthroplasty. J Bone Joint Surg Am. 2006; 88:1223–30.
5. Ryan DJ, Yoshihara H, Yoneoka D, Zuckerman JD. Blood transfusion in primary total shoulder arthroplasty: incidence, trends, and risk factors in the United States from 2000 to 2009. J Shoulder Elb Surg. 2015;24(5):760.
6. Schumer RA, Chae JS, Markert RJ, Sprott D, Crosby LA. Predicting transfusion in shoulder arthroplasty. J Shoulder Elb Surg. 2010;19:91–6.
7. Sperling JW, Duncan SF, Cofield RH, Schleck CD, Harmsen WS. Incidence and risk factors for blood transfusion in shoulder arthroplasty. J Shoulder Elb Surg. 2005;14:599–601.
8. Kandil A, Griffin JW, Novicoff WM, Brockmeier SF. Blood transfusion after total shoulder arthroplasty: which patients are at high risk? Int J Shoulder Surg. 2016 Apr-Jun;10(2):72–7.
9. Carson JL, Grossman BJ, Kleinman S, Tinmouth AT, Marques MB, Fung MK, et al. Red blood cell transfusion: a clinical practice guideline from the AABB. Ann Intern Med. 2012;157:49–58.
10. National Heart, Lung, and Blood Institute. What are the risks of a blood transfusion? 2012. https://www.nhlbi.nih.gov/health/health-topics/topics/bt/risks. Accessed 05 May 2017.
11. Grier AJ, Bala A, Penrose CT, Seyler TM, Bolognesi MP, Garrigues GE. Analysis of complication rates following perioperative transfusion in shoulder arthroplasty. J Shoulder Elbow Surg. 2017. pii: S1058–2746(16)30612–7.
12. Kopanidis P, Hardidge A, McNicol L, Tay S, McCall P, Weinberg L. Perioperative blood management programme reduces the use of allogenic blood transfusion in patients undergoing total hip and knee arthroplasty. J Orthop Surg Res. 2016;11:28.
13. Moonen AF, Neal TD, Pilot P. Perioperative blood management in elective orthopaedic surgery. A critical review of the literature. Injury. 2006;37(Suppl 5):S11–6.
14. Mannucci PM. Hemostatic drugs. N Engl J Med. 1998;339:245–53.
15. Alshryda S, Sarda P, Sukeik M, Nargol A, Blenkinsopp J, Mason JM. Tranexamic acid in total knee replacement: a systematic review and meta-analysis. J Bone Joint Surg Br. 2011;93:1577–85.
16. Chen S, Wu K, Kong G, Feng W, Deng Z, Wang H. The efficacy of topical tranexamic acid in total hip arthroplasty: a meta-analysis. BMC Musculoskelet Disord. 2016;17:81. https://doi.org/10.1186/s12891-016-0923-0.
17. Sukeik M, Alshryda S, Haddad FS, Mason JM. Systematic review and meta-analysis of the use of tranexamic acid in total hip replacement. J Bone Joint Surg Br. 2011;93:39–46.
18. Yang ZG, Chen WP, Wu LD. Effectiveness and safety of tranexamic acid in reducing blood loss in total knee arthroplasty: a meta-analysis. J Bone Joint Surg Am. 2012;94:1153–9.
19. Friedman RJ, Gordon E, Butler RB, Mock L, Dumas B. Tranexamic acid decreases blood loss after total shoulder arthroplasty. J Shoulder Elb Surg. 2016;25(4):614–8.
20. Gillespie R, Shishani Y, Joseph S, Streit JJ, Gobezie R. Neer award 2015: a randomized, prospective evaluation on the effectiveness of tranexamic acid in reducing blood loss after total shoulder arthroplasty. J Shoulder Elb Surg. 2015;24(11):1679–84.
21. Sun CX, Zhang L, Mi LD, Du GY, Sun XG, He SW. Efficiency and safety of tranexamic acid in reducing blood loss in total shoulder arthroplasty: a systematic review and meta-analysis. Med (Baltimore). 2017;96(22):e7015. https://doi.org/10.1097/MD.0000000000007015.
22. Kirsch JM, Bedi A, Horner N, Wiater JM, Pauzenberger L, Koueiter DM, et al. Tranexamic acid in shoulder arthroplasty: a systematic review and meta-analysis. JBJS Rev. 2017 Sep;5(9):e3. https://doi.org/10.2106/JBJS.RVW.17.00021.
23. Pauzenberger L, Domej MA, Heuberer PR, Hexel M, Grieb A, Laky B, et al. The effect of intravenous tranexamic acid on blood loss and early post-operative pain in total shoulder arthroplasty. Bone Joint J. 2017 Aug;99-B(8): 1073–9.
24. Kim SH, Jung WI, Kim YJ, Hwang DH, Choi YE. Effect of tranexamic acid on hematologic values and blood loss in reverse Total shoulder arthroplasty. Biomed Res Int. 2017;2017:9590803. https://doi.org/10.1155/2017/9590803.
25. Higgins JP, Altman DG, Gøtzsche PC, Jüni P, Moher D, Oxman AD, Savovic J, Schulz KF, Weeks L, Sterne JA. Cochrane bias methods group. Cochrane Statistical Methods Group The Cochrane Collaboration's tool for assessing risk of bias in randomised trials BMJ. 2011;343:d5928.
26. Higgins JP, Green S. Cochrane Handbook for Systematic Reviews of Interventions Version 5.1.0. The Cochrane Collaboration. 2011. http://www.cochrane-handbook.org. Accessed 15 Aug 2017.
27. Wells GA, Shea B, O'Connell D, Peterson J, Welch V, Losos M, et al. The Newcastle-Ottawa scale (NOS) for assessing the quality of nonrandomised

studies in meta-analyses. Ottawa Hospital Research Institute; 2014. http://www.ohri.ca/programs/clinical_epidemiology/oxford.asp. Accessed 15 Aug 2017.
28. Higgins JP, Thompson SG. Quantifying heterogeneity in a meta-analysis. Stat Med. 2002;21:1539–58.
29. Higgins JP, Thompson SG, Deeks JJ, Altman DG. Measuring inconsistency in meta-analyses. BMJ. 2003;327:557–60.
30. DerSimonian R, Laird N. Meta-analysis in clinical trials. Control Clin Trials. 1986;7:177–88.
31. Hozo SP, Djulbegovic B, Hozo I. Estimating the mean and variance from the median, range, and the size of a sample. BMC Med Res Methodol. 2005;5:13.
32. Moher D, Liberati A, Tetzlaff J, Altman DG, PRISMA Group. Preferred reporting items for systematic reviews and meta-analyses: the PRISMA statement. PLoS Med. 2009;6(7):e1000097. https://doi.org/10.1371/journal.pmed.1000097.
33. Abildgaard JT, McLemore R, Hattrup SJ. Tranexamic acid decreases blood loss in total shoulder arthroplasty and reverse total shoulder arthroplasty. J Shoulder Elb Surg. 2016 Oct;25(10):1643–8.
34. Vara AD, Koueiter DM, Pinkas DE, Gowda A, Wiater BP, Wiater JM. Intravenous tranexamic acid reduces total blood loss in reverse total shoulder arthroplasty: a prospective, double-blinded, randomized, controlled trial. J Shoulder Elb Surg. 2017;26:1383–9.
35. Nuttall GA, Brost BC, Connis RT, Gessner JS, Harrison CR, Miller RD, et al. Practice guidelines for perioperative blood transfusion and adjuvant therapies: an updated report by the American Society of Anesthesiologists Task Force on perioperative blood transfusion and adjuvant therapies. Anesthesiology. 2006 Jul;105(1):198–208.
36. Shin YS, Yoon JR, Lee HN, Park SH, Lee DH. Intravenous versus topical tranexamic acid administration in primary total knee arthroplasty: a meta-analysis. Knee Surg Sports Traumatol Arthrosc. 2016; https://doi.org/10.1007/s00167-016-4235-6.
37. Chen Y, Chen Z, Cui S, Li Z, Yuan Z. Topical versus systemic tranexamic acid after total knee and hip arthroplasty: a meta-analysis of randomized controlled trials. Med (Baltimore). 2016 Oct;95(41):e4656. https://doi.org/10.1097/MD.0000000000004656.
38. Kim TK, Chang CB, Koh IJ. Practical issues for the use of tranexamic acid in total knee arthroplasty: a systematic review. Knee Surg Sports Traumatol Arthrosc. 2014 Aug;22(8):1849–58.
39. Nishihara S, Hamada M. Does tranexamic acid alter the risk of thromboembolism after total hip arthroplasty in the absence of routine chemical thromboprophylaxis? Bone Joint J. 2015 Apr;97-B(4):458–62.

2

Silver-coated modular Mega-endoprostheses in salvage revision arthroplasty after periimplant infection with extensive bone loss

Dirk Zajonz[1,3†], Undine Birke[1†], Mohamed Ghanem[1], Torsten Prietzel[2,3], Christoph Josten[1,3], Andreas Roth[1] and Johannes K.M. Fakler[1*]

Abstract

Background: Hip and knee replacements in patients with bone defects after infection correlates with high rates of reinfection. In this vulnerable patient population, the prevention of reinfection is to be considered superordinate to the functionality and defect bridging. The use of silver coating of aseptic implants as an infection prophylaxis is already proven; however, the significance of these coatings in septic reimplantation of large implants is still not sufficiently investigated.

Methods: In a retrospective analysis, 34 patients who have been treated with a modular mega-endoprosthesis after a cured bone infection of the lower limb (femur or tibia) have been evaluated. One group with 14 patients (NSCG: non silver- coated group) was supplied with the non silver- coated implants: MML München- Lübeck™ modular endoprosthesis system (AQ Implants, Ahrensburg, Germany) or MUTARS® Modular Universal Tumor And Revision System (Implantcast GmbH, Buxtehude, Germany). The other group with 20 patients (SCG: silver- coated group) was supplied with the silver- coated system of MUTARS®. In addition to the clinical findings and the patients' histories, specifically the reinfection rates, the patients' mobility was assessed using the New Mobility Score (NMS, by Parker and Palmer).

Results: The median follow-up period was 72 months, ranging from 6 to 267 months. The dropout rate was 5.8%. The reinfection rate after healed reinfection in SCG was 40% (8/20), in NSCG 57% (8/14), $p = 0.34$; $\alpha = 0.05$. The time for reinfection was, on average, 14 months (1–72 months) in SCG and 8 months (1–48 months) in the NSCG ($p = 0.61$; $\alpha = 0.05$). The two groups showed no differences in the NMS.

Conclusion: With this retrospective analysis, it can be determined that the rate of reinfection of modular mega-endoprostheses on the hip and knee joint after healed periprosthetic joint infection (PJI) can be reduced by the use of silver coated implants. The time until reinfection can also be delayed by utilizing silver coated implants. Due to the low number of cases of this highly specific patient population, no statistical significance could be determined. A positive effect, however, can be assumed through the use of silver coatings in mega-endoprostheses after an infectious situation.

Keywords: Periimplant infection, Modular mega-endoprostheses, Silver-coated implants, Bone defects, Reinfection

* Correspondence: Johannes.fakler@medizin.uni-leipzig.de
†Equal contributors
[1]Department of Orthopaedic Surgery, Trauma Surgery and Plastic Surgery, University Hospital Leipzig, Liebigstrasse 20, D-04103 Leipzig, Germany
Full list of author information is available at the end of the article

Background

Hip and knee replacements are among the most common surgical procedures worldwide [1]. In response to demographic changes, the number of endoprosthetic surgeries is constantly increasing. For example, the number of total hip arthroplasties (THA) carried out in the U.S. rose by a factor of 2.5 from 200,216 in 1993 to 497,419 in 2005. In that same period, the amount of primary total knee arthroplasties (TKA) grew 1.7-fold from 135,992 to 237,645 [1–3]. With primary arthroplasty on the rise, cases of revision arthroplasty are also set to increase [4, 5]. Correlating with the number of endoprosthetic surgeries, the total amount of complications are also increasing; although, primary endoprostheses result in fewer than 10% of cases being problematic [6]. Because of this, surgeons specialising in endosprosthetics are faced with increasingly challenging situations in which conventional prosthesis systems are not sufficient, i.e. large defect situations after implant loosening with major osteolysis, periprosthetic fractures with extensive osseous substance defects, or periprosthetic infections and pseudarthrosis (non-union). A clinically established approach is the use of modular mega-endoprosthetic systems [7, 8]. The majority of experiences with this approach have been obtained through tumour surgery [9, 10]. Since modular mega-endoprosthesis systems can be modified intraoperatively, they enable solutions even in complex cases where only unsatisfactory resection arthroplasty or amputation were previously possible [4, 7, 11]. The conditions for using modular mega-endoprostheses must, however, be strictly verified. There are numerous differences when comparing primary arthroplasty with mega-endoprostheses: the implant's larger surface area, the greater surgical access, the frequently longer duration of surgery, and the relatively higher blood loss. Also, multi-morbidity is less prevalent in patients receiving a primary arthroplasty; therefore, implantation of modular endoprostheses is associated with higher complication rates [4, 7, 12].

This is particularly the case with PJI with an implanted mega-endoprosthesis, of which a high percentage lead to ablative surgery or even death. The infection rate of modular mega-endoprostheses is stated in the literature as 4–36% [3, 13–15]. In the case of reinfections, it can rise up to 40% [4]. A possible solution is the silver coating of the endoprosthesis. Various in vitro studies have shown that silver coatings effectively inhibit or even prevent the formation of biofilms on metal surfaces of different bacteria [16, 17]. Recently, silver coating of medical devices, such as external fixation pins, heart valves, endotracheal tubes, and cardiac and urinary catheters, has been shown to reduce infection rates [18–20]. Furthermore, several clinical studies have confirmed the positive effects of silver coatings in preventing infections in endoprostheses [21–23]. This seems to be a probable method of preventing infection in particularly complex defect cases, where cured bone infections of the lower extremity are supplied with a modular mega-endoprosthesis. The aim of this study is to retrospectively evaluate patients who have been treated with a modular mega-endoprosthesis after a cured bone infection of the lower limb. The difference in the outcomes, particularly with regards to the reinfection rate, will be shown between silver- coated and non silver-coated implants.

Methods

Prior to the start of the investigation, the local university's ethics committee was consulted, and after examination, a positive vote was issued. The vote-number of the audit authority was 355/16-ek. Written, informed consent was obtained from all study participants, including consent for publication of the results. The diagnosis of periprosthetic infection was provided based on the international consensus for the diagnosis of periprosthetic joint infection.

Zajonz et al. [3] as reinfection or recurrence developed, a clinical and microbiological recurrence of local periprosthetic joint infections was defined, according to the antibiotic-free period and the absence of clinical symptoms for at least 6 weeks [3, 4]. Until 1999, β-lactam antibiotics (mainly ampicillin) were used as perioperative antibiotic prophylaxis. As of 1999, 2-generation cephalosporins (mainly cefuroxime) were used. Glindamycin was used in allergies.

To select the patient cohort, all patients who had been fitted with a modular endoprosthesis of the lower extremity at our hospital between September 1994 and December 2014 were retrospectively identified. Patients' data was collected based on their archived records and electronic files in IS-H SAP (Siemens AG Healthcare Sector, Erlangen, Germany), as well as radiological findings and images from SIENET MagicWeb/ACOM (Siemens AG Healthcare Sector, Erlangen, Germany). All available data was acquired from our patient documentation system. All patients were invited to and consulted for a clinical follow-up. Patients who did not appear for a follow-up were interviewed by telephone. The patients who could not be examined either in person or by telephone made contact with their family doctors. In addition to the clinical findings and the patient's history, the NMS was used as an assessment of mobility [24].

From the patient population, a total of 36 patients with implanted modular endoprostheses after cured infections were identified. Due to inadequate documentation, 2 patients were excluded. From these 34 patients, two groups were formed. One group (NSCG: non silver- coated group) with 14 patients, 8 of whom were supplied with the non- silver- coated system: MML München- Lübeck™ modular endoprosthesis system (AQ Implants, Ahrensburg, Germany) and 6 with non- silver- coated system MUTARS®

Modular Universal Tumor And Revision System (Implantcast GmbH, Buxtehude, Germany) [4]. Figure 1 of those, 3 were knee and 11 were hip endoprostheses. The other group (SCG: silver- coated group) consisted of 20 patients, all of whom were supplied with the silver- coated system MUTARS® Modular Universal Tumor And Revision System (Implantcast GmbH, Buxtehude, Germany). This group consisted of 7 knee and 13 hip endoprostheses. Figure 2 All patients had an infection of the lower extremity (prosthesis infection, infection osteosynthesis, and secondary infections after a periprosthetic fracture), which was treated with either spacer implantation or removal of the material (Girdlestone arthroplasty). The handlingof the infection was carried out for all patients on the basis of the standards for treatment of periprosthetic joint infections according to the current guidelines of our hospital. In all patients, the infected implants were removed and reimplantation took place after infectious conditioning. An antibiotic treatment was administered under microbiotic and pharmaceutical stewardship.

Statistical analysis was performed using the spreadsheet software Microsoft Excel (Microsoft Corporation, Redmond, USA). Both examination groups are normally distributed and not connected. Both groups were normally distributed, as determined by optical analysis of the distribution pattern. For the same variance, the *t*-test for two unconnected samples was used to calculate significance. The chi-square test according to Pearson was used for nonlinear test variables, with the level of significance being set at 5% (α = 0.05). Statistical advice from a mathematician has been sought.

Results

The median follow-up period was 72 months, ranging from 6 to 267 months (SCG: 72 months (6–114) and NSCG: 74 months (18–267)). In two patients, no further information could be obtained despite extensive research (telephone consultation, written inquiry, consultation with the family physician). Thus, the drop out rate was 5.8%. Due to the lengthy follow-up period, 13 patients had already passed away prior to the latest follow-up examination. Extensive examination of the remaining patients (consultation with family members and doctors, as well as file analysis) proved there was no reinfection to be found; all patients had died of other causes (pulmonary embolism, tumor progression, cardiac genesis, age-related multimorbidity). In these patients, the last file entry in our hospital was defined as the follow-up time.

The patient specifics of the two groups, such as age, gender, and secondary diseases, are presented in Table 1. There was no significant difference between the groups in any of the features. Additionally, there was no fundamental difference in the treatment regime between the two groups. The individual treatment strategy (antibiosis, number of revisions, Spacer vs. Girdelestone) had been adapted to accommodate the specific situation of each patient. The specifics for the infection repair before reimplantation are shown in Table 2. There was no significant difference between the groups in any of the features either. The observed bacteria in the groups are shown in Table 3. The reinfection rate after healed reinfection in SCG was 40% (8/20). In the NSCG, it was 57% (8/14). A statistically significant difference was not detectable (p = 0.97; α =0.05). The time for reinfection was, on average, 14 months (1–72 months) in SCG and 8 months (1–48 months) in the NSCG (p = 0.61; α =0.05). In both groups, 37% (3/8) showed a germinal change to initial infection. The two groups showed no differences in the NMS, used as an assessment for mobility. The exact distribution is shown in Table 4.

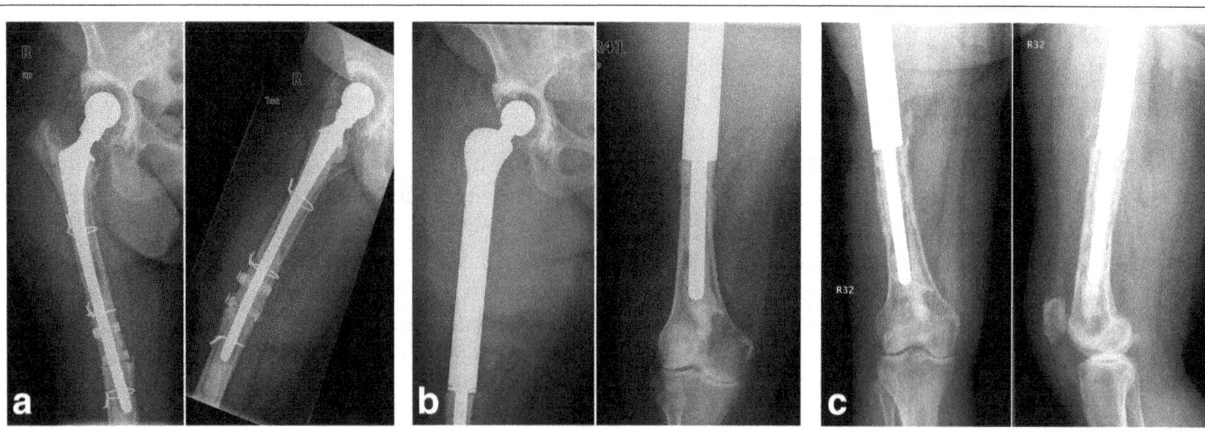

Fig. 1 Anterior-posterior and lateral X-rays of the right hip with thigh of a 78-year-old woman with **a** a total hip arthroplasty (THA) after multiple revisions and acute periprosthetic fracture with implant loosening **b** after implantation of a proximal femur replacement and intraoperative detection of staphylococci with the clinical presentation of a PJI with implant-preserved revision and antibiosis **c** after 14 months, a chronic infection with increasing loosening of the implants

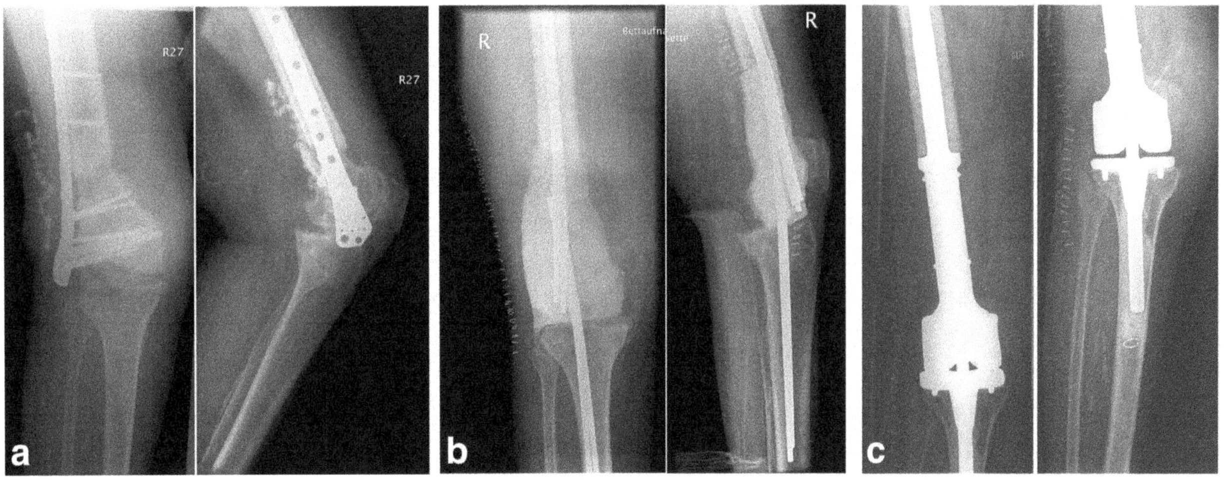

Fig. 2 Anterior-posterior and lateral X-rays of the right knee with thigh of a 74-year-old woman with **a** infected pseudoarthrosis of the right distal femur after plate osteosynthesis of a supracondylar femur fracture **b** resection of the distal femur and implantation of an intramedullary cement spacer **c** after implantation of a silver- coated distal femoral replacement endoprosthesis (System MUTARS® Modular Universal Tumor And Revision System, Implantcast GmbH, Buxtehude, Germany)

Discussion

Periprostetic joint infections of mega-endoprostheses remain a serious complication in orthopedic surgery [4]. Furthermore, reinfection is an escalating problem with revision surgery in patients who suffered from infections associated with primary endoprosthetic replacement of the knee and hip joint. These patients may need multiple revision surgeries and in some cases, even amputation [4, 7, 9]. Many different approaches to treatment have been pursued. Nevertheless, the reinfection rate is still around 40% [4]. One approach to therapy is the use of silver coated implants. Since ancient times, people have been aware of the antimicrobial effect of various metals (i.e. silver and copper), but the exact methodology has yet to be investigated. The reason for the antimicrobial potency of the different ions appears to be the oligodynamic effect [25]. First, clinical trials from an orthopedic background were carried out through animal experiments. Gosheger et al. investigated the infection rates and the side effects of silver- coated implants (MUTARS) versus titanium implants in rabbits. The silver group showed significantly lower infection rates (7% versus 47%, $p < 0.05$) in comparison with the titanium group [26]. Usually, the non-scientific press emphasizes the toxic effect caused by the release of silver ions from silver-coated implants; however, the concentrations of silver in the blood in both the animal and human trials did not reach toxic levels. Even in histopathological investigations of the tissues, histological changes of the organs could not be determined. In conclusion, silver-coated mega-endoprostheses allow a release of silver, without any presentation of local or systemic side-effects [26, 27]. In clinical research, Hardes et al. showed a substantial reduction of periprosthetic infection of mega-endoprostheses in patients with bone sarcoma from 17.6% (51 patients) in the titanium group to 5.9% (74 patients) in the silver group over a 5-year period [20]. Also, a recent study by Grosso et al. showed a significant reduction in PJI with the use of silver-impregnated occlusive dressing in over 1100 primary endoprostheses on the hip and knee (1,58% to 0,33%, $p = 0.03$). These studies, however, deal with previously uninfected areas. Despite extensive literature research, work dealing with the PJI rate after pre-existing infections in endoprostheses, especially mega-endoprostheses, could not be found. Only Wafa and colleagues reported their experiences in a case-control study of the incidence of early periprosthetic infection with silver-treated endoprostheses in high-risk

Table 1 Patient specifics of the groups, such as sex, median age (min-max), diabetes, immunosuppression due to medication, peripheral arterial disease, malignant tumour, anticoagulation, and rheumatism, are presented

	Silver- coated group SCG)	non silver-coated Group (NSCG)	Statistical significance (α = 0.05)
Femal sex	55% (11/20)	57% (8/14)	0.91
Median Age (min-max)	74 (46–83)	69 (35–87)	0.36
Diabetes	45% (9/20)	42% (6/14)	0.91
Drug immunosuppression	5% (1/20)	7%(1/14)	0.80
Peripheral arterial disease, PAD	10% (2/20)	0	0.21
Malignomas	0	14% (2/14)	0.08
Anticoagulation	30%(6/20)	28%(4/14)	0.93
Rheumatism	5%(1/20)	7%(1/14)	0.85

Table 2 Specifics for the infection repair before reimplantation, such as multiple-stage prosthesis replacement with bone cement spacer or temporary girdlestone, as well as one-stage prosthesis replacement, number of revisions up to reimplantation (median; min -max), time until reimplantation after initiation of infection therapy in months, reimplantation time in minutes, time spent in hospital for treatment, C- reactive protein (CRP) at discharge (mg/dl), Leukocytes at discharge (10exp9)

Median (min -max)	Silver- coated group (SCG)	non silver-coated Group (NSCG)	Statistical significance (α = 0.05)
Multiple-stage prosthesis replacement (bone cement spacer)	16/20 (80%)	10/14 (71%)	0.81
Multiple-stage prosthesis replacement (temporary girdlestone)	2/20 (10%)[a]	1/14 (7%)	0.71
One-stage prosthesis replacement	4/20 (20%)	3/14 (21%)	0.61
Number of revisions up to reimplantation (median; min -max)	4 (0–10)	4 (0–7)	0.19
Time to reimplantation after initiation of infection therapy in months	3 (0–10)	4 (0–24)	0.28
Reimplantation time in minutes	188 (128–236)	193 (122–277)	0.51
Time spent in the hospital for infectious treatment	22 (10–139)	32 (14–158)	0.74
C- reaktive proteine (CRP) at discharge (mg/dl)	17.5 (4.3–89)	18.2 (1.5–89)	0.39
Leukocytes at discharge (10exp9)	7 (5–10.5)	6,6 (4.7–10)	0.92

[a]In two cases, both temporary Girdlestone situations and cement spacer therapy were used

patients (primary reconstructions, one-stage revisions and two-stage revisions for infection) [28]. In this study, the overall post-operative infection rate of the silver-coated group was 11.8%, in contrast to the 22.4% for the control group (p = 0.033). Wafa concluded that silver-treated implants were particularly useful in two-stage revisions for infection and in those patients with incidental positive cultures at the time of the prosthetic's implantation. Debridement with antibiotic treatment and retention of the implant appeared to be more successful with silver-coated implants [28]. Especially in cases of treated PJI, the reinfection rate with non-silver coated endoprostheses was 20%, whereas, it reached up to 40% with mega-endoprostheses. Based on the available analysis and the successful results in aseptic endoprostetics, a positive effect in PJI can also be assumed. Similarly in our analysis, there was a reduction of PJI from 57% to 40% through the use of silver coatings. However, these results were not statistically significant, due largely to the low number of cases of this highly specific patient population. Additionally, the time until reinfection was almost twice as long in the SCG compared to the NSCG (14 vs. 8 months). It is striking that in our study, mostly *Staphylococcus aureus*, specifically 25% of which was MRSA, was found as the initial germ in the SCG. Table 2 It is known that PJI with MRSA due to an aggressive biofilm has a significantly higher failure rate than other non-resistant germs. Thus, the lower SCG reinfection rate can be given more importance in this difficult germination. It can therefore be assumed that the formation of a biofilm in silver coating will be at least reduced, if not prevented. Hazer et al. could also show this effect in the rabbit model [29]. A significant difference in the germ spectrum was not established between the two groups. Exact statements regarding the germination parameters are only possible to a limited extent due to the small case number. It is noticeable that in both groups, a change of the germination had occurred in one third of the patients. This indicates the presence of mixed infections or superinfections, which is not unusual for this vulnerable patient population [4]. The coating had no effect on the

Table 3 Observed bacteria in the groups (MRSA: methicillin resistant *Staphylococcus aureus*)

Bacteria	Silver- coated group (SCG)	non silver-coated Group (NSCG)
Staphylococcus aureus	8 /20 (40%)	2/14 (14%)
of this MRSA	5/20 (25%)	0
Coagulase negative staphylococci	7/20 (35%)	4/14 (28%)
of this *Staphylococcus epidermidis*	2/20 (10%)	4/14 (21%)
Enterococci	6/20 (30%)	4/14 (21%)
Pseudomonas	3/20 (15%)	1/14 (7%)
Escherichia coli	4/20 (20%)	1/14 (7%)
without germination	4/20 (20%)	5/14 (35%)
mixed infections	12/20 (60%)	4/14 (28%)

Table 4 New Mobility Score (Parker and Palmer) as assessment for mobility of the two groups (SCG vs. NSCG) and statistical significance

Mobility	Silver- coated group (SCG)	Non silver-coated Group (NSCG)	Statistical significance (α = 0.05)
Able to get about the houase	2 (1–2)	2 (0–3)	0.95
Able to get aout of the house	2 (0–2)	2 (0–2)	0.42
Able to go shopping	1 (0–2)	1,5 (0–2)	0.41
Total score	5 (1–6)	5,5 (0–7)	0.50

In each subgroup, a maximum of 3 points (3 no difficulties, 2 with an aid, 1 with help from another person, and 0 not at all) can be achieved. A maximum score of 9 points can be achieved germination specimen in our investigation. There are no valid statements in prior research regarding this issue.

Limitations

A disadvantage of this study is the low number of cases, which is a highly specific and rare patient population. Therefore, only tendencies, rather than statistically valid statements, are possible. The inhomogeneity of the treatment is also seen as a limitation, whereby the treatment of PJI is always case-dependent; nevertheless, this can be put into perspective by the comparable treatment modalities (Tables 1 and 2) and the same standards in treatment. Due to the long study period of 6 years (median 72 months) and the advanced age of many of the patients, a significant number had already died. Due to the retrospective survey occurring over a long period of time, details of the survey also got lost (antibiotics, sampling, etc).

Conclusion

Through this retrospective analysis, it can be determined that the rate of reinfection of modular mega-endoprostheses on the hip and knee joint after healed PJI can be reduced through the use of silver coated implants. The time until reinfection can also be prolonged using silver coated implants. Due to the low number of cases of this highly specific patient population, no statistical significance could be determined; however, a positive effect can be assumed from the use of silver coatings in mega-endoprostheses after an infection develops.

Abbreviations

MRSA: Methicillin resistant *Staphylococcus aureus*; NMS: New Mobility Score; NSCG: Non silver- coated group; PJI: Periprosthetic joint infection; SCG: Silver-coated group; THA: Total hip arthroplasty; TKA: Total knee arthroplasty

Acknowledgements

We acknowledge support from the German Research Foundation (DFG) and University Hospital Leipzig within the programme of Open Access Publishing. We would like to thank Prof. Th. Kahn, Department of Diagnostic and Interventional Radiology, for providing the radiographs. We also thank Anna Martinez for the linguistic revision of the manuscript.

Funding

This study was funded by German Research Foundation (DFG) and the University Hospital Leipzig within the programme of Open Access Publishing. The funding body had no role in designing the study, collecting, analysing and interpreting the data, or in writing the manuscript.

Authors' contributions

DZ analysed and interpreted the patient data and was a major contributor in writing the manuscript. UB carried out the data collection and contributed significantly to the preparation of the manuscript. MG, TP, CJ, AR and JMF were mainly responsible for the treatment of the patients and contributed as assistants to the preparation of the work. SG was responsible for the microbiological analysis and JMF initiated the work and was supervised considerably. All authors read and approved the final manuscript.

Consent for publication

All participating patients gave written, informed consent in the treatment contract, the study and in the publication of the anonymised data.

Competing interests

The authors declare that they have no competing interests.

Author details

[1]Department of Orthopaedic Surgery, Trauma Surgery and Plastic Surgery, University Hospital Leipzig, Liebigstrasse 20, D-04103 Leipzig, Germany. [2]Department of Orthopaedics and Trauma Surgery, HELIOS Clinic Blankenhain, Wirthstrasse 5, D-99444 Blankenhain, Germany. [3]ZESBO – Zentrum zur Erforschung der Stuetz- und Bewegungsorgane, Semmelweisstrasse 14, D-04103 Leipzig, Germany.

References

1. Mota REM, Tarricone R, Ciani O, Bridges JFP, Drummond M. Determinants of demand for total hip and knee arthroplasty: a systematic literature review. BMC Health Serv Res. 2012;12:225. doi:10.1186/1472-6963-12-225.
2. Tian W, DeJong G, Brown M, Hsieh C-H, Zamfirov ZP, Horn SD. Looking upstream: factors shaping the demand for postacute joint replacement rehabilitation. Arch Phys Med Rehabil. 2009;90:1260–8. doi:10.1016/j.apmr.2008.10.035.
3. Zajonz D, Wuthe L, Tiepolt S, Brandmeier P, Prietzel T, Salis-Soglio GF v, et al. Diagnostic work-up strategy for periprosthetic joint infections after total hip and knee arthroplasty: a 12-year experience on 320 consecutive cases. Patient Saf Surg. 2015;9:20. doi:10.1186/s13037-015-0071-8.
4. Zajonz D, Zieme A, Prietzel T, Moche M, Tiepoldt S, Roth A, et al. Periprosthetic joint infections in modular endoprostheses of the lower extremities: a retrospective observational study in 101 patients. Patient Saf Surg. 2016;10:6. doi:10.1186/s13037-016-0095-8.
5. Ascherl R. Infection management of megaimplants. Orthopade. 2010;39:980–93. doi:10.1007/s00132-009-1570-z.
6. Malchau H, Herberts P, Eisler T, Garellick G, Soderman P. The Swedish Total hip replacement register. J Bone Joint Surg Am. 2002;84-A(Suppl 2):2–20.
7. Salis-Soglio G v, Ghanem M, Meinecke I, Ellenrieder M, Klinger H-M, Kirchhoff C. The modular endoprosthetic system Munich-Luebeck (MML): potential applications and results in the lower extremities. Orthopade. 2010;39:960–7. doi:10.1007/s00132-009-1569-5.
8. Fakler JK, Hase F, Bohme J, Josten C. Safety aspects in surgical treatment of pathological fractures of the proximal femur - modular endoprosthetic replacement vs. intramedullary nailing. Patient Saf Surg. 2013;7:37. doi:10.1186/1754-9493-7-37.
9. Kotz R. Tumor endoprosthesis in malignant bone tumors. Orthopade. 1993;22:160–6.
10. Morris HG, Capanna R, Campanacci D, Del Ben M, Gasbarrini A. Modular endoprosthetic replacement after total resection of the femur for malignant tumour. Int Orthop. 1994;18:90–5.
11. Foo LSS, Hardes J, Henrichs M, Ahrens H, Gosheger G, Streitburger A. Surgical difficulties encountered with use of modular endoprosthesis for limb preserving salvage of failed allograft reconstruction after malignant tumor resection. J Arthroplast. 2011;26:744–50. doi:10.1016/j.arth.2010.06.011.
12. Anagnostakos K, Kohn D. Megaprostheses of the knee joint. Orthopade. 2010;39:949–59. doi:10.1007/s00132-009-1565-9.
13. Pala E, Trovarelli G, Calabro T, Angelini A, Abati CN, Ruggieri P. Survival of modern knee tumor megaprostheses: failures, functional results, and a comparative statistical analysis. Clin Orthop Relat Res. 2015;473:891–9. doi:10.1007/s11999-014-3699-2.
14. Sevelda F, Schuh R, Hofstaetter JG, Schinhan M, Windhager R, Funovics PT. Total femur replacement after tumor resection: limb salvage usually achieved but complications and failures are common. Clin Orthop Relat Res. 2015;473:2079–87. doi:10.1007/s11999-015-4282-1.
15. Capanna R, Scoccianti G, Frenos F, Vilardi A, Beltrami G, Campanacci DA. What was the survival of megaprostheses in lower limb reconstructions after tumor resections? Clin Orthop Relat Res. 2015;473:820–30. doi:10.1007/s11999-014-3736-1.
16. Cheng H, Li Y, Huo K, Gao B, Xiong W. Long-lasting in vivo and in vitro antibacterial ability of nanostructured titania coating incorporated with silver nanoparticles. J Biomed Mater Res A. 2014;102:3488–99. doi:10.1002/jbm.a.35019.

17. Qin H, Cao H, Zhao Y, Zhu C, Cheng T, Wang Q, et al. Vitro and in vivo anti-biofilm effects of silver nanoparticles immobilized on titanium. Biomaterials. 2014;35:9114–25. doi:10.1016/j.biomaterials.2014.07.040.
18. Kollef MH, Afessa B, Anzueto A, Veremakis C, Kerr KM, Margolis BD, et al. Silver-coated endotracheal tubes and incidence of ventilator-associated pneumonia: the NASCENT randomized trial. JAMA. 2008;300:805–13. doi:10.1001/jama.300.7.805.
19. Tobin EJ, Bambauer R. Silver coating of dialysis catheters to reduce bacterial colonization and infection. Ther Apher Dial. 2003;7:504–9.
20. Hardes J, Eiff C von , Streitbuerger A, Balke M, Budny T, Henrichs MP, et al. Reduction of periprosthetic infection with silver-coated megaprostheses in patients with bone sarcoma. J Surg Oncol 2010;101:389–395. doi:10.1002/jso.21498.
21. Alt V. Antimicrobial coated implants in trauma and orthopaedics-a clinical review and risk-benefit analysis. Injury. 2016; doi:10.1016/j.injury.2016.12.011.
22. Schmolders J, Koob S, Schepers P, Pennekamp PH, Gravius S, Wirtz DC, et al. Lower limb reconstruction in tumor patients using modular silver-coated megaprostheses with regard to perimegaprosthetic joint infection: a case series, including 100 patients and review of the literature. Arch Orthop Trauma Surg. 2017;137:149–53. doi:10.1007/s00402-016-2584-8.
23. Wilding CP, Cooper GA, Freeman AK, Parry MC, Jeys L. Can a silver-coated arthrodesis implant provide a viable alternative to above knee amputation in the unsalvageable, infected Total knee arthroplasty? J Arthroplast. 2016; 31:2542–7. doi:10.1016/j.arth.2016.04.009.
24. Parker MJ, Palmer CRA. New mobility score for predicting mortality after hip fracture. J Bone Joint Surg Br. 1993;75:797–8.
25. Donati F, Di Giacomo G, Ziranu A, Spinelli S, Perisano C, Rosa MA, Maccauro G. Silver coated prosthesis in oncological limb salvage surgery reduce the infection rate. J Biol Regul Homeost Agents. 2015;29:149–55.
26. Gosheger G, Hardes J, Ahrens H, Streitburger A, Buerger H, Erren M, et al. Silver-coated megaendoprostheses in a rabbit model–an analysis of the infection rate and toxicological side effects. Biomaterials. 2004;25:5547–56. doi:10.1016/j.biomaterials.2004.01.008.
27. Hardes J, Ahrens H, Gebert C, Streitbuerger A, Buerger H, Erren M, et al. Lack of toxicological side-effects in silver-coated megaprostheses in humans. Biomaterials. 2007;28:2869–75. doi:10.1016/j.biomaterials.2007.02.033.
28. Wafa H, Grimer RJ, Reddy K, Jeys L, Abudu A, Carter SR, Tillman RM. Retrospective evaluation of the incidence of early periprosthetic infection with silver-treated endoprostheses in high-risk patients: case-control study. Bone Joint J. 2015;97-B:252–7. doi:10.1302/0301-620X.97B2.34554.
29. Hazer DB, Sakar M, Dere Y, Altinkanat G, Ziyal MI, Hazer B. Antimicrobial effect of polymer-based silver nanoparticle coated pedicle screws: experimental research on biofilm inhibition in rabbits. Spine (Phila Pa 1976). 2016;41:E323–9. doi:10.1097/BRS.0000000000001223.

3

Interview based malnutrition assessment can predict adverse events within 6 months after primary and revision arthroplasty

Christoph Ihle[1], Christoph Weiß[1], Gunnar Blumenstock[2], Ulrich Stöckle[1], Björn Gunnar Ochs[3], Christian Bahrs[1], Andreas Nüssler[1*] and Anna Janine Schreiner[1]

Abstract

Background: Being at risk for malnutrition can be observed among hospitalized patients of all medical specialties. There are only few studies in arthroplasty dealing with defining and assessing malnutrition as such a potentially risk. This study aims to identify the risk for malnutrition following primary (pAP) and revision arthroplasty (rAP) (1) using non-invasive interview based assessment tools and to analyze effects on clinical outcome (2) and quality of life (3).

Methods: A consecutive series of hospitalized patients of a Department of Arthroplasty at a Level 1 Trauma Center in Western Europe was observed between June 2014 and June 2016. Patients were monitored for being at risk for malnutrition at hospital admission (T1) and 6 months post surgery (T2) by non-invasive interview based assessment tools (NRS 2002, SF-MNA, MNA). Adverse events, length of hospital stay and quality of life (HRQL, SF-36) were monitored.

Results: 351 (283 pAP/ 68 rAP) patients were included. At T1, 13.4% (47) / 23.9% (84) / 27.4% (96) and at T2 7.3% (18) / 17.1% (42) / 16.0% (39) of all patients were at risk for malnutrition regarding NRS/SF-MNA/MNA. Prevalence of malnutrition risk was higher in rAP (22.1–29.4%) compared to pAP (11.3–26.9%). Patients being at risk for malnutrition showed prolonged hospitalization (NRS 14.5 to 12.5, SF-MNA 13.7 to 12.4, MNA 13.9 to 12.3 days, $p < 0.05$), delayed mobilization (NRS 2.1 to 1.7, SF-MNA 1.8 to 1.7, MNA 1.9 to 1.7 days), lower values in HRQL and more adverse events.

Conclusions: There is a moderate to high prevalence of risk for malnutrition in arthroplasty that can easily be assessed through interview based screening tools. Being at risk for malnutrition can reduce the clinical outcome following pAP and rAP. Patients with an impaired nutritional status show reduced values in physical and mental aspects of HRQL. Non-invasive interview-based nutritional assessment can predict adverse events in primary and revision total arthroplasty and can therefore help identifying patients at risk before surgery.

Keywords: Malnutrition, Arthroplasty, Interview based assessment, NRS 2002, MNA, SF-MNA

* Correspondence: andreas.nuessler@gmail.com
[1]Siegfried Weller Institute for Trauma Research, BG Trauma Center Tübingen, Eberhard Karls University Tübingen, Schnarrenbergstrasse 95, 72076 Tübingen, Germany
Full list of author information is available at the end of the article

Background

Impaired nutritional status can be observed among hospitalized patients across all medical specialties with prevalence rates between 20 and 61% [1, 2]. Several studies have shown the substantial importance of malnutrition and its impact on clinical results [3, 4]. Higher age as well as disease- and lifestyle associated circumstances are risk factors for developing nutritional deficiencies [5]. It is an increasing problem with relevant consequences regarding medical as well as socio-economic aspects due to higher complication rates and prolonged hospitalization accompanied by demographic changes resulting in higher costs for hospitals and health insurances [3, 6]. The relevance is underlined by an increasing number of publications in the past years, especially the latest ESPEN (European Society for Clinical Nutrition and Metabolism) publications and definitions [7, 8]. Nevertheless, there is still little information concerning the nutritional status of hospitalized orthopedic and trauma patients [9, 10]. The prevalence of malnutrition is estimated between 9 and 39% in orthopedic patients undergoing arthroplasty [9]. Studies so far used controversially discussed invasive biomarkers, e.g. albumin, to show that malnutrition is associated with delayed wound healing, periprosthetic joint infections, prolonged length of hospital stay and re-mobilization as well as increased mortality in patients undergoing total hip and knee replacement [9, 11–14].

There are different screening tools to evaluate patients' probability of being nutritionally at risk. Depending on the used screening method, the prevalence of malnutrition in geriatric patients suffering hip related fractures ranges between 32 and 60% [15–17] and was analyzed as an independent factor of 12-month mortality [18]. ESPEN recognizes the NRS 2002 as well as the SF-MNA as risk screening tools to be used in hospital, elderly care and community settings [8]. Besides the risk screening tools named above, blood markers for malnutrition like albumin, total leucocyte count and transferrin are in controversial discussion [14, 19–21]. However, the relevance of patient assessment at risk for malnutrition in a large and prospectively evaluated case series comparing NRS 2002, SF-MNA and MNA side-by-side as established non-invasive interview based screening tools in patients undergoing primary and revision arthroplasty documented from the time point of hospital admission following six months after hospital dismissal does not exist so far. In contrast to other medical specialties, malnutrition in arthroplasty is partially underreported and needs further evidence, especially regarding evaluation, clinical application of scoring systems and health related quality of life.

Methods

Study population

The study protocol was approved by the local ethics committee (193/2014BO2) and registered at the German Clinical Trials Register according to WHO standard (DKRS00006192). Written consent of the ethics committee of the medical university of Tübingen is available. All included subjects gave their informed written consent. The study was conducted according to the guidelines for reporting of observational studies in Epidemiology (STROBE) [22].

A consecutive series of hospitalized patients of a supraregional Department of Arthroplasty at a Level 1 Trauma Center in Western Europe was observed between June 2014 and June 2015. All patients who agreed to participate in the study and were hospitalized for more than two nights were included. Minors, patients suffering from dementia, with insufficient knowledge of the study language and incapability to answer the questions due to severe health conditions were excluded. Patients at the Intensive Care Unit were generally excluded as being defined as patients with severe health conditions.

The patients were checked for their nutritional status respectively for being at risk for malnutrition at the time of their hospital admission one day prior to operation (T1). Three interview-based, internationally approved and well-established assessment tools were used for the assessment: The Nutritional Risk Screening (NRS 2002), the Mini Nutritional Assessment (MNA) as well as the Short Form MNA (SF-MNA) were administered to all patients. To evaluate the generic quality of life, SF-36 questionnaire was used.

All comorbidities and further information concerning patients' health and general conditions were collected using a standardized protocol. The diagnoses were self-reported and depended on previously diagnoses and/or taken medication. Adverse events and further general patient data were captured out of our hospital information system after discharge. These data were used for further statistical evaluation as well. All interview based assessments were repeated 6 months after surgery (T2). The assessment was carried out by eight independent observers. Observer bias was avoided by preceding standardized observer training for two weeks in groups of two with frequently changing partners.

Nutritional risk screening (NRS 2002)

Nutritional Risk Screening (NRS 2002) by Kondrup et al. is an international well-established interview-based assessment tool describing the risk for malnutrition in hospitalized patients [23]. It has been used in several clinical trials of different medical fields so far and is recommended by the European Society for Clinical Nutrition and Metabolism (ESPEN) [7]. Being nutritionally at risk is defined as a NRS-Score ≥ 3 whereas a regular nutrition state is implied by a NRS < 3. Besides registering weight loss within the last 3 months, patient age and the severity of illness are included in this score [7].

Mini nutritional assessment (MNA)

The Mini Nutritional Assessment (MNA) was developed and validated by the Nestlé Nutrition Institute during studies between 1991 and 1993 in the United States of America and France [24]. Briefly, the application of the MNA is recommended for elderly patients over 65 years. We applied it to all patients of our study. It can be downloaded for free on the internet (http://www.mna-elderly.com). It is a well-established screening tool for malnutrition and has been used in several clinical trials so far. Being at risk of malnutrition is implied by MNA ≤ 11 points. The score includes amongst others Body Mass Index (BMI), behavior concerning food and recent weight loss.

Short form mini nutritional assessment (SF-MNA)

The SF-MNA (Mini Nutritional Assessment Short-Form) was also developed by Nestlé and is available at the internet (http://www.mna-elderly.com) [25, 26]. Briefly, being nutritionally at risk is defined between a range of 0–7 points. The SF-MNA is applied to elderly patients over 65 years. It is also a well-established assessment tool and of easy and fast application with good accuracy for assessing risk for malnutrition. Next to weight loss within the last 3 months, BMI, mobility and severity of illness are included in this score.

Health related quality of life (SF-36 questionnaire)

To describe Health Related Quality of Life (HRQL) the SF-36 questionnaire was used [27]. We used the interview-based version of this tool consisting of 36 questions. Based on these questions' values, eight scales describing physical and mental health can be assessed. The physical part is represented by Physical Functioning (PF), Role Physical (RP), Bodily Pain (BP) and General Health (GH). Vitality (VT), Social Functioning (SF), Role Emotional (RE) and Mental Health (MH) describe the mental aspect of HRQL. Usually regular scoring is performed first (RS, 0–100 points). Physical and mental component summary scores (PSC and MCS) can be achieved by transformation of the summary scores and is a widespread method [28–30].

Clinical outcome and patient data

Clinical outcome was described through adverse events, length of stay (LOS) and mobilization after primary or revision arthroplasty. Postoperative mobilization was defined as safe walking on crutches out of bed. This information was captured out of the rehabilitation protocol of the clinical information system. Patient data (comorbidities, number of daily medication etc.) were captured out of the digital clinical information system after patients' discharge.

Adverse events

Adverse events were monitored at two points of time - during hospital stay and at T2 for the period of 6 months following primary or revision arthroplasty excluding adverse events having already occurred during hospitalization. All adverse events weighted equally. Major adverse events were defined as death, infections, wound healing disorders, further operations and thrombosis. Minor adverse events were postoperative anemia and postoperative electrolyte imbalance with therapeutic necessity and delayed removal of drains more than two days following surgery.

Statistics

Evaluated scales and scores were quantitative or semi-quantitative parameters in the present study. They were described as mean and standard deviation, minimum and maximum, as well as quartiles. Normality was tested with the Kolmogorov-Smirnov-Test. Nominally and ordinally scaled values were displayed in counts and percentages. Contingency tables were used to compare two of each of these values and the chi-square-test was applied for testing association. The drop-out analysis was performed with the t-test for independent samples for the variables age and BMI and with cross-tabulations with chi-quadrat-statistics for the variables sex, alcohol consumption and understanding of the study language. The tests were two sided with a significance level of 5%. An alpha adjustment for multiple testing was not applied. The results were interpreted accordingly. Statistical analysis was performed with IBM SPSS Statistics 23 (SPSS Inc., IBM Company Chicago, IL, USA) and with JMP 13 (SAS, SAS Institute, Cary, NC, USA).

Results

Patient characteristics and general information

A patient flow chart is presented in Fig. 1. 351 arthroplasty patients were included in the present study for statistical analysis. The whole group can be divided in the subgroup of primary arthroplasty (pAP, $n = 283$) and revision arthroplasty (rAP, $n = 68$). There was no relevant statistical difference in patient age between the subgroups with a mean age of all patients of 67.9 ± (28–91) years ($p = 0.69$). Women outnumbered men in both subgroups. According to the World Health Organization (WHO 2004) our study population can be classified as predominantly pre-obese regarding BMI (25.0–29.9) without noticeable statistical differences regarding the subgroups pAP and rAP ($p = 0.61$).

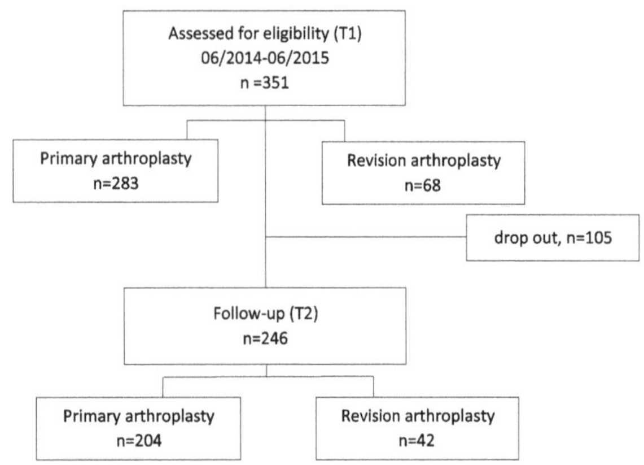

Fig. 1 Patient flow chart according to STROBE standards

Follow-up

Addressing an expected loss to follow-up, a drop-out-analysis was performed. Based on the drop-out-analysis of all eligible and assessed 351 patients (T1), a follow-up of 70,1% ($n = 246$) was achieved without any relevant statistical differences between the group with a total follow-up (T2) and the group lost to follow-up after T1 regarding nutritional status, sex, BMI and age. Nevertheless, there was a statistical difference regarding "language skills of the study language". Statistically significant more patients who quit the study after T1 showed reduced skills of the study language. In detail, the follow-up was 72,1% ($n = 204$) for the primary arthroplasty group (pAP) respectively 61,8% ($n = 42$) for the revision arthroplasty group (rAP). The question of drop out needn't to be included in further analysis according to missing statistical differences between the two groups.

Prevalence of malnutrition in primary and revision arthroplasty

At the time of hospital admission (T1), 13.4% ($n = 47$) / 23.9% ($n = 84$) / 27.4% ($n = 96$) of all patients were at risk for malnutrition according NRS, SF-MNA, and MNA, respectively.

Among pAP patients 11.3% ($n = 32$) / 23.3% ($n = 66$), and 26.9% ($n = 76$) were at risk for malnutrition according to NRS, SF-MNA, and MNA respectively. In the group of rAP patients 22.1% ($n = 15$), 26.5% ($n = 18$), and 29.4% ($n = 20$) were at risk for malnutrition according to NRS, SF-MNA, and MNA respectively. Based on the three different tools we found the highest prevalence of malnutrition when applying the MNA assessment tool in patients undergoing revision arthroplasty.

At the time of follow-up (T2), we found that among all study subjects 7.3% (n = 18), 17.1% ($n = 42$), and 16.0% ($n = 39$) were still at risk for malnutrition regarding NRS, SF-MNA, and MNA respectively.

Among pAP patients, we found at T2 5.9% ($n = 12$), 16.2% ($n = 33$), and 15.4% ($n = 31$) were at risk for malnutrition according to NRS, SF-MNA, and MNA respectively. In the group of rAP patients 14.3% ($n = 6$), 21.4% ($n = 9$), and 19.1% ($n = 8$) according to the three assessment tools respectively. At T2 the highest prevalence of malnutrition risk was assessed by SF-MNA tool. Nevertheless, there was a clear reduction of the risk of malnutrition within six months (from T1 to T2) in all groups. This was not statistically significant, most likely due to small sample sizes.

Malnutrition and quality of life

HRQL for the whole study population is presented in Fig. 2 at both time points of evaluation. Part one shows the values of HRQL in all eight dimensions for the whole study population as well as the two subgroups pAP and rAP at T1. Part two describes the development of HRQL six months after surgery for the above mentioned three groups. A significant pre- to postoperative (T1 to T2) improvement of HRQL can be found in all eight dimensions for the overall collective ($p < 0.001$). Part three shows the eight SF-36 dimensions according to the nutritional scores respectively the nutritional status (with or without risk for malnutrition) at T1. HRQL is preoperatively decreased for both nutritional groups (with or without risk for malnutrition), especially for PF, RP, BP, VT and RE. Moreover, patients being at risk for malnutrition before surgery show statistically significant lower values - according mainly to SF-MNA and MNA - in all physical (PF, RP, BP, GH) as well as mental dimensions (SF, RE, MH) in comparison to those with a regular nutritional status. Part 4 describes HRQL according to patients' nutritional status postoperatively. All 8 dimensions show an increase for both nutritional groups (with or without risk for malnutrition) after surgery. In comparison to the preoperative SF-36 results, the values of the patients with risk for malnutrition are adjusting to the values of the patients with a regular nutritional status, but BP and GH are still statistically significant lower for patients being at risk for malnutrition ($p = 0.02$ respectively $p = 0.001$ according to SF-MNA) than for patients without being at risk.

In summary, patients being at risk for malnutrition show lower values in each dimension of HRQL before and after surgery in comparison to patients with a regular nutritional status regarding the physical as well as mental aspects of SF-36. Improvements after arthroplasty can be found in both nutritional groups in all dimensions with a persisting but closer gap between the values of patients at risk for malnutrition and those with a regular nutritional status.

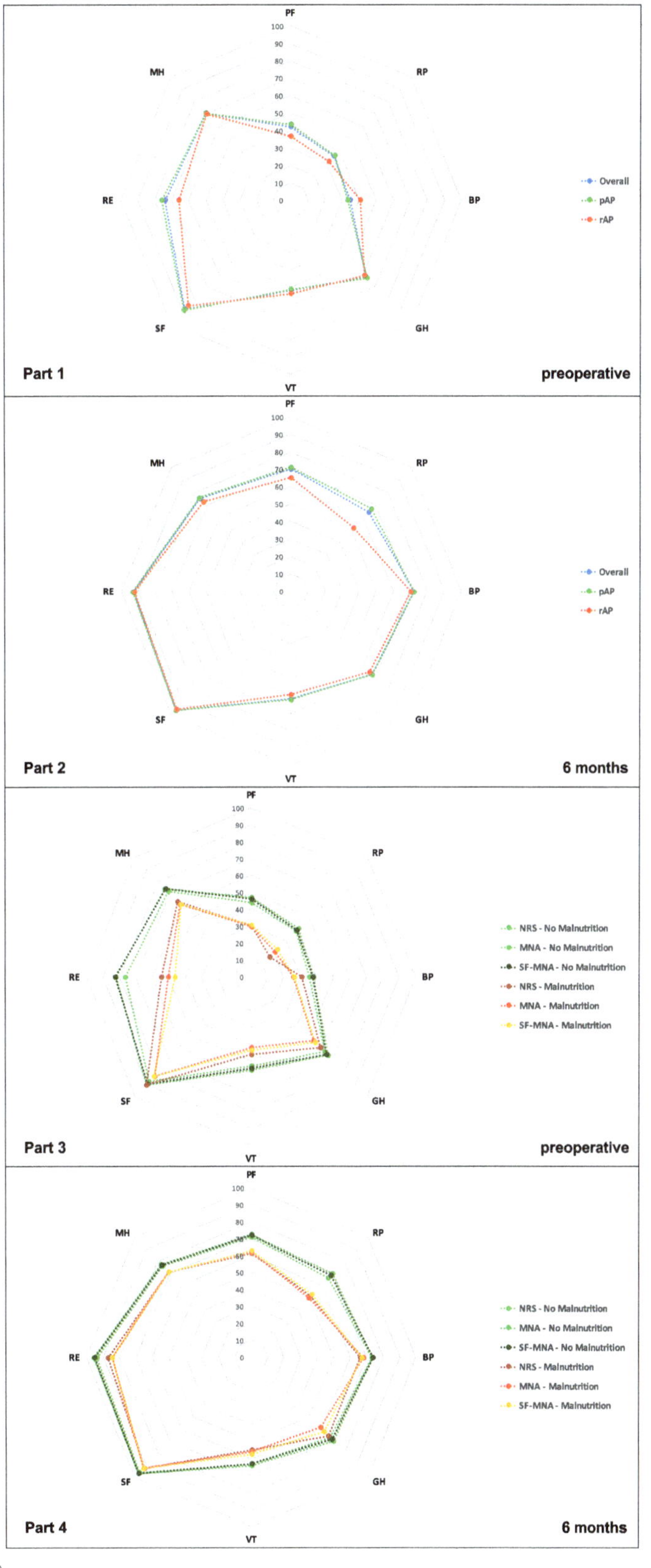

Fig. 2 (See legend on next page.)

(See figure on previous page.)
Fig. 2 Health related quality of life in primary and revision arthroplasty comparing different nutritional status. Part 1 and 2: Figure two part one and two describe the values of health related quality of life at hospital admission and six months following surgery in all eight SF-36 dimensions comparing primary arthroplasty (pAP), revision arthroplasty (rAP) and the whole study population (overall). A pre- to postoperative improvement of HRQL can be found according to all eight dimensions. Part 3 and 4: Part three and four show the eight SF-36 dimensions of the whole study population according to all three nutritional scores comparing the nutritional status (Malnutrition vs. No Malnutrition) at hospital admission and six months following surgery. HRQL is preoperatively decreased. Patients being at risk for malnutrition before surgery show statistically significant lower values in physical (PF, RP, BP, GH) as well as mental dimensions (SF, RE, MH). In comparison to the preoperative SF-36 results, the values of the patients with risk for malnutrition are adjusting to the values of the patients with a regular nutritional status. PF: Physical Functioning; RP: Role Physical; BP: Bodily Pain; GH: General Health; VT: Vitality; SF: Social Functioning; RE: Role Emotional; MH: Mental Health; pAP: Primary Arthroplasty; rAP: Revision Arthroplasty; HRQL: Health related quality of life

HRQL in relation to nutritional scores

Regarding the relation of nutritional scores at T1 und SF-36 at T2, the MNA shows a statistically significant effect in almost all dimensions (p: PF 0.02 / RP 0.016 / GH 0.004 / VT 0.022 / RE 0.006 / MH 0.044). The SF-MNA unfolded a statistical significance for RE (p = 0.018) and MH (p = 0.04). The NRS showed no statistically significant difference in any dimension.

Clinical outcome

LOS and mobilization

The average LOS was 12.7 ± 3.65 (6–33) days. Mean LOS was 12.1 ± 2.7 (6–31) days for the pAP group respectively 15.31 ± 5.52 (8–33) days for the rAP group. Mobility in all patients was achieved 1.74 ± 0.79 (1–7) days after arthroplasty was performed. It took 1.7 ± 0.6 (1–5) days in the pPA group respectively 2.12 ± 1.11 (1–7) days in the rAP group until postoperative mobilization could be obtained out of bed.

All Patients assessed at T1 at risk for malnutrition showed a highly statistically significant prolonged length of hospital stay for all assessment tools (p-value NRS, SF-MNA, and MNA: 0.006, 0.001, and 0.0001, respectively). In parallel, we found that mobilization after surgery was equally statistically significant delayed compared to patients with a regular nutritional status according to NRS (p = 0.012). LOS and mobilization divided according to the different nutritional scores are shown in Table 1.

Incidence of adverse events in primary and revision arthroplasty during hospitalization

The incidence and subdivision of adverse events regarding all patients and regarding pAP and rAP is demonstrated in Table 2. Adverse events divided according to the different nutritional scores and according the above mentioned groups are shown in Table 3. Patients being at risk for malnutrition according to interview based assessment tools showed a higher incidence of all adverse events (minor and major) before and after arthroplasty compared to patients with a regular nutritional status. The highest prevalence of adverse events was found when patients were assessed by the NRS assessment tool.

Discussion

Our study could show a moderate to high prevalence of 13 to 27% being at risk for malnutrition in arthroplasty patients prior to surgery. The main findings of the present study were that being at risk for malnutrition results in suboptimal postoperative clinical outcome. Based on our data, prolonged hospitalization, delayed mobilization after surgery, more adverse events and reduced health related quality of life have to be expected in these patients. Non-invasive interview-based nutritional assessment can predict adverse events in primary and revision total arthroplasty and can therefore help identifying patients at risk before surgery.

The aim of this study was to determine the prevalence of risk for malnutrition in hospitalized patients undergoing primary and revision arthroplasty and to analyze its clinical effects up to 6 months after surgery. Moreover, we wanted to evaluate the relation between impaired nutritional status and health related quality of life as well as to determine which screening tool is useful in daily clinical practice. Based on our data, being at risk for malnutrition according to NRS-, SF-MNA-, and MNA assessment results clearly in suboptimal clinical outcomes. Independently of the assessment tool used, the risk for malnutrition was associated with prolonged hospitalization, more wound healing disorders, more

Table 1 Length of hospital stay (LOS) and Mobilization in relation to NRS, SF-MNA and MNA

NRS				
Risk for malnutrition / no risk		+	–	p
all	Hospitalization (LOS, days)	14.5 ± 5.3	12.5 ± 3.2	0.006
all	Mobilization (days after surgery)	2.1 ± 1.0	1.7 ± 0.7	0.012
SF-MNA		T1		
Risk for malnutrition / no risk		+	–	p
all	Hospitalization (LOS, days)	13.7 ± 3.9	12.4 ± 3.5	0.001
all	Mobilization (days after surgery)	1.8 ± 0.9	1.7 ± 0.7	0.267
MNA		T1		
Risk for malnutrition / no risk		+	–	p
all	Hospitalization (LOS, days)	13.9 ± 4.3	12.3 ± 3.3	0.001
all	Mobilization (days after surgery)	1.9 ± 1.0	1.7 ± 0.6	0.189

Table 2 Incidence of major (grey) and minor adverse events in primary and revision arthroplasty

	all		pAP		rAP	
No adverse events T1	62.1% (218)		66.4% (188)		44.1% (30)	
No adverse events T2	89.1% (219)		91.2% (186)		78.6% (33)	
Adverse events T1	37.9% (133)		33.6% (95)		55.9% (38)	
Adverse events T2	10.9% (27)		8.8% (18)		21.4% (9)	
Infection T1	3 / 351	0.9%	1 / 283	0.4%	2 / 68	2.9%
Infection T2	8 / 246	3.3%	5 / 204	2.5%	3 / 42	7.1%
Wound healing disorder T1	3 / 351	0.9%	2 / 283	0.7%	1 / 68	1.5%
Wound healing disorder T2	2 / 246	0.8%	2 / 204	1.0%	0 / 42	0.0%
Further operations T1	5 / 351	1.4%	2 / 283	0.7%	3 / 68	4.4%
Further operations T2	1 / 246	0.4%	1 / 204	0.5%	0 / 42	0.0%
Thrombosis T1	1 / 351	0.3%	0 / 283	0.0%	1 / 68	1.5%
Thrombosis T2	2 / 246	0.8%	2 / 204	1.0%	0 / 42	0.0%
Minor adverse events T1	121 / 351	34.5%	90 / 283	31.8%	31 / 68	45.6%
Minor adverse events T2	14 / 246	5.7%	8 / 204	3.9%	6 / 42	14.3%

adverse events and reduced health related quality of life compared to patients with a regular nutritional status. NRS tool identified patients being at risk for malnutrition that were associated with higher rates of adverse events superior compared to the other used tools.

As the risk for malnutrition was significantly reduced in all patients, as well as in pAP and rAP after operative treatment, arthroplasty obviously reduced the pain level, improved the mobility, and ameliorated the initial impaired nutritional status. Nevertheless, our data shows that being at risk for malnutrition is a relevant risk factor for several aspects of a diminished clinical outcome that seems to be undervalued so far in clinical routine. Non-invasive interview-based nutritional assessment can predict adverse events in primary and revision total arthroplasty and can therefore help identifying patients at risk before surgery. To our knowledge, this is the first study analyzing these results for primary as well as revision arthroplasty with the focus on interview based assessment and HRQL in a prospective and huge cohort. The moderate to high prevalence of 13–27% of risk for malnutrition found in our study corresponds with the predominant data presented in a recent review which reports a scope from 9 to 39% with other studies showing incidences as high as 50% [9]. Thomas et al. reported a prevalence of 24.1% of patients at risk for malnutrition according to NRS in elective surgery [2]. This is similar to the finding of Nicholson et al. who defined malnutrition by albumin levels and total lymphocyte count (TLC). The authors concluded from their data a prevalence of 30% in elective THA compared to 86% in trauma THA of malnutrition [20].

Jensen et al. and Golladay et al. reported delayed wound healing, persistent drainage and prosthetic joint infection in orthopedic patients as the most common complications in association with malnutrition [9, 11]. Other studies reviewing and/or defining malnutrition by low transferrin, total lymphocyte count or albumin also describe the following associated complications in arthroplasty: wound complications, extended length of stay and periprosthetic joint infection [20, 31, 32]. Besides, re-admission and further complications such as postoperative hematoma, seroma, renal complications and pneumonia are described [31]. All these findings are in line with our results. As far as we know there has not been an evaluation of HRQL in arthroplasty patients with an impaired nutrition status so far. We could recently show that traumatology and orthopedic patients show lower values in each dimension of SF-36 [16]. Our current results confirm these findings especially for arthroplasty patients. The applied assessment tools in our study have proven to be useful and easy to use according to our data. We and others compared various nutritional assessment tools in elderly trauma patients (NRS, SF-MNA and MUST) with hip fractures [15, 33]. Koren-Hakim et al. reported that only the SF-MNA could predict readmission and mortality besides detecting malnutrition while the other two assessment tools did not [33]. Considering our results, it becomes obvious that the application of different nutritional scores unfolds with similar general and comparable results but with emphasis on different key aspects. In the opinion of the authors, there is an advantage in some scores assessing the following aspects in patients undergoing arthroplasty.

- Risk of malnutrition: MNA, SF-MNA superior to NRS
- Mobilization: NRS

Table 3 All Adverse events in relation to NRS, SF-MNA and MNA

NRS		T1			T2		
Risk for malnutrition / no risk		+	–	p	+	–	p
all	Adverse events	53.2% (25)	35.5% (108)		22.6% (7)	9.3% (20)	
	No adverse events	46.8% (22)	64.5% (196)	0.02	77.4% (24)	90.7% (195)	0.03
	n total	*47*	*304*		*31*	*215*	
pAP	Adverse events	40.6% (13)	32.7% (82)		13.6% (3)	8.2% (15)	
	No adverse events	59.4% (19)	67.3% (169)	0.37	86.4% (19)	91.8% (167)	0.40
	n total	*32*	*251*		*22*	*182*	
rAP	Adverse events	80.0% (12)	49.1% (26)		44.4% (4)	15.2% (5)	
	No adverse events	20.0% (3)	50.9% (27)	0.03	55.6% (5)	84.8% (28)	0.06
	n total	*15*	*53*		9	*33*	
SF-MNA		T1			T2		
Risk for malnutrition / no risk		+	–	p	+	–	p
all	Adverse events	46.4% (39)	35.2% (94)		17.9% (10)	8.9% (17)	
	No adverse events	53.6% (45)	64.8% (173)	0.06	82.1% (46)	91.1% (173)	0.06
	n total	*84*	*267*		*56*	*190*	
pAP	Adverse events	39.4% (26)	31.8% (69)		12.8% (6)	7.6% (12)	
	No adverse events	60.6% (40)	68.2% (148)	0.25	87.2% (41)	92.3% (145)	0.28
	n total	*66*	*217*		*47*	*157*	
rAP	Adverse events	72.2% (13)	50.0% (25)		44.4% (4)	15.2% (5)	
	No adverse events	27.8% (5)	50.0% (25)	0.10	55.6% (5)	84.8% (28)	0.06
	n total	*18*	*50*		*9*	*33*	
MNA		T1			T2		
Risk for malnutrition / no risk		+	–	p	+	–	p
all	Adverse events	49.0% (47)	33.7% (86)		17.5% (11)	8.7% (16)	
	No adverse events	51.0% (49)	66.3% (169)	0.01	82.5% (52)	91.3% (167)	0.06
	n total	*96*	*255*		*63*	*183*	
pAP	Adverse events	43.2% (33)	29.9% (62)		15.1% (8)	6.6% (10)	
	No adverse events	56.8% (43)	70.1% (145)	0.03	8.9% (45)	93.4% (141)	0.06
	n total	*76*	*207*		*53*	*141*	
rAP	Adverse events	70.0% (14)	50.0% (24)		30.0% (3)	18.8% (6)	
	No adverse events	30.0% (6)	50.0% (24)	0.13	70.0% (7)	81.2% (26)	0.45
	n total	*20*	*48*		*10*	*32*	

- Adverse events: NRS superior to MNA and SF-MNA
- HRQL: MNA superior to SF-MNA

There are some limitations of the present study. One limitation is the high drop out rate of our cohort. To avoid statistical bias and misinterpretation of the data additional drop out analysis was carried out. More patients, in the group that did not finish the whole assessment, showed reduced skills of the study language. In our opinion, this is the main reason for a drop out rate of nearly 30%. Because of missing statistical differences this aspect was not included in further statistical analysis 6 months after surgery. In contrast to the majority of the few available studies investigating malnutrition in arthroplasty, biomarkers such as Albumin and Pre-Albumin were not quantified in our study. On the one hand, the discussion concerning the use of biomarkers in this context is not yet concluded. Morey et al. recently put into question the values of serum albumin level and TLC as a surrogate marker of malnutrition for predicting wound complications in total knee arthroplasty [21]. In contrast, Nelson et al. described an association of low albumin levels with complications after total knee arthroplasty and Yi et al. an association of nutritional biomarkers with acute postoperative infection [34, 35].

On the other hand, there are no studies so far that concentrate on the evaluation of being at risk for malnutrition by validated and widespread used non-invasive scoring systems in primary as well as in revision arthroplasty. The applied assessment tools in our study however have been approved several times in different medical fields and are globally recommended to identify patients being at risk for malnutrition in a non-invasive way [36]. Interview based assessment is an easy to handle tool and can be well integrated into daily clinical setting [15]. Based on our data and in agreement with studies in trauma and other medical specialties, NRS, SF-MNA and MNA are valuable tools for assessing patients at risk for malnutrition and may be used to predict clinical outcomes and HRQL [36, 37]. Regarding the use of MNA and SF-MNA there is a limitation concerning patients' age as these scores are recommended for patients older than 65 years [38, 39]. We used these scores nevertheless, as they are well established screening tools. Furthermore, a majority of 65,8% ($n = 231$) of our patients were older than 65 years. Another point of discussion is that the primary and revision AP groups differ in quantity. This fact corresponds with the distribution of arthroplasty patients in general, but it could be interesting to evaluate a larger patient groups undergoing revision arthroplasty as they show a higher prevalence of risk for malnutrition according to our data. Besides serum markers and standardized scoring tools there are also anthropometric measurements as optional surrogate marker for malnutrition [31, 32]. However, these parameters are at least under debate or questioned to identify marginal or acute nutritional deficiency and might be better used as additional indicators for chronic changes in the nutritional status [31, 32]. In our opinion, a screening tool for malnutrition should be fast, non-invasive, economical, applied to all medical fields of a single clinic, and easy to handle in daily clinical routine. After a first screening for malnutrition by interview-based assessment tools, invasive procedures such as biomarkers and anthropometric measurements can be helpful to give additional information and strengthen the diagnosis.

In summary, our study has clearly shown, that there is a moderate to high prevalence of risk for malnutrition in arthroplasty that can easily be assessed through interview based screening tools. This should be integrated as a standard procedure in clinical routine to be able to evaluate patients' risk for malnutrition as well as the accompanying risks regarding the clinical outcome already before arthroplasty takes place. Several studies have highlighted the necessity to routinely screen patients to detect their risk for malnutrition [9, 40]. Although there is only 7.3% to 29.4% of all cases that have a risk for malnutrition, all tested assessment tools can clearly identify these cases and initiate a possible perioperative intervention such as using oral nutritional supplements. The precise prediction of cases with a risk for malnutrition has most likely also an economical effect, since only the cases of a risk for malnutrition are subject of an interventional therapy and not all patients. In contrast to general or trauma surgery there are so far no studies evaluating this kind of intervention. Compared to trauma patients there is even the chance to substitute elective arthroplasty patients before surgery. Furthermore, the discussion of the use and significance of biomarkers should be continued.

Conclusions

The prevalence for being at risk for malnutrition for patients undergoing primary or revision arthroplasty is between 7.3% to 29.4% according to our data. Patients with an impaired nutritional status show reduced values in physical and mental aspects of HRQL. The risk for malnutrition results in suboptimal clinical outcomes regarding especially adverse events, length of stay, mobilization and wound healing. Non-invasive interview-based nutritional assessment can predict adverse events in primary and revision total arthroplasty and can therefore help identifying patients at risk before surgery.

Abbreviations

ESPEN: European Society for Clinical Nutrition and Metabolism; HRQL: Health Related Quality of Life; LOS: Length of Stay; MNA: Mini Nutritional Assessment; NRS: Nutritional Risk Screening; pAP: Primary Arthroplasty; rAP: Revision Arthroplasty; SF-36: Short Form 36; SF-MNA: Short Form Mini Nutritional Assessment; STROBE: Strengthening the reporting of observational studies in epidemiology; THA: Total Hip Arthroplasty; TKA: Total Knee Arthroplasty

Acknowledgements

We want to thank Svetlana Gasimova (Translator) for proofreading the manuscript and the whole "Nutrition Working Group" of the BG Trauma Center Tübingen, especially Barbara Zirn for participating in data collection. We want to thank Julia Grünwald for initial statistical guidance.

Funding

The study was partially supported by Oskar Helene Heim Foundation and intramural funding by the BG Trauma Center Tübingen, Germany. Our study sponsors have (1) no involvement in the study design; (2) collection, analysis and interpretation of data; (3) the writing of the manuscript; (4) the decision to submit the manuscript for publication.

Authors' contributions

GB analyzed the patient data and revised the manuscript regarding statistical aspects. CI and AJS were the major contributor in writing the manuscript. AN and US made substantial contributions to conception and design. CB and GO analyzed and interpreted the patient data. CI, AJS and CW were involved in data collection and writing the manuscript. All authors read and approved the final manuscript. AN, CB, GO, US revised the manuscript critically for important intellectual content.

Consent for publication
Not applicable.

Competing interests
The authors declare that they have no competing interests.

Author details
[1]Siegfried Weller Institute for Trauma Research, BG Trauma Center Tübingen, Eberhard Karls University Tübingen, Schnarrenbergstrasse 95, 72076 Tübingen, Germany. [2]Department of Clinical Epidemiology and Applied Biometry, Eberhard Karls University Tübingen, Silcherstrasse 5, 72076 Tubingen, Germany. [3]Department of Orthopedics and Trauma Surgery, Medical Center, Albert-Ludwigs-University of Freiburg, Faculty of Medicine, Freiburg, Germany.

References
1. Pirlich M, Schutz T, Norman K, Gastell S, Lubke HJ, Bischoff SC, et al. The German hospital malnutrition study. Clin Nutr (Edinburgh, Scotland). 2006; 25(4):563–72.
2. Thomas MN, Kufeldt J, Kisser U, Hornung HM, Hoffmann J, Andraschko M, et al. Effects of malnutrition on complication rates, length of hospital stay, and revenue in elective surgical patients in the G-DRG-system. Nutr (Burbank, Los Angeles County, Calif). 2016;32(2):249–54.
3. Loser C. Malnutrition in hospital: the clinical and economic implications. Dtsch Arztebl Int. 2010;107(51–52):911–7.
4. Pirlich M, Schutz T, Kemps M, Luhman N, Burmester GR, Baumann G, et al. Prevalence of malnutrition in hospitalized medical patients: impact of underlying disease. Dig Dis (Basel, Switzerland). 2003;21(3):245–51.
5. Lambert C, Nussler A, Biesalski HK, Freude T, Bahrs C, Ochs G, et al. Age-dependent risk factors for malnutrition in traumatology and orthopedic patients. Nutr (Burbank, Los Angeles County, Calif) 2017;37:60–67.
6. Felder S, Lechtenboehmer C, Bally M, Fehr R, Deiss M, Faessler L, et al. Association of nutritional risk and adverse medical outcomes across different medical inpatient populations. Nutr (Burbank, Los Angeles County, Calif). 2015;31(11–12):1385–93.
7. Cederholm T, Barazzoni R, Austin P, Ballmer P, Biolo G, Bischoff SC, et al. ESPEN guidelines on definitions and terminology of clinical nutrition. Clin Nutr (Edinburgh, Scotland). 2017;36(1):49–64.
8. Cederholm T, Bosaeus I, Barazzoni R, Bauer J, Van Gossum A, Klek S, et al. Diagnostic criteria for malnutrition - an ESPEN consensus statement. Clin Nutr (Edinburgh, Scotland). 2015;34(3):335–40.
9. Golladay GJ, Satpathy J, Jiranek WA. Patient optimization-strategies that work: malnutrition. J Arthroplast. 2016;31(8):1631–4.
10. Jensen JE, Jensen TG, Smith TK, Johnston DA, Dudrick SJ. Nutrition in orthopaedic surgery. J Bone Joint Surg Am volume. 1982;64(9):1263–72.
11. Jensen JE, Smith TK, Jensen TG, Dudrick SJ, Butler JE, Johnston DA. The frank Stinchfield award paper. Nutritional assessment of orthopaedic patients undergoing total hip replacement surgery. The Hip. 1981:123–35.
12. Del Savio GC, Zelicof SB, Wexler LM, Byrne DW, Reddy PD, Fish D, et al. Preoperative nutritional status and outcome of elective total hip replacement. Clin Orthop Relat Res. 1996;326:153–61.
13. Bohl DD, Shen MR, Kayupov E, Cvetanovich GL, Della Valle CJ. Is hypoalbuminemia associated with septic failure and acute infection after revision Total joint arthroplasty? A study of 4517 patients from the National Surgical Quality Improvement Program. J Arthroplast. 2016;31(5):963–7.
14. Huang R, Greenky M, Kerr GJ, Austin MS, Parvizi J. The effect of malnutrition on patients undergoing elective joint arthroplasty. J Arthroplast. 2013;28(8 Suppl):21–4.
15. Ihle C, Bahrs C, Freude T, Bickel M, Spielhaupter I, Wintermeyer E, Stollhof L, Grünwald L, Ziegler P, Pscherer S, Stöckle U, Nussler A. Malnutrition in Elderly Trauma Patients - Comparison of Two Assessment Tools. Z Orthop Unfall. 2017;155(2):184 93. https://doi.org/10.1055/s-0042-116822.
16. Ihle C, Freude T, Bahrs C, Zehendner E, Braunsberger J, Biesalski HK, et al. Malnutrition - an underestimated factor in the inpatient treatment of traumatology and orthopedic patients: a prospective evaluation of 1055 patients. Injury. 2017;48(3):628–36.
17. Goisser S, Schrader E, Singler K, Bertsch T, Gefeller O, Biber R, et al. Malnutrition according to mini nutritional assessment is associated with severe functional impairment in geriatric patients before and up to 6 months after hip fracture. J Am Med Dir Assoc. 2015;16(8):661–7.
18. Bell JJ, Pulle RC, Crouch AM, Kuys SS, Ferrier RL, Whitehouse SL. Impact of malnutrition on 12-month mortality following acute hip fracture. ANZ J Surg. 2016;86(3):157–61.
19. Bohl DD, Shen MR, Kayupov E, Della Valle CJ. Hypoalbuminemia independently predicts surgical site infection, pneumonia, length of stay, and readmission after Total joint arthroplasty. J Arthroplast. 2016;31(1):15–21.
20. Nicholson JA, Dowrick AS, Liew SM. Nutritional status and short-term outcome of hip arthroplasty. J Orthop Surg (Hong Kong). 2012;20(3):331–5.
21. Morey VM, Song YD, Whang JS, Kang YG, Kim TK. Can serum albumin level and Total lymphocyte count be surrogates for malnutrition to predict wound complications after Total knee arthroplasty? J Arthroplast. 2016;31(6):1317–21.
22. von Elm E, Altman DG, Egger M, Pocock SJ, Gotzsche PC, Vandenbroucke JP. The strengthening the reporting of observational studies in epidemiology (STROBE) statement: guidelines for reporting observational studies. Lancet (London, England). 2007;370(9596):1453–7.
23. Kondrup J, Rasmussen HH, Hamberg O, Stanga Z. Nutritional risk screening (NRS 2002): a new method based on an analysis of controlled clinical trials. Clin Nutr (Edinburgh, Scotland). 2003;22(3):321–36.
24. Vellas B, Guigoz Y, Garry PJ, Nourhashemi F, Bennahum D, Lauque S, et al. The mini nutritional assessment (MNA) and its use in grading the nutritional state of elderly patients. Nutr (Burbank, Los Angeles County, Calif). 1999; 15(2):116–22.
25. Donini LM, Poggiogalle E, Molfino A, Rosano A, Lenzi A, Rossi Fanelli F, et al. Mini-nutritional assessment, malnutrition universal screening tool, and nutrition risk screening tool for the nutritional evaluation of older nursing home residents. J Am Med Dir Assoc. 2016;17(10):959.e11–8.
26. Lera L, Sanchez H, Angel B, Albala C. Mini nutritional assessment short-form: validation in five Latin American cities. SABE study. J Nutr Health Aging. 2016;20(8):797–805.
27. Tarlov AR, Ware JE Jr, Greenfield S, Nelson EC, Perrin E, Zubkoff M. The medical outcomes study. An application of methods for monitoring the results of medical care. JAMA. 1989;262(7):925–30.
28. Saier T, Minzlaff P, Feucht MJ, Lammle L, Burghoff M, Ihle C, et al. Health-related quality of life after open-wedge high tibial osteotomy. Knee Surg Sports Traumatol Arthrosc. 2015;25(3):934–42.
29. Rainer TH, Yeung JH, Cheung SK, Yuen YK, Poon WS, Ho HF, et al. Assessment of quality of life and functional outcome in patients sustaining moderate and major trauma: a multicentre, prospective cohort study. Injury. 2014;45(5):902–9.
30. Ihle C, Ateschrang A, Grunwald L, Stockle U, Saier T, Schroter S. Health-related quality of life and clinical outcomes following medial open wedge high tibial osteotomy: a prospective study. BMC Musculoskelet Disord. 2016;17:215.
31. Ellsworth B, Kamath AF. Malnutrition and Total Joint Arthroplasty. J Nat Sci. 2016;2(3):e179.
32. Cross MB, Yi PH, Thomas CF, Garcia J, Della Valle CJ. Evaluation of malnutrition in orthopaedic surgery. J Am Acad Orthop Surg. 2014; 22(3):193–9.
33. Koren-Hakim T, Weiss A, Hershkovitz A, Otzrateni I, Anbar R, Gross Nevo RF, et al. Comparing the adequacy of the MNA-SF, NRS-2002 and MUST nutritional tools in assessing malnutrition in hip fracture operated elderly patients. Clin Nutr (Edinburgh, Scotland). 2016;35(5):1053–8.
34. Nelson CL, Elkassabany NM, Kamath AF, Liu J. Low albumin levels, more than morbid obesity, are associated with complications after TKA. Clin Orthop Relat Res. 2015;473(10):3163–72.
35. Yi PH, Frank RM, Vann E, Sonn KA, Moric M, Della Valle CJ. Is potential malnutrition associated with septic failure and acute infection after revision total joint arthroplasty? Clin Orthop Relat Res. 2015;473(1):175–82.
36. Raslan M, Gonzalez MC, Dias MC, Nascimento M, Castro M, Marques P, et al. Comparison of nutritional risk screening tools for predicting clinical outcomes in hospitalized patients. Nutrition. 2010;26(7–8):721–6.

4

Incidence of total hip or knee replacement due to osteoarthritis in relation to thyroid function: a prospective cohort study (The Nord-Trøndelag Health Study)

Alf Inge Hellevik[1,2*], Marianne Bakke Johnsen[3,6], Arnulf Langhammer[1], Anne Marie Fenstad[4], Ove Furnes[4,5], Kjersti Storheim[3,6], John Anker Zwart[3,6], Gunnar Flugsrud[2] and Lars Nordsletten[2,6]

Abstract

Background: To study whether thyroid function was associated with risk of hip or knee replacement due to primary osteoarthritis.

Methods: In a prospective cohort study, data from the second and third survey of the Nord-Trøndelag Health Study were linked to the Norwegian Arthroplasty Register in order to identify total hip or knee replacement as a result of primary osteoarthritis.

Results: Among 37 891 participants without previously known thyroid disease we recorded 978 total hip replacements (THRs) and 538 total knee replacements (TKRs) during a median follow-up time of 15.7 years. The analyses were adjusted for sex, age, BMI (body mass index), smoking, physical activity and diabetes. We did not find any association between TSH (thyroid stimulating hormone) and THR or TKR due to osteoarthritis. Neither were changes in TSH over time, or overt hypo- or hyperthyroidism, associated with incidence of THR or TKR.

Conclusion: No association was found between thyroid function and hip or knee joint replacement due to osteoarthritis.

Keywords: Thyroid function, Thyroid stimulating hormone, Osteoarthritis, Hip joint replacement, Knee joint replacement

Background

Osteoarthritis in the hip and knee is a major health problem and leads to significant morbidity [1]. Several drugs have been evaluated, but so far only exercise has been found to effectively prevent or delay the onset of osteoarthritis [2, 3]. This finding emphasizes the importance of identifying modifiable risk factors. Thyroid hormones play a role in the remodelling and maintenance of bone, and recent studies also indicate the potential importance of thyroid hormones in joints and articular cartilage [4]. Genetic studies have suggested that deiodinase-regulated local availability of the active thyroid hormone triiodothyronine (T3) plays an important role in cartilage maintenance and repair [5]. Further data have indicated that increased intracellular T3 availability increases the risk of osteoarthritis, leading to the hypothesis that reduced tissue T3 availability protects joints from development of osteoarthritis [6]. A phase III clinical trial investigating the use of eprotirome, a thyroid receptor β-agonist, for treatment of hypercholesterolemia [7], was terminated due to indications of dose related articular cartilage damage in dogs which had been treated with eprotirome for 12 months [8]. This was surprising, as eprotirome is a liver-specific thyroid receptor β-agonist, but it indicates that thyroid hormones influence cartilage [9] and could play a role in the pathogenesis of osteoarthritis.

* Correspondence: alf.hellevik@ntnu.no
[1]The HUNT Research Centre, Department of Public Health and Nursing, Faculty of Medicine and Health Sciences, Norwegian University of Science and Technology (NTNU), Levanger, Norway
[2]Division of Orthopaedic Surgery, Oslo University Hospital, Oslo, Norway
Full list of author information is available at the end of the article

No prospective population studies have investigated the association between thyroid function and osteoarthritis. An older cross-sectional study did not find any association between radiological knee osteoarthritis and thyroid status measured by thyroid stimulating hormone (TSH) [10]. In this prospective cohort study of 37 891 individuals without previously known thyroid disease, the aim was to assess whether thyroid function was associated with subsequent risk of hip or knee replacement due to primary osteoarthritis.

Methods

In the Nord-Trøndelag Health Study (HUNT) all inhabitants of Nord-Trøndelag county ≥ 20 years of age were invited to participate in three surveys: HUNT1 (1984–1986), HUNT2 (1995–1997) and HUNT3 (2006–2008) [11]. This study only included data from the HUNT2 and HUNT3 surveys, as the HUNT1 study did not collect blood samples. HUNT2 had 65 237 participants (69.5% of those invited), and HUNT3 had 50 807 participants (54.1% of those invited) [12].

In HUNT2, TSH was measured in 35 269 persons; in all women over 40 years old, in a random 50% sample of men over 40 years old and in a random 5% sample of participants aged 20–40 years. In HUNT3, TSH was measured in all 49 179 participants. We included 35 269 participants from HUNT2 and 13 132 new participants with TSH measurements from HUNT3. In persons that participated in both HUNT2 and HUNT3, baseline measurements from HUNT2 were used in the main analyses. Among these 48 401 individuals, 10 510 were excluded from analysis (Fig. 1). The exclusion criteria included self-reported thyroid disease (hypothyroidism, hyperthyroidism, goitre, other thyroid disease, use of levothyroxine, carbimazole, previous thyroid surgery or radioiodine therapy) ($n = 3895$), missing information on BMI ($n = 364$), missing information on smoking ($n = 962$), previous THR or TKR ($n = 644$), missing date of operation ($n = 99$), emigration during baseline measurements period ($n = 1$) or self-reported osteoarthritis at baseline ($n = 4545$). Thus, a total of 37 891 people (22 714 women and 15 177 men) were eligible for follow-up in this study. Each participant contributed person-years from baseline (either between August 1995 and June 1997 or between October 2006 and June 2008) until a THR or TKR due to osteoarthritis, THR or TKR due to other causes, migration, death or end of follow-up (December 31, 2013), whichever occurred first.

Measurements

The participants filled out a self-administered questionnaire, including history of thyroid disease [13]. The survey also included measurements of height and weight by trained personnel. Weight was measured while the participants were wearing light clothing without shoes.

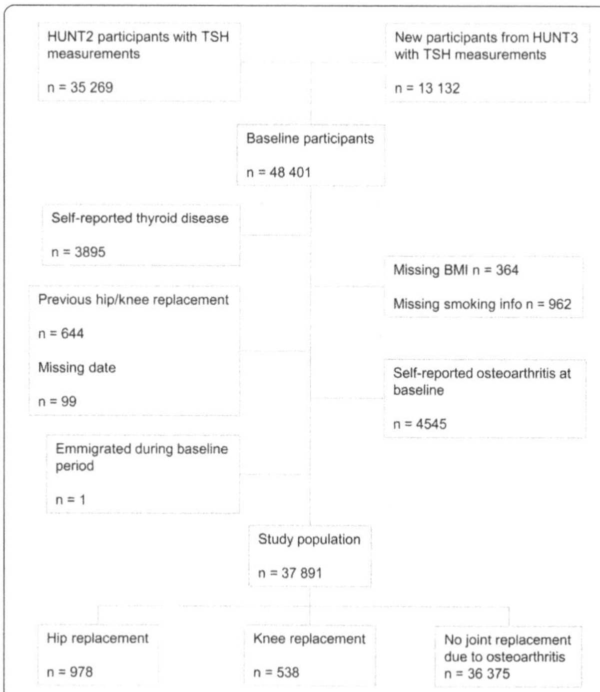

Fig. 1 Flowchart (TSH: Thyroid stimulating hormone)

BMI was calculated as weight in kilograms divided by squared height in metres.

A non-fasting venous blood sample was drawn from each participant. Concentrations of TSH, free thyroxine (fT4) and total triiodothyronine (T3) in HUNT2 were measured at the Hormone Laboratory, Aker University Hospital, Oslo, using DELFIA hTSH Ultra (sensitivity, 0.03 mU/L; and total analytic variation <5%), DELFIA fT4 (total analytic variation <7%), and AutoDELFIA T3 (total analytic variation <5%), all from Wallac Oy, Turku, Finland. In HUNT3, serum TSH and fT4 were measured at Levanger Hospital, Levanger, Norway, using Architect cSystems ci8200 (sensitivity, 0.01 mU/l; and a total analytic variation <5%), and Architect cSystems ci8200 (total analytic variation <6%), respectively, both from Abbott, Clinical Chemistry, USA. The measurement methods of TSH in HUNT2 and HUNT3 have previously been compared, with similar results [14], and agreement expressed by Bland-Altman [15] did not reveal any obvious pattern or deviations. The Norwegian population is considered to have sufficient iodine intake [16], and reference range for clinically normal TSH was defined as 0.50 to 3.5 mU/l based on previous publications from this population [13].

Covariates

The covariates were chosen based on previous literature, and had to be associated with both thyroid function and osteoarthritis. We mapped possible casual pathways between all variables using a directed acyclic graph model (DAG) (Appendix) to visually identify possible confounding pathways [17]. Based on this DAG-model, the possible confounders included in this analysis were sex, age (continuous), BMI (continuous), current smoking status (never, former or current), diabetes (yes or no) and physical activity. Physical activity was categorized by duration of light physical activity (none, <1, 1–2, ≥3 h/week), and/or duration of hard physical activity (none, <1, 1–2, ≥3 h/week). The physical activity questions have been previously validated among men, where especially hard physical activity correlated well with more objective measures [18]. These two variables were combined into one physical activity variable indicating intensity and duration: None (no activity), medium (≤2 h/week light physical activity and/ or < 1 h/week hard physical activity), hard (≥ 3 h/week light physical activity and/or ≥ 1 h/week hard physical activity).

Osteoarthritis at baseline was based on an affirmative answer to the question: "Has a doctor ever said that you have/have had osteoarthritis?" from HUNT2 participants, and "Have you had or do you have osteoarthritis?" from HUNT3 participants.

Outcome

In this study, primary total hip or knee replacement was considered to be a surrogate measure of severe osteoarthritis; and we used primary total hip or knee replacement due to primary osteoarthritis as outcome. The 11-digit identification numbers assigned to every Norwegian citizen enabled linkage to the Norwegian Arthroplasty Register (NAR). For each arthroplasty performed, the orthopaedic surgeon submits a standardized form containing information about the patient, the diagnosis that led to the arthroplasty, the procedure and the type of implant used [19]. NAR was established in 1987 and includes all artificial joints from 1994 onwards. The completeness of hip and knee replacement registration is over 95% [20].

Statistical methods

The participants were placed in five categories according to their TSH level: One category indicating hyperthyroid function (<0.50 mU/l); three categories within the clinical reference range (0.50–1.49, 1.5–2.49 and 2.5–3.5 mU/l); and one category indicating hypothyroid function (≥3.5 mU/l) [21]. Hazard ratios (HRs) of THR or TKR by category of TSH were estimated using a Cox proportional hazards model with 95% confidence interval (CI); TSH 1.5–2.49 mU/l was chosen as a reference. TSH was also analysed as both a continuous variable, and as log-transformed continuous TSH. The HRs were adjusted for age, sex, BMI and smoking. An additional analysis also adjusted for physical activity and diabetes. We treated THR and TKR both as separate outcomes and combined in one outcome variable of total joint replacement (TJR).

A sub-analysis included only persons that participated in both HUNT2 and HUNT3 ($n = 19\ 397$). TSH levels at HUNT3 were then subtracted from the TSH levels in HUNT2 to estimate the change in TSH during the intervening decade. Information on the other baseline covariates was taken from HUNT3. Among these participants a total of 7740 were excluded due to self-reported thyroid disease ($n = 2744$), missing information on BMI ($n = 108$), missing information on smoking ($n = 621$), previous THR or TKR ($n = 928$), missing date of operation ($n = 29$) or self-reported osteoarthritis at baseline ($n = 3310$). Thus, a total of 11 657 people were eligible for this sub-analysis. This sub-population was also used in an analysis that investigated whether the results changed when those who had started on thyroid medication after baseline in HUNT2 were excluded.

In a sensitivity analysis people were divided into two groups, one with biochemically manifest (overt) hypothyroidism (defined as TSH >4.0 mU/L combined with fT4 < 8.0 pmol/L), and the other with overt hyperthyroidism (defined as TSH <0.10 mU/L and fT4 > 20.0 pmol/L and/or total T3 > 2.7 nmol/L). This classification by overt hypo- or hyperthyroidism was made possible by the fT4 measurements taken in people whose TSH levels were <0.20 mU/l or >4.0 mU/l in HUNT2, and in people whose levels were <0.10 mU/l or >3.0 mU/l in HUNT3. Total T3 was only available in HUNT2 and only measured if TSH levels were <0.20mU/L.

Two additional analyses were performed on the baseline population: First, we investigated the association between TSH level (categorical) and self-reported osteoarthritis at baseline by using a logistic regression model, adjusting for sex, age, BMI, smoking, physical activity and diabetes. Second, we compared the incidence rate of THR or TKR in participants with and without self-reported thyroid disease at baseline using Fisher's Exact test. After excluding participants with missing information on BMI and smoking, previous THR or TKR, missing date of operation or self-reported osteoarthritis at baseline, 2955 participants reported thyroid disease.

Proportional hazards assumptions were evaluated by Schoenfeld residuals tests. They showed proportional hazards on all covariates, except for age. Thus we did an additional stratified analysis on age, but it did not show different results (data not shown). Age was therefore kept as a continuous variable in all our analyses. All statistical analyses were two-sided with a significance level of $p < 0.05$. The analyses were performed using Stata 14.0/SE (StataCorp LP, College Station, TX, USA).

Results

Of the 37 891 participants, 908 (2.4%) had low TSH (<0.50 mU/l) indicating hyperthyroid function, and 2307 (6.1%) had high TSH (≥3.6 mU/l) indicating hypothyroid function (Table 1). Among the women, 6.9% had high TSH, compared to 4.8% of men. Participants with high TSH were generally older and were less likely to be current smokers than participants in the reference group (TSH 1.5–2.4 mU/l). No clear trend was seen in relation to physical activity.

In total, 978 received THR and 538 received TKR during a median follow-up time of 15.7 years (mean 12.3 years). At baseline, the mean age was 50.7 years (SD 15.8), and the mean ages at THR and TKR were 69.5 years (SD 8.9) and 69.4 years (SD 8.4), respectively.

TSH level did not influence the risk of THR or TKR in the unadjusted analysis or the analysis adjusted for gender, age, BMI and smoking (Table 2). Neither additional adjustment for physical activity and diabetes (Table 2), nor collapsing the outcome variable into total joint replacement (TJR) (Table 3), altered these results. Analyses using TSH as a continuous variable did not show any association between TSH and THR or TKR (Fig. 2). Additional log-transformation of TSH as a continuous variable did not significantly change these results (data not shown).

In a separate analysis studying the change in TSH (delta-TSH) during the time between HUNT2 and HUNT3, 11 657 participants were included. Of these, 200 received THR and 102 received TKR during a mean follow-up time of 6.1 years. No association was seen between changes in TSH and risk of THR or TKR (Fig. 3). Additional adjustment for baseline TSH did not substantially alter these results. The same sub-population was also used to identify persons with no thyroid disease or treatment at baseline in HUNT2 who still had no thyroid disease or treatment at HUNT3. However, no association between TSH and THR (HR 1.00, 95% CI 0.97–1.02) or TKR (HR 0.98, 95% CI 0.94–1.03) was found.

In a sensitivity analysis neither overt hypo- nor hyperthyroid function was found to influence the risk of THR or TKR, (HR 0.91, 95% CI 0.40–2.04) and (HR 2.01, 95% CI 0.75–5.4) respectively. Also, no association was found between overt hypothyroid function and TKR (HR 1.03, 95% CI 0.38–2.78). There were no cases of TKR amongst the overtly hyperthyroid, so no analysis could be performed in this subgroup.

In additional analyses on the baseline population, there was no association between TSH levels and self-reported osteoarthritis at baseline (data not shown). Those with self-reported thyroid disease at baseline had an incidence rate of 0.0027 THR per person-year and 0.0015 TKR per person-year. Our main study population (excluding those with self-reported thyroid disease) had an incidence rate of 0.0021 THR per person-year and 0.0012 TKR per person-year. This gave and incidence rate ratio of 1.28 (95% CI 1.04–1.56) for THR, and 1.27 (95% CI 0.95–1.95) for TKR, and indicated a slightly higher incidence rate for THR in those with self-reported thyroid disease, but no significant difference in the incidence rate for TKR, compared to participants without self-reported thyroid disease.

Discussion

In this large prospective study we did not find any association between thyroid function and the risk of THR or

Table 1 Study population characteristics in relation to thyroid stimulating hormone (TSH) categories

	Serum TSH										Total	
	<0.50		*0.50–1.49*		*1.5–2.49*		*2.5–3.49*		*≥3.5*			
Participants (%)	908	(2.4)	17675	(46.7)	13228	(34.9)	3773	(10.0)	2307	(6.1)	37891	
Women (%)	651	(2.9)	10405	(45.8)	7738	(34.1)	2346	(10.3)	1574	(6.9)	22714	(60.0)
Men (%)	257	(1.7)	7270	(47.9)	5490	(36.2)	1427	(9.4)	733	(4.8)	15177	(40.0)
Age (SD)	50.7	(16.7)	48.2	(15.3)	51.6	(15.6)	54.9	(15.9)	58.3	(15.3)	50.7	(15.8)
BMI (SD)	25.9	(4.4)	26.1	(4.1)	26.8	(4.2)	27.1	(4.4)	27.2	(4.5)	26.5	(4.2)
Smoking status (%)												
Never	335	(36.9)	6778	(38.3)	6080	(46.0)	1869	(49.5)	1167	(50.6)	16229	(42.8)
Former	236	(26.0)	4683	(26.5)	3768	(28.5)	1120	(29.7)	723	(31.3)	10530	(27.8)
Current	337	(37.1)	6214	(35.2)	3380	(25.5)	784	(20.8)	417	(18.1)	11132	(29.4)
Physical activity (%) (missing = 6826)												
Low	46	(6.5)	862	(6.0)	719	(6.6)	232	(7.4)	151	(8.2)	2010	(6.5)
Medium	371	(52.8)	7226	(49.9)	5454	(50.0)	1555	(49.7)	921	(50.1)	15527	(50.0)
High	286	(40.7)	6394	(44.1)	4738	(43.4)	1344	(42.9)	766	(41.7)	13528	(43.6)
Diabetes (%) (missing = 56)	55	(6.1)	613	(3.5)	559	(4.2)	173	(4.6)	115	(5.0)	1515	4.0

Table 2 Association between TSH categories and hip or knee replacement due to osteoarthritis

TSH (mU/L)	Persons (n)	Cases (n)	HR[a]	(95% CI)	HR[b]	(95% CI)	HR[c]	(95% CI)
THR								
< 0.50	908	21	0.98	(0.63–1.53)	0.99	(0.64–1.53)	1.04	(0.63–1.69)
0.50–1.49	17675	411	0.93	(0.81–1.08)	1.07	(0.93–1.24)	1.09	(0.94–1.28)
1.5–2.49	13228	359	1	Reference	1	Reference	1	Reference
2.5–3.49	3773	105	0.98	(0.79–1.22)	0.85	(0.68–1.05)	0.88	(0.69–1.11)
> 3.5	2307	82	1.22	(0.96–1.55)	0.96	(0.76–1.22)	0.98	(0.75–1.27)
TKR								
< 0.50	908	14	1.26	(0.73–2.16)	1.32	(0.76–2.26)	1.33	(0.74–2.4)
0.50–1.49	17675	224	0.97	(0.80–1.18)	1.15	(0.95–1.40)	1.12	(0.91–1.37)
1.5–2.49	13228	191	1	Reference	1	Reference	1	Reference
2.5–3.49	3773	64	1.12	(0.84–1.48)	0.94	(0.71–1.25)	0.88	(0.65–1.20)
> 3.5	2307	45	1.24	(0.90–1.72)	0.98	(0.70–1.35)	0.87	(0.61–1.25)

(*THR* total hip replacement, *TKR* total knee replacement)
[a]Unadjusted
[b]Adjusted for age, sex, BMI and smoking
[c]Adjusted for age, sex, BMI, smoking, physical activity and diabetes

TKR due to osteoarthritis. Neither were changes in TSH over time, or overt hypo- or hyperthyroidism, associated with incidence of THR or TKR.

Few previous population studies have investigated the association of thyroid function with risk of osteoarthritis. In 1996, a cross-sectional study of 577 men and 798 women found no evidence of a significant association between current thyroid status and either chondrocalcinosis or osteoarthritis [10]. However, that study only investigated prevalent osteoarthritis with a concurrent serum TSH concentration and could not take into account development in TSH or later treatment for abnormal thyroid function. Since our study could use data from both the second and third waves of the HUNT-survey, we were able to investigate the development of TSH over a median time of 11.2 years (SD 0.6). Change in TSH over time was however not associated with osteoarthritis development resulting in the need for joint replacement.

Previous or current thyroid disease at baseline was an exclusion criterion in our study. Nonetheless, all participants with TSH levels suggesting hypothyroid or hyperthyroid function may have received medical treatment for thyroid disease during the follow-up period, as participants with biochemical indication of pathological thyroid function were recommended to contact their general practitioners [22]. This could have weakened any association between TSH and osteoarthritis. We therefore did a sub-analysis of persons that participated in both HUNT2 and HUNT3, and excluded participants that reported use of thyroid medication or thyroid disease in HUNT3. This did not significantly alter the results.

Our findings must be interpreted in relation to recent genetic studies on intracellular T3 availability in joint cartilage. There has been an increased interest in the effect of deiodinase polymorphisms on osteoarthritis [5]. Iodothyronine deiodinases represent a family of proteins involved in local homeostasis of thyroxine (T4) and triiodothyronine (T3). Three deiodinases have been described and, of these, the deiodinase type 2 (D2) and deiodinase type 3 (D3) are

Table 3 Association between TSH categories and total joint replacement (TJR) in the hip or knee due to osteoarthritis

TSH (mU/L)	Persons (n)	Cases (n)	HR[a]	(95% CI)	HR[b]	(95% CI)	HR[c]	(95% CI)
<0.50	908	35	1.08	(0.77–1.52)	1.10	(0.78–1.55)	1.15	(0.79–1.67)
0.50–1.49	17675	635	0.95	(0.84–1.06)	1.10	(0.98–1.23)	1.10	(0.97–1.25)
1.5–2.49	13228	550	1	Reference	1	Reference	1	Reference
2.5–3.49	3773	169	1.03	(0.87–1.22)	0.88	(0.74–1.05)	0.88	(0.73–1.06)
>3.5	2307	127	1.23	(1.01–1.49)	0.97	(0.80–1.17)	0.94	(0.76–1.16)

[a]Unadjusted
[b]Adjusted for age, sex, BMI and smoking
[c]Adjusted for age, sex, BMI, smoking, physical activity and diabetes

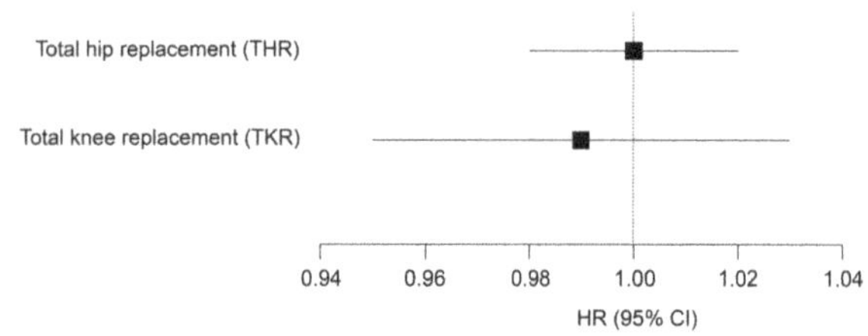

Fig. 2 Association between continuous TSH and total hip replacement (THR) or total knee replacement (TKR) due to osteoarthritis. (Adjusted for age, sex, BMI, smoking, physical activity and diabetes)

detected in bone and cartilage. D2 plays a major role in conversion of T4 to biologically active T3 [23] and thus upregulates local T3 levels. Deiodinase type 3 (D3) is the main T3-inactivating enzyme and consequently downregulates the local T3 levels. T3 is considered an important regulator of chondrocyte cell growth and differentiation in the endochondral growth plate [24]. Local T3 availability, regulated by the opposite functions of D2 and D3, may be a determinant of osteoarthritis development. D2 has been reported to be upregulated in the cartilage of joints affected by osteoarthritis compared to joints unaffected by osteoarthritis [25, 26]. However, it is not known if this is a result of the ongoing osteoarthritis process, or a reflection of the underlying disease pathway. Taken together, these findings suggest that deiodinase regulated local availability of T3 in chondrocytes is a possible factor in the pathophysiology of osteoarthritis [27, 28]. Since our study did not find any association between circulating TSH, T3/T4 levels and osteoarthritis, it is conceivable that the serum thyroid hormone levels may be independent of local intracellular T3 levels in joints. Another possible explanation could be that polymorphism in the gene coding for D2 creates a predisposition for non-optimal bone shape [29, 30], leading to increased risk of osteoarthritis independent of local thyroid hormone levels.

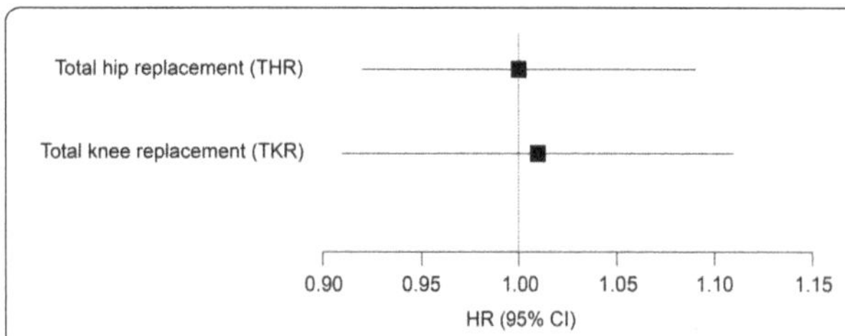

Fig. 3 Association between change in TSH (delta TSH) and total hip replacement (THR) or total knee replacement (TKR) due to osteoarthritis. (Adjusted for age, sex, BMI and smoking)

Strengths and limitations

Our study included over 37 000 persons without known thyroid disease at baseline, and in most cases thyroid function was measured many years prior to joint replacement. To the best of our knowledge, this is the first prospective population study addressing the association between thyroid function and joint replacement due to primary osteoarthritis. The prospective design and longitudinal data on TSH measurements are strengths of this study. By excluding participants with self-reported osteoarthritis at baseline it was possible to differentiate between risk of osteoarthritis development and progression.

Our study used joint replacement due to primary osteoarthritis as a surrogate measure of severe osteoarthritis. Validation of the osteoarthrosis diagnosis from the Norwegian Arthroplasty Register has not been done in an unselected population [31]. However, the Danish hip Arthroplasty Registry has reported a positive predictive value of 85% regarding primary hip osteoarthritis diagnosis [32], and it is likely that these results are comparable to the Norwegian Arthroplasty Register. The advantage of using joint replacement as a proxy for osteoarthritis is its unambiguous connection with disease burden of osteoarthritis compared to other osteoarthritis definitions, e.g., radiographic criteria, symptom criteria or osteoarthritis defined by self-reported diagnosis [33]. However, this outcome measure is still limited in some respects, most importantly, that patients' health status and potential comorbidities influence orthopaedic surgeons' choices regarding operative treatment. Secondly, persons with moderate osteoarthritis who engage in demanding physical activities could be more motivated to have surgery than less active persons. Persons who are generally inactive may be less motivated to have surgery even if they have more severe osteoarthritis. This could give a healthy patient selection bias with corresponding underestimation of the effect of thyroid function.

Previous injuries increase the risk of knee osteoarthritis [34, 35], but only joint replacements due to primary/idiopathic osteoarthritis were included in our study. We did not have direct information on previous injury, but we excluded all cases in which the operating surgeon reported that the knee joint replacement was due to sequela from fracture, ligament injury, meniscal injury, infection, rheumatoid arthritis or ankylosing spondylitis.

The interrelationship between BMI and thyroid function is complex and BMI could be treated as either a confounder or a mediator in our model [36]. The reason we chose to define it as a confounder was that we wanted to investigate the direct effect of thyroid function on joint replacement, independent of BMI. Potential confounding by other unmeasured factors could not be excluded. But these factors should then be associated with both thyrotropin level and osteoarthritis. Therefore, we did not adjust for level of education in this study (Appendix).

The participation rate in the HUNT-surveys was fairly high compared to most other surveys, but there is always a potential risk of selection bias that cannot be adjusted for in the statistical analysis [37]. Blood samples were not drawn at a set time of the day, and it is known that other factors like exercise and sleep deprivation influence TSH levels [38]. This might have led to non-differential classification bias, thus weakening any associations. We also only had data on fT4 and T3 in subpopulations. Therefore, the absolute numbers of participants with overt hypo- or hyperthyroidism were small, reducing the power to detect any association between them and euthyroid subject and should thus be interpreted with caution.

This study focused on the relationship between thyroid function and osteoarthritis. However, there may also be an association between autoimmune thyroid disease and osteoarthritis [39]. As thyroid autoantibody not necessarily correlate with thyroid function, an association between thyroid function and osteoarthritis trough autoimmune factors could be missed in our study.

The exclusion of participants who reported hypo- or hyperthyroidism in their answers regarding use of treatment or medication might have caused misclassification since radioiodine is used in the treatment of cancer and T4 in the medical treatment of goitre. However, these treatments are infrequent, and it is unlikely that they substantially altered our results.

In the analysis comparing incidence rate of THR in people with and without self-reported thyroid disease we found a small, but significant, increased risk of THR in people reporting thyroid disease. And since we excluded participants with self-reported thyroid disease, this might have led to an underestimation of the effect on THR. We therefore did an additional analysis including those with self-reported thyroid disease: This showed no association between TSH levels and THR in a Cox-regression model (data not shown), and thus confirmed the findings from the primary analysis.

Conclusion

In this prospective study of 37 891 participants without previously known thyroid disease, we did not find that thyroid function was associated with risk of hip or knee joint replacement due to osteoarthritis. Neither did we find any association between TSH development over time and risk of hip or knee joint replacement due to osteoarthritis.

Appendix

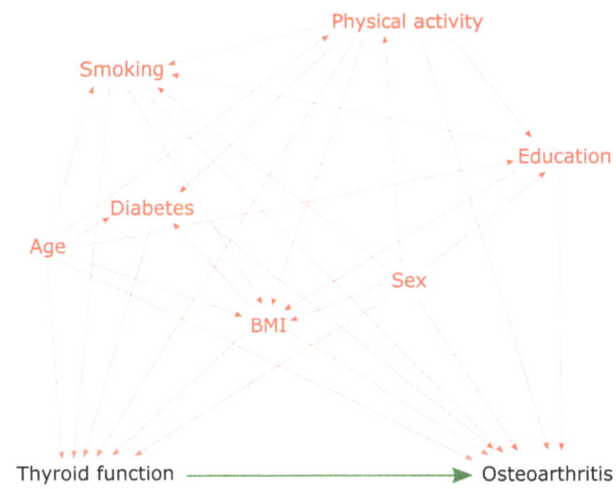

Fig. 4 Direct Acyclic Graph (DAG) – analysis. Figure showing possible casual pathways between variables

Abbreviations

BMI: Body mass index; D2: Deiodinase type 2; D3: Deiodinase type 3; DAG: Directed acyclic graph; fT4: Free thyroxine; HR: Hazard ratio; HUNT: The Nord-Trøndelag Health study; NAR: Norwegian Arthroplasty Register; OA: Osteoarthritis; SD: Standard deviation; T3: Triiodothyronine; T4: Thyroxine; THR: Total hip replacement; TKR: Total knee replacement; TSH: Thyroid stimulating hormone

Acknowledgements

The Nord-Trøndelag Health Study is a collaborative effort of the Faculty of Medicine, Norwegian University of Science and Technology; the Norwegian Institute of Public Health; and the Nord-Trøndelag County Council. The Norwegian Arthroplasty Register is owned by the Norwegian Orthopedic Association and administered by the Orthopedic Department at Haukeland University Hospital, Bergen, Norway.

Funding

This study was supported by research grants from the Liaison Committee between the Central Norway Regional Health Authority (RHA) and the Norwegian University of Science and Technology (NTNU), the Dr. Egil Kjeldaas foundation (Lege Egil Kjeldaas legat), the Norwegian Orthopaedic Association and Levanger Hospital, Nord-Trøndelag Hospital Trust. The funding sources had no involvement in the study design, the collection, analysis or interpretation of data, writing the paper or the decision to submit the paper for publication.

Authors' contributions

AL conceived of the idea for this study. AIH participated in the study concept and design, obtained funding, performed the analysis, interpreted the data and drafted the manuscript. LN, MBJ, AL, GBF, OF, KS and JAZ were involved in the conception and design of the study. OF was also involved in the collection of hip and knee replacement data. AMF contributed statistical expertise. All the authors revised the manuscript for important intellectual content and approved the final version of the manuscript.

Competing interests

The authors declare that they have no competing interests.

Consent for publication

Not applicable.

Author details

[1]The HUNT Research Centre, Department of Public Health and Nursing,

Faculty of Medicine and Health Sciences, Norwegian University of Science and Technology (NTNU), Levanger, Norway. [2]Division of Orthopaedic Surgery, Oslo University Hospital, Oslo, Norway. [3]Research and Communication Unit for Musculoskeletal Health, Division of Clinical Neuroscience, Oslo University Hospital, Oslo, Norway. [4]The Norwegian Arthroplasty Register, Department of Orthopedic Surgery, Haukeland University Hospital, Bergen, Norway. [5]Department of Clinical Medicine, Institute of Medicine and Dentistry, University of Bergen, Bergen, Norway. [6]Faculty of Medicine, University of Oslo, Oslo, Norway.

References

1. Vos T, Flaxman AD, Naghavi M, Lozano R, Michaud C, Ezzati M, Shibuya K, Salomon JA, Abdalla S, Aboyans V, et al. Years lived with disability (YLDs) for 1160 sequelae of 289 diseases and injuries 1990-2010: a systematic analysis for the Global Burden of Disease Study 2010. Lancet. 2012;380(9859):2163–96.
2. Goldring MB, Berenbaum F. Emerging targets in osteoarthritis therapy. Curr Opin Pharmacol. 2015;22:51–63.
3. Svege I, Nordsletten L, Fernandes L, Risberg MA. Exercise therapy may postpone total hip replacement surgery in patients with hip osteoarthritis: a long-term follow-up of a randomised trial. Ann Rheum Dis. 2015;74(1):164–9.
4. Williams GR. Thyroid Hormone Actions in Cartilage and Bone. European Thyroid J. 2013;2(1):3–13.
5. Verloop H, Dekkers OM, Peeters RP, Schoones JW, Smit JW. Genetics in endocrinology: genetic variation in deiodinases: a systematic review of potential clinical effects in humans. Eur J Endocrinol. 2014;171(3):R123–135.
6. Waung JA, Bassett JH, Williams GR. Adult mice lacking the type 2 iodothyronine deiodinase have increased subchondral bone but normal articular cartilage. Thyroid. 2015;25(3):269–77.
7. Ladenson PW, Kristensen JD, Ridgway EC, Olsson AG, Carlsson B, Klein I, Baxter JD, Angelin B. Use of the thyroid hormone analogue eprotirome in statin-treated dyslipidemia. N Engl J Med. 2010;362(10):906–16.
8. Sjouke B, Langslet G, Ceska R, Nicholls SJ, Nissen SE, Ohlander M, Ladenson PW, Olsson AG, Hovingh GK, Kastelein JJ. Eprotirome in patients with familial hypercholesterolaemia (the AKKA trial): a randomised, double-blind, placebo-controlled phase 3 study. Lancet Diabetes Endocrinol. 2014;2(6):455–63.
9. Lammel Lindemann J, Webb P. Sobetirome: the past, present and questions about the future. Expert Opin Ther Targets. 2016;20(2):145–9.
10. Chaisson CE, McAlindon TE, Felson DT, Naimark A, Wilson PW, Sawin CT. Lack of association between thyroid status and chondrocalcinosis or osteoarthritis: the Framingham Osteoarthritis Study. J Rheumatol. 1996;23(4):711–5.
11. HUNT home page [http://www.ntnu.no/hunt]. Accessed 15 Nov 2016
12. Krokstad S, Langhammer A, Hveem K, Holmen TL, Midthjell K, Stene TR, Bratberg G, Heggland J, Holmen J. Cohort Profile: the HUNT Study, Norway. Int J Epidemiol. 2013;42(4):968–77.
13. Bjoro T, Holmen J, Kruger O, Midthjell K, Hunstad K, Schreiner T, Sandnes L, Brochmann H. Prevalence of thyroid disease, thyroid dysfunction and thyroid peroxidase antibodies in a large, unselected population. The Health Study of Nord-Trondelag (HUNT). Eur J Endocrinol. 2000;143(5):639–47.
14. Svare A, Nilsen TI, Bjoro T, Asvold BO, Langhammer A. Serum TSH related to measures of body mass: longitudinal data from the HUNT Study, Norway. Clin Endocrinol (Oxf). 2011;74(6):769–75.
15. Bland JM, Altman DG. Statistical methods for assessing agreement between two methods of clinical measurement. Lancet. 1986;1(8476):307–10.
16. Kapelrud H, Frey H, Theodorsen L. [Excretion of iodine in the urine. A study from 6 different Norwegian districts in 1985]. Tidsskr Nor Laegeforen. 1987; 107(15):1320–1. 1317.
17. Suttorp MM, Siegerink B, Jager KJ, Zoccali C, Dekker FW. Graphical presentation of confounding in directed acyclic graphs. Nephrol Dial Transplant. 2015;30(9):1418–23.
18. Kurtze N, Rangul V, Hustvedt B-E, Flanders WD. Reliability and validity of self-reported physical activity in the Nord-Trøndelag Health Study (HUNT 2). Eur J Epidemiol. 2007;22(6):379 87.
19. Havelin LI, Engesaeter LB, Espehaug B, Furnes O, Lie SA, Vollset SE. The Norwegian Arthroplasty Register: 11 years and 73,000 arthroplasties. Acta Orthop Scand. 2000;71(4):337–53.
20. Espehaug B, Furnes O, Havelin LI, Engesaeter LB, Vollset SE, Kindseth O. Registration completeness in the Norwegian Arthroplasty Register. Acta Orthop. 2006;77(1):49–56.
21. Hellevik AI, Asvold BO, Bjoro T, Romundstad PR, Nilsen TI, Vatten LJ. Thyroid function and cancer risk: a prospective population study. Cancer Epidemiol Biomarkers Prev. 2009;18(2):570–4.
22. HUNT databank [https://hunt-db.medisin.ntnu.no/hunt-db/]. Accessed 15 Nov 2016.
23. Kohrle J. Local activation and inactivation of thyroid hormones: the deiodinase family. Mol Cell Endocrinol. 1999;151(1-2):103–19.
24. Robson H, Siebler T, Stevens DA, Shalet SM, Williams GR. Thyroid hormone acts directly on growth plate chondrocytes to promote hypertrophic differentiation and inhibit clonal expansion and cell proliferation. Endocrinology. 2000;141(10):3887–97.
25. Bos SD, Bovee JV, Duijnisveld BJ, Raine EV, van Dalen WJ, Ramos YF, van der Breggen R, Nelissen RG, Slagboom PE, Loughlin J, et al. Increased type II deiodinase protein in OA-affected cartilage and allelic imbalance of OA risk polymorphism rs225014 at DIO2 in human OA joint tissues. Ann Rheum Dis. 2012;71(7):1254–8.
26. Meulenbelt I, Bos SD, Chapman K, van der Breggen R, Houwing-Duistermaat JJ, Kremer D, Kloppenburg M, Carr A, Tsezou A, Gonzalez A, et al. Meta-analyses of genes modulating intracellular T3 bio-availability reveal a possible role for the DIO3 gene in osteoarthritis susceptibility. Ann Rheum Dis. 2011;70(1):164–7.
27. Waung JA, Bassett JH, Williams GR. Thyroid hormone metabolism in skeletal development and adult bone maintenance. Trends Endocrinol Metab. 2012; 23(4):155–62.
28. Bay-Jensen AC, Slagboom E, Chen-An P, Alexandersen P, Qvist P, Christiansen C, Meulenbelt I, Karsdal MA. Role of hormones in cartilage and joint metabolism: understanding an unhealthy metabolic phenotype in osteoarthritis. Menopause. 2013;20(5):578–86.
29. Waarsing JH, Kloppenburg M, Slagboom PE, Kroon HM, Houwing-Duistermaat JJ, Weinans H, Meulenbelt I. Osteoarthritis susceptibility genes influence the association between hip morphology and osteoarthritis. Arthritis Rheum. 2011;63(5):1349–54.
30. Meulenbelt I, Min JL, Bos S, Riyazi N, Houwing-Duistermaat JJ, van der Wijk HJ, Kroon HM, Nakajima M, Ikegawa S, Uitterlinden AG, et al. Identification of DIO2 as a new susceptibility locus for symptomatic osteoarthritis. Hum Mol Genet. 2008;17(12):1867–75.
31. Engesaeter IO, Lehmann T, Laborie LB, Lie SA, Rosendahl K, Engesaeter LB. Total hip replacement in young adults with hip dysplasia: age at diagnosis, previous treatment, quality of life, and validation of diagnoses reported to the Norwegian Arthroplasty Register between 1987 and 2007. Acta Orthop. 2011;82(2):149–54.
32. Pedersen A, Johnsen S, Overgaard S, Soballe K, Sorensen HT, Lucht U. Registration in the danish hip arthroplasty registry: completeness of total hip arthroplasties and positive predictive value of registered diagnosis and postoperative complications. Acta Orthop Scand. 2004;75(4):434–41.
33. Kim C, Nevitt MC, Niu J, Clancy MM, Lane NE, Link TM, Vlad S, Tolstykh I, Jungmann PM, Felson DT, et al. Association of hip pain with radiographic evidence of hip osteoarthritis: diagnostic test study. BMJ. 2015;351:h5983.
34. Oiestad BE, Holm I, Engebretsen L, Aune AK, Gunderson R, Risberg MA. The prevalence of patellofemoral osteoarthritis 12 years after anterior cruciate ligament reconstruction. Knee Surg Sports Traumatol Arthrosc. 2013;21(4):942–9.
35. Murphy L, Schwartz TA, Helmick CG, Renner JB, Tudor G, Koch G, Dragomir A, Kalsbeek WD, Luta G, Jordan JM. Lifetime risk of symptomatic knee osteoarthritis. Arthritis Rheum. 2008;59(9):1207–13.
36. Pearce EN. Thyroid hormone and obesity. Curr Opin Endocrinol Diabetes Obes. 2012;19(5):408–13.
37. Holmen J, Midthjell K, Krüger O, Langhammer A, Holmen TL, Bratberg G, Vatten LG. L-LP: The Nord-Trøndelag Health Study 1995-97 (HUNT 2): Objectives, contents, methods and participation. Norsk Epidemiologi. 2003;13(1):19–32.
38. Surks MI, Goswami G, Daniels GH. The thyrotropin reference range should remain unchanged. J Clin Endocrinol Metab. 2005;90(9):5489–96.
39. Soy M, Guldiken S, Arikan E, Altun BU, Tugrul A. Frequency of rheumatic diseases in patients with autoimmune thyroid disease. Rheumatol Int. 2007; 27(6):575–7.

5

Glenoid morphology in light of anatomical and reverse total shoulder arthroplasty: a dissection- and 3D-CT-based study in male and female body donors

Sandra Mathews[1*†], Marco Burkhard[2†], Nabil Serrano[1,2], Karl Link[1,2], Martin Häusler[1,2], Nakita Frater[1], Ingeborg Franke[2], Helena Bischofberger[2], Florian M. Buck[3,4], Dominic Gascho[5], Michael Thali[5], Steffen Serowy[6], Magdalena Müller-Gerbl[7], Gareth Harper[8], Ford Qureshi[9], Thomas Böni[1,10], Hans-Rudolf Bloch[11], Oliver Ullrich[2], Frank-Jakobus Rühli[1†] and Elisabeth Eppler[2,6,7†]

Abstract

Background: Placement of the glenoid baseplate is of paramount importance for the outcome of anatomical and reverse total shoulder arthroplasty. However, the database around glenoid size is poor, particularly regarding small scapulae, for example, in women and smaller individuals, and is derived from different methodological approaches. In this multimodality cadaver study, we systematically examined the glenoid using morphological and 3D-CT measurements.

Methods: Measurements of the glenoid and drill hole tunnel length for superior baseplate screw placement were recorded to define size of the glenoid and the distance to the scapular notch on cadaveric specimens. Glenoid angles were determined on both, 3D-CT-scans of the thoraxes using the Friedman method and on subsequently isolated scapulae from 18 male and female donors (average 84 years, range 60–98 years).

Results: Mean glenoid height was 36.6 mm ± 3.6, and width 27.8 mm ± 3.1 with a significant sex dimorphism ($p \leq 0.001$): in males, glenoid height 39.5 mm ± 3.5, and width 30.3 mm ± 3.3, and in females, glenoid height 34.8 mm ± 2.2, and width 26.2 mm ± 1.6. The average distance from the superior screw entry to its exit in the scapular notch measured by calliper was 27.2 mm ± 6.0 with a sex difference: in males, 29.4 mm ± 5.7, and in females, 25.8 mm ± 5.9 mm with a minimum recorded distance of 15 mm. Measured by CT, the mean inclination angle for male and female donors combined was 13.0° ± 7.0, and the ante-/retroversion angle −1.0° ± 4.0°.

Conclusion: This study is one of the first to combine dissection, including drill holes, with anatomical measurements and radiological data. In some women and smaller individuals, smaller baseplates should be selected. The published safe zone of 20 mm is generally feasible for superior screw placement, however, in small patients this distance may be substantially shorter than expected and start as of 13 and 15 mm, respectively. No correlation between glenoid height or width with the length of our drilling canal towards the scapular notch was found. Preoperative CT-based treatment planning to determine version and inclination angles is recommended.

Keywords: Anatomical and reverse total shoulder arthroplasty, Suprascapular nerve, Screw placement, Glenoid cavity, Anteversion angle, Retroversion angle, Inclination angle, Dissection study

* Correspondence: sandra.mathews@iem.uzh.ch
†Equal contributors
[1]Institute of Evolutionary Medicine (IEM), University of Zurich, Winterthurerstrasse 190, CH-8057 Zurich, Switzerland
Full list of author information is available at the end of the article

Background

Anatomical (TSA) and reverse total shoulder arthroplasty (RTSA) are effective treatment options for multiple disorders of the shoulder [1–4]. For long-term successful management, optimal positioning of the components is crucial [2, 5]. Implanting the glenoid component in an anatomical position is a challenge, which may explain the high rates of glenoid component loosening. This has been ascribed to limited bone stock of the available glenoid, the lack of reliable landmarks to determine the position of the blade of the scapula intra-operatively, and the poor understanding of the anatomical position, which shows great patient-specific variability. Surgeons may tend to aim for a 'standard' position of so-called neutral orientation of the glenoid component [6, 7].

Thus, orthopaedic surgeons emphasize a need for better understanding of the glenoid morphology to ensure proper sizing and correct placement of prosthetic components [8]. In particular, the consideration of glenoid size is of high relevance for long-term osseous integration [2, 9, 10]. Recent findings showed that small baseplates improve primary stability of the glenoid component in small glenoids [9], but published data for small glenoids for example in women are limited.

Furthermore, choice of inclination, version and rotation of the prosthetic glenoid component is mandatory for stability, a painless range of motion and to prevent impingement [5, 6, 11]. Thus, preoperative CT-based investigation is increasingly used to optimize pre-operative planning [12–15], but may not be easily accessible in all instances.

Nerve injury after RTSA has been reported with an incidence of 0.5-2.9% depending on the surgical approach [1, 16]. For implanting the glenoid component, there is a specific concern for the suprascapular nerve as it travels through the suprascapular notch where it is vulnerable to damage by the superior baseplate screw [17, 18]. Functional consequences of suprascapular nerve injury may be considered as minor since patients undergoing RTSA reportedly already have little function of the rotator cuff [19], but chronic pain and weakness may necessitate further medical intervention [18, 20, 21]. Furthermore, in patients with an intact rotator cuff, favourable influence of the rotator cuff has been reported for the range of motion and dynamic stabilisation of the anatomic and reverse total shoulder prosthesis [22, 23].

Data from human cadavers and/or scapular bones are essential to enhance knowledge of the glenoid anatomy in a representative elderly male and female population. Some studies have been conducted using isolated scapular bones [24–32], and anatomical studies are excellent tools to investigate safe drilling distances. However, such studies have been mainly directed to the posterior aspect of the scapula to optimise interventions such as the Bankart and Latarjet procedures and rotator cuff repair [2, 27, 33–40].

In a recent study on the Latarjet procedure [2], a safe zone for placement of graft-fixing screws was proposed as an approximately 2 cm-wide area medial to the glenoid rim, similar to previous suggestions for a safe zone of 2 cm in the posterior glenoid neck at the level of the supraglenoid tubercle [37]. In another study, injuries to the suprascapular nerve of up to 6% have been reported during surgery for shoulder instability, such as rotator cuff repair, [39, 40]. The median distance between glenoid and suprascapular nerve in the spinoglenoid region, measured on anatomic shoulder specimens, was 12 mm (range 6–15 mm) and 19 mm (range 11–23 mm) depending on shoulder rotation [34].

Even less data are available with regard to safe screw placement for (reverse) total shoulder arthroplasty [7], and only a few and methodologically divergent studies have used human cadavers to address the issue of safe screw placement for total or reverse shoulder arthroplasty so far [16, 17, 19, 39, 41, 42].

Furthermore, whilst a few anatomical studies have performed drill hole experiments, they did not take into account the sex dimorphism of the scapula [17, 19, 42], particularly as many patients undergoing total shoulder arthroplasty are women [4, 43]. In another study, morphological and radiological data were combined with drill hole experiments for screw placement, however the study was based on a historical bone collection, which may not accurately represent the anatomy of patients being treated today [41]. Thus, in the present study, we provide further data on the anatomical dimensions and inclination of the glenoid using an elderly cohort of body donors with a mixed sex ratio representative of patients undergoing total shoulder arthroplasty.

In our study we hypothesized that glenoid height and width might predict the distance to the scapular notch to facilitate and increase the safety of intraoperative drill hole placement. To allow comparison of the morphological measurements with routine preoperative treatment planning, 3D-CT measurements of version and inclination angles were additionally performed. To the best of our knowledge, this is one of the first studies using such a comprehensive approach.

Methods

Design of the study

Glenoid height and width were determined in a cadaver dissection study searching for potential predictors for the distance from the glenoid to the scapular notch. To gather further information relevant to anatomical and reverse total arthroplasty, the glenoid angles were also measured. To allow comparison with published data, which are predominantly recorded on isolated bones from anthropological and forensic collections (e.g., [26, 44]), the scapulae were subsequently extracted and orientated in a fixation device (similar to a previous method, [26]). In the present study, both anthropologists and anatomists measured glenoid angles and additional distances to broaden the database in the published literature. A radiologist experienced in orthopaedics performed 3D-CT measurements of version and inclination angles using the method of Friedman [45].

Body donors

The study was performed on formalin-embalmed cadavers from the institutional body donation programme at the University of Zurich (http://www.anatomy.uzh.ch/de/koerperspende.html) subsequent to the 2nd year curricular dissection course for medical bachelor students. Prior to dissection, cadavers were routinely CT-scanned at the Institute of Forensic Medicine for teaching purposes, as is increasingly becoming established practice in anatomy courses (e.g., [46]). The study was approved by the Zurich Cantonal Ethics Committee (KEK ZH-Nr. 2014–0303). The study included the thoraces from 11 female and 7 male body donors, with an average age of 84 years (range: 60–98 years). All body donors gave informed consent for research, which the authors herewith gratefully acknowledge.

Cadaver dissection and in situ measurements of distances

After exposure of the glenohumeral joint by the deltopectoral approach, maximal length and width of the glenoid were determined after Martin and Saller [47] as is commonly used intraoperatively (see: Fig. 1). In brief, a line (height) was drawn from the most cranial point of the glenoid cavity (Point A, Fig. 1) to the most caudal point (Point B, Fig. 1), and another line (width) from the most dorsal point of the glenoid rim (Point C, Fig. 1) to the most ventral point (Point D, Fig. 1). In a next step, the metal back glenoid L1 (SMR reverse shoulder prosthesis Systema Multiplana Randelli, provided by Lima Corporate SA, Italy) was selected according to the glenoid size (Small-R: $n = 14$ in 7 female donors, Standard: $n = 22$ in 11 donors, 7 males, 4 females). The central peg hole (Point F, Fig. 1) was designated at the appropriate position according to the recommendations by the manufacturer [48] for clinical practice. During surgery, special instruments are used to determine the correct position of the central K-wire, which is positioned before drilling the central peg hole of the metal back after preoperative determination of the center of the glenoid by CT scan. By analogy in our study, the intersection of the two lines (height and width) was constructed to determine the position of the central peg hole (Point F, Fig. 1). For the baseplate superior screw drilling procedure, the corresponding position of the superior screw entry point was designated 1 cm above the central peg hole at the 12-o'clock position (Point E, Fig. 1) for use as the origin of the drilling canal for the superior screw towards the suprascapular notch (Point H, Fig. 2a). All drillings were performed by the same two investigators (K.L, M.B.) according to instructions of an experienced shoulder surgeon (H.R.B.). Relevant distances between the glenoid and the scapular notch (see Fig. 2a,b) as well as the distance of the supraglenoid tubercle to the screw entry (Fig. 1a,b) were recorded with a calliper (Fig. 2c) to the nearest 1 mm. All measurements were taken repeatedly and recorded by the same three investigators (K.L., M.B., S.M.) as described [49]. The suprascapular notch was dissected to identify the suprascapular nerve and blood vessels (Fig. 1b).

Measurements of glenoid angles on isolated scapular bones

After disarticulation, extraction and removal of soft tissue, the scapulae were orientated in a fixation device. The inclination angle α (Fig. 3a) and the ante-/retroversion angle

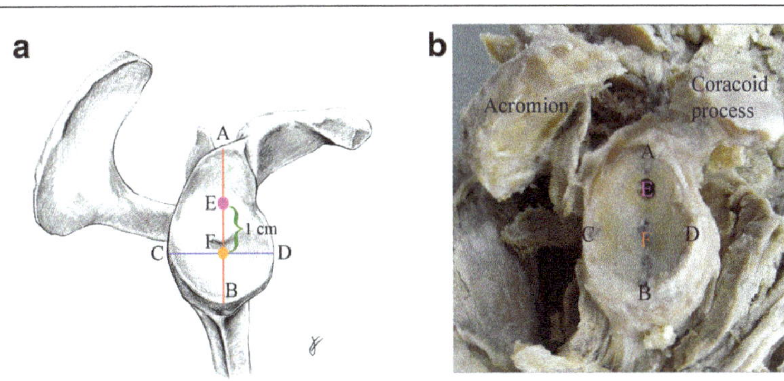

Fig. 1 Schematic **a** and photographic **b** depictions of landmarks for measurements in a right scapula, lateral view. *A* Most cranial point of the glenoid cavity. *B* Most caudal point of the glenoid cavity. *C* Most dorsal point of the glenoid rim. *D* Most ventral point of the glenoid rim. *E* Drill hole entry. *F* Central peg hole

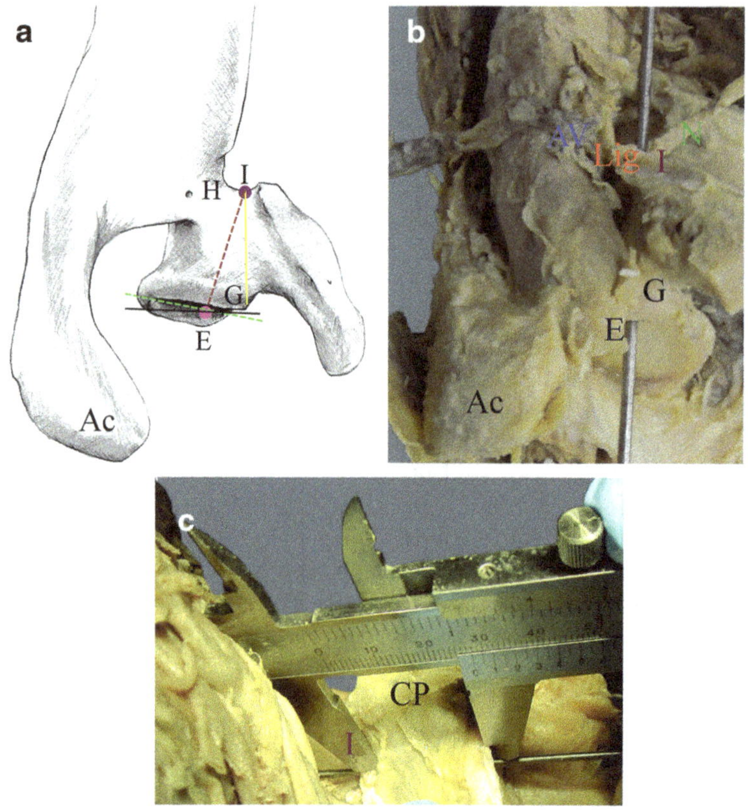

Fig. 2 Schematic **a** and photographic **b** depictions of landmarks for measurements in a right scapula from a cranial view. **a** *Dotted violet line* designates the drilling canal. **b** Drill hole as depicted with a probe. **c** Photograph from a ventral view showing drill hole measurements using a calliper. *E* Drill hole entry. *I* Drill hole exit. *G* Supraglenoid tubercle. *Ac* Acromion. *CP* Coracoid process. *N* Suprascapular nerve. *AV* Suprascapular artery and vein. *Lig* Superior transverse scapular ligament. *Green line* designates the ante-/retroversion angle perpendicular to the glenoid inclination (*black line*)

β (Fig. 3b) were measured by experienced anthropologists (S.M., N.F.) assisted by an experienced gross anatomist (K.L.) and the average result was taken as described previously [50]. In brief, a geometrical triangle was adjusted on the dorsal side below the spine from the root of the spine (J, see Fig. 3a) to the most posterior point at the glenoid rim (C). Another geometrical triangle was placed from the supraglenoid (A) to the infraglenoid (B) tubercle. The angle γ between these 2 axes was measured (Fig. 3a) and from this, the inclination angle α was calculated by the formula: $\alpha = \gamma - 90°$. The ante-/retroversion angle β (Fig. 3c) was determined perpendicular to glenoid inclination, and the angles were recorded as (−) for retroversion and (+) for anteversion similar to 3D-CT-reconstructed measurements [51]. A probe was adjusted from root of the spine (J) along the supraspinous fossa towards the supraglenoid tubercle (A). A geometrical triangle was used to designate the intersecting point between the perpendiculars from the supraglenoid tubercle (A) to the middle of the line traversing the glenoid (C to D). From this, the angle μ was measured between the axes of these two lines. To allow comparison with the CT scan, the ante-/retroversion angle β had to be calculated: in a first step, the angle δ was calculated by the formula: $\delta = 180° - \mu$, and in a next step, the ante-/retroversion angle β was converted by the formula: $\beta = \delta - 90°$.

Measurements of glenoid angles by CT scan analysis

The CT scans of the cadavers were performed on a 128-slice CT scanner (Somatom Definition Flash, Siemens Medical Solutions, Forchheim, Germany). The reconstruction parameters were 120 kV, 500 reference mAs dose modulation (CAREdose4D™, Siemens Medical Solutions), and 0.6 mm slice thickness with 0.4 mm increments with a hard kernel in the osseous windows. Reconstructions were made in a small field of view adapted to the shoulder. The DICOM files were transferred to OSIRIX™ (Pixmeo SARL, Bernex, Switzerland). In the 3D multiplanar reconstruction mode, a plane of the scapula was defined by the midpoint of the root of the scapular spine (J, Fig. 3b), the centre of the glenoid (F) and the most distal point of the inferior scapula angle (K) as previously described [52]. Measurements were performed by a radiologist experienced in orthopaedics (F.M.B.) using established techniques [15, 53].

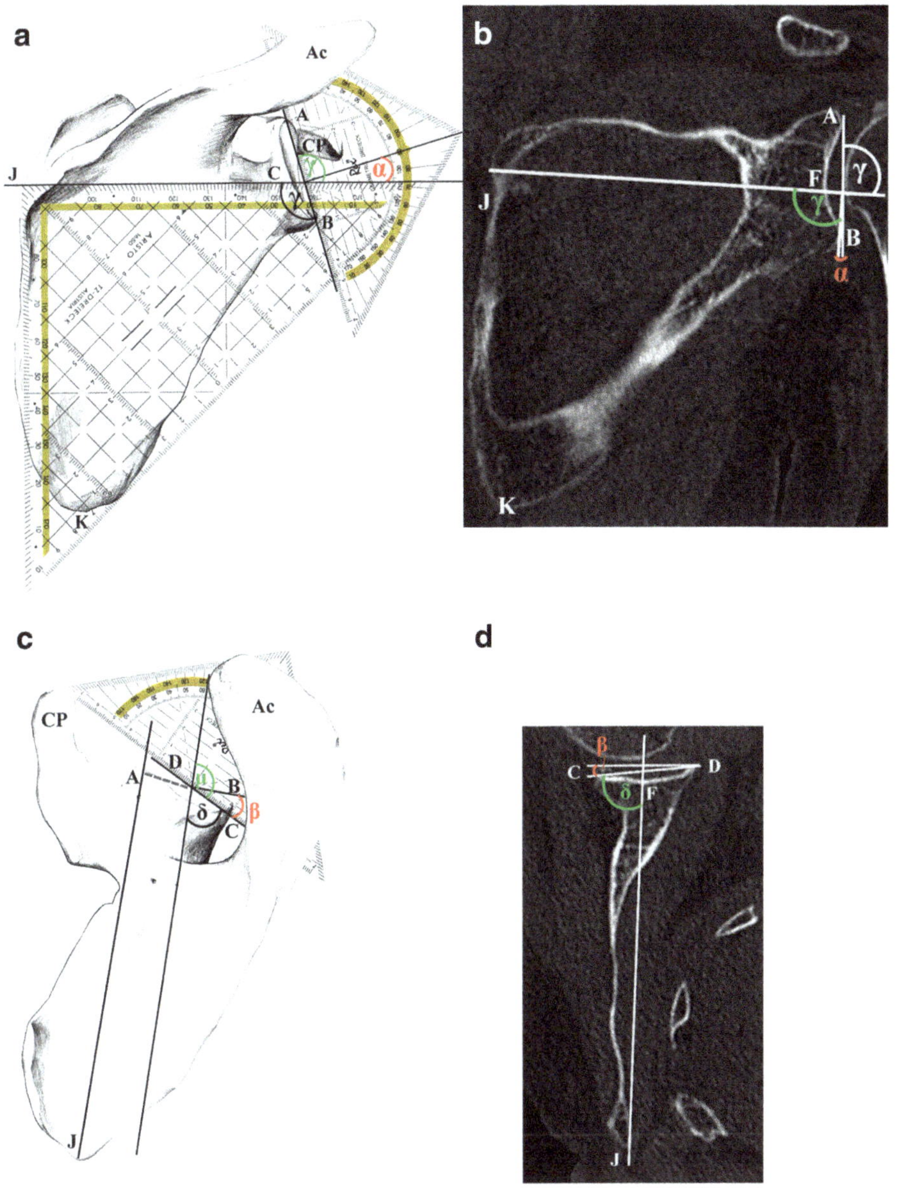

Fig. 3 Measurements of glenoid angles using bones (**a**, **c**) and 3D-CT-reconstructions (**b**, **d**). **a** For determination of the inclination angle α, a geometrical triangle was adjusted on the dorsal side below the spine running from root of the spine (*J*) to the most posterior point at the glenoid rim (*C*). Another geometrical triangle was placed running from the supraglenoid (*A*) to the infraglenoid (*B*) tubercle. The angle γ (*green*) between these 2 axes was measured and from this, the inclination angle α (*red*) calculated by the formula: α = γ - 90°. **b** On the CT scan, the inclination angle α was determined in the coronal plane. *A* line was drawn from the root of the spine (*J*) to the midpoint of the glenoid cavity (*F*). A second line was drawn through the most cranial (*A*) and caudal (*B*) points of the glenoid rim. Angle γ (*green*) was measured between the axes of these two lines in the caudal direction. From this, the glenoid angle α (*red*) was calculated by the formula α = γ - 90°. **c** A geometrical triangle was used to designate the intersecting point between the perpendicular starting at *A* (extrapolation of the dotted line) to the middle of the line between *C* to *D*. From this, the angle μ (*green*) was measured between the axes of these two lines. In a next step, the angle δ was calculated by the formula: δ = 180°- μ and then the ante-/retroversion angle β (*red*) was converted by the formula: β = δ - 90°. **d** On the CT scan, the ante-/retroversion angle β was determined in the transversal plane according to Friedman [45]. A line was drawn through the root of the spine (*J*) to the midpoint of the glenoid cavity (*F*). A second line was drawn through the most posterior (*C*) and anterior (*D*) points of the glenoid rim. Angle δ (*green*) was measured between the axes of these two lines in the sagittal direction and from this, angle β (*red*) was calculated by the formula: β = δ - 90°. *Ac* Acromion, *CP* coracoid process

The inclination angle α was determined in the coronal plane (Fig. 3b). In brief, a line was drawn through the root of the scapular spine (J) to the midpoint of the glenoid cavity (F). A second line was drawn through the most cranial (A, see Fig. 3b) and caudal (B) points of the glenoid rim. Angle γ was measured between the axes of these two lines in the caudal direction. For comparison of the CT data with the angle α in the extracted scapulae (Fig. 3a) and with published data, the angle γ was converted by the formula $\alpha = \gamma - 90°$.

The ante-/retroversion angle β was determined in the transversal plane (Fig. 3d) according to the method by Friedman et al. [45]. In brief, a line was drawn through the root of the scapular spine (J) to the midpoint of the glenoid cavity (F). A second line was drawn through the most posterior (C) and anterior (D) points of the glenoid rim. Angle δ was measured between the axes of these two lines in the sagittal direction (Fig. 3d). For comparison with the angle β in the extracted scapulae (Fig. 3c) and published data, the angle β had to be calculated by the formula: $\beta = \delta - 90°$. Negative values indicate retroversion, positive values indicate an anteversion of the glenoid.

Statistics

For statistical calculations, Microsoft Excel and IBM SPSS 23 were used. Data were examined by Shapiro-Wilk test to check for normal distribution and calculating Pearson's correlation coefficient (r). Significances were calculated with 2-tailed Student's *t*-test. A significance level $p < 0.05$ was considered statistically significant.

Results

Measurements of the glenoid cavity

For both, male and female samples combined (Table 1), the average maximum height of the glenoid (A-B, Fig. 1a,b) was 36.6 mm ± 3.6 mm (range 31.0-43.6 mm), and width (C-D, Fig. 1a,b) was 27.8 mm ± 3.1 mm (range 23.5-34.7 mm) with a significant sex dimorphism ($p \leq 0.001$). In males (Table 2), the glenoid height was 39.5 mm ± 3.5 mm (range 33.5-43.6 mm) and width 30.3 mm ± 3.3 mm (range 24.5-34.7 mm), and in females (Table 2), the glenoid height was 34.8 mm ± 2.2 mm (range 31.0-38.3 mm) and width 26.2 mm ± 1.6 mm (range 23.5-29.3 mm). Glenoid height and width correlated with each other (correlation r = 0.90).

Measurement of the distances

For both, male and female samples combined, the length of the drilling canal (E-I, Fig. 2a, b) measured externally via calliper (Fig. 2c) was 27.2 mm ± 6.0 mm (range 15.0-37.5 mm). In detail, in males, the distance from the entry point of the superior screw to its exit in the scapular notch (E-I, Fig. 2a, b) was 29.4 mm ± 5.7 mm (range 18.4-37.5 mm), and in females 25.8 mm ± 5.9 mm (range 15.0-33.9 mm) however, these distances were not significantly different from each other. The distance from the supraglenoid tubercle to the superior screw exit in the scapular notch (G-I, Fig. 2a, b) was 26.8 mm ± 6.5 mm (range 14.0-37.0 mm) with a significant sex difference ($p < 0.05$). In detail, in males, the distance from the supraglenoid tubercle to the screw exit in the scapular notch (E-I, Fig. 2a, b) was 29.6 mm ± 5.9 mm (range 19.3-37.0 mm), and in females 25.0 mm ± 6.3 mm (range 14.0-32.8 mm). Further distances are summarized in Tables 1 and 2. The distance from the entry point of the superior screw to its exit in the scapular notch (E-I) did not significantly correlate with the glenoid height (correlation $r = 0.31$) and width (correlation $r = 0.28$).

Measurements of glenoid angles

The average inclination angle (Fig. 3a, b) from male and female donors combined was 13.0° ± 7.0° (range −3.0° - 26.0°) as determined by 3D-CT (Fig. 3b). When measured on orientated fixed skeletal specimens (Fig. 3a), it was 5.0° ± 3.0° (range 0.5° - 13.5°). The average ante-/retroversion angle (Fig. 3c,d) from male and female donors combined was −1.0° ± 4.0° (range −10.0° - 10.0°) as determined by 3D-CT (Fig. 3d). When measured on orientated fixed skeletal specimens (Fig. 3c), it was −3.5° ± 4.0° (range −13.5 - 3.5). Data separated by sex are listed in Table 2. For measurements on the extracted scapulae, no significant interobserver error was found, but significant differences were observed between CT and morphological measurements: $p \leq 0.001$ for inclination angles, and $p \leq 0.01$ and $p \leq 0.001$, respectively, for the ante-/retroversion angles.

Table 1 Measurements in cadaveric specimens from male and female donors combined

Measurement	Landmarks (from-to)	Average (mm)	SD (mm)	Range (mm)
Glenoid height	A-B	36.6	3.6	31.0-43.6
Glenoid width	C-D	27.8	3.1	23.5-34.7
Supraglenoid tubercle to superior screw (entrance)	G-E	13.2	3.4	7.0-20.3
Supraglenoid tubercle to scapular notch (centre caudal)	G-H	32.7	2.8	26.0-39.0
Superior screw entrance and exit	E-I	27.2	6.0	15.0-37.5
Supraglenoid tubercle to superior screw exit in suprascapular notch	G-I	26.8	6.5	14.0-37.0

SD standard deviation

Table 2 Measurements of scapulae and scapula angles sorted by sex

	Sex	N	Mean (mm)	SD (mm)	Range (mm)
Glenoid height***	m	14	39.5	3.5	33.5-43.6
	f	22	34.8	2.2	31.0-38.3
Glenoid width***	m	14	30.3	3.3	24.5-34.7
	f	22	26.2	1.6	23.5-29.3
Supraglenoid tubercle to superior screw (entrance)*	m	14	14.9	3.6	8.0-20.3
	f	22	12.1	2.8	7.0-17.1
Supraglenoid tubercle to scapular notch (centre caudal)*	m	14	33.9	3.2	27.5-39.0
	f	22	32.0	2.3	26.0-35.0
Superior screw entrance and exit	m	14	29.4	5.7	18.4-37.5
	f	22	25.8	5.9	15.0-33.9
Supraglenoid tubercle to superior screw exit in suprascapular notch*	m	14	29.6	5.9	19.3-37.0
	f	22	25.0	6.3	14.0-32.8
Inclination CT	m	14	15.0	8.0	−3-26.0
	f	22	12.0	6.0	1.0-26.0
Inclination scapular bone	m	14	5.0	3.0	1.5-13.5
	f	22	4.0	3.0	0.5-9.0
Ante-/retroversion angle CT	m	14	0	3.0	−5.0-6.0
	f	22	−1.0	5.0	−10.0-10.0
Ante-/retroversion angle scapular bone	m	14	−3,5	4.5	−13.5-3.5
	f	22	−4.0	4.0	−10.5-3.5

SD standard deviation
***indicates a *P* value < 0.001
**indicates a *P* value < 0.01
*indicates a *P* value < 0.05 as statistically calculated with *t*-test and Pearson correlation

Discussion

In this multimodality approach, we measured the glenoid fossa and its distance from the scapular notch. A few studies on human cadavers have addressed the issue of safe screw placement for total shoulder arthroplasty so far (Table 3) using baseplates with 3 [41] or 4 screws [9, 17, 19, 42] with different orientations of the baseplate and drilling canal, respectively. Although 4 screw holes offer the advantage of good fixation, the required drilling procedures may cause further bone loss and thus weaken the construct even more [19, 41].

In the present study, we used a 2-screw system and laid special emphasis on the superior screw. In all cases, we used standard or small glenosphere baseplates to determine the drilling hole. The origin of the drilling canal for the superior screw towards the suprascapular notch was designated at the 12-o'clock position in a centrally orientated peg glenosphere as recommended by the

Table 3 Comparison of distances from the present study in male and female donors combined (for further details see Tables 1 and 2) with published data using drilling experiments on human cadaver specimens. Please note that the respective distances can be estimated only very roughly due to the different approaches of the published data. BP: baseplate

Study	Glenoid height (mm)	Glenoid width (mm)	Superior screw entrance and exit (drilling canal, mm)
Present study	36.6 (range 31–43.6)	27.8 (range 23.5-34.7)	27.2 (range 15–37.5)
DiStefano et al. [19]	39.5 ± 2.6	31 ± 2.5	Optimal screw length 35 ± 8 depending on angulation, inferior BP inclination
Molony et al. [17]	No data	No data	Screw length 36.6 (range 32–42)
Hart et al. [42]	No data	No data	29.3 (13–43) 1-o'clock position
Chae et al. [9]	25 mm BP: 32.6 ± 2.5 29 mm BP: 32.1 ± 2.4	25 mm BP: 23.3 ± 2.0 29 mm BP: 23.3 ± 1.7	25 mm BP: 32 ± 6.4 29 mm BP: 25.4 ± 5.8

manufacturer. In our study, length of the drilling canal showed an average for both sexes combined of 27.2 mm (29.4 mm in males, 25.8 mm in females) with a calliper adjusted to the probe within the drilling canal (Fig. 2c). These results are shorter than reported by other groups (see Table 3), but resemble more the proposed optimal length of 29 mm (range 18–29 mm) for the ideal screw position as calculated from CT-simulations [41], and correlate for female to the published mean length of 25.4 mm in the female subgroup of 29 mm baseplate (see Table 3) in another study [9].

To allow comparison with other studies from different countries, we expanded our measurements to the distance from the supraglenoid tubercle to the center of the scapular notch. Our data from Switzerland had an average of 32.7 mm, which is similar to that of 31 mm from Italy [27], 33 mm from Turkey [54] and Germany [2] and of 30 mm [37] and 34.2 mm [39], from the USA. Slightly shorter distances of 28.7-29.1 mm were found in a study from India [32] and Kenya with a range of 27.3-30.1 mm depending on the scapular notch type [55] and of 29 mm (23–35 mm) from Japan [38].

In a study on the Latarjet procedure [2], distances of 33 mm (range 31–35 mm) between the suprascapular nerve and 3 reference points along the glenoid rim were measured, including the supraglenoid tubercle, of which the latter could be used for comparison with our average of 32.7 mm. Nevertheless, it has to be noted that in our investigated Middle European population, the distance between screw entry and suprascapular notch was little as 15 mm in females. To the best of our knowledge a similar short distance of 13 mm has only been previously reported in a single study [42], but without providing further data regarding the specimens used. Also a recent clinical study has emphasised the increasing use of small baseplates [56]. This would mean that the proposed safe distance of 20 mm described above might entail a potential risk in some smaller individuals, or individuals from other populations, or particularly in women. Thus, more studies are needed to investigate the sex dimorphism of scapular size in males and females.

Integration of CT and/or MRI scans in planning shoulder arthroplasty is therefore generally recommended.

In the present study, glenoid size showed an average height of 39.5 mm and width of 30.3 mm for males, and height of 34.8 mm and width of 26.2 mm for females. We had hypothesized that glenoid height and width should correlate with each other, which we herewith confirm. However, no correlation was found between glenoid height or width, and the length of the drilling canal towards the scapular notch.

The glenoids measured in the present study affirm the described sex difference [25]. Similar data from Middle Europe showed a glenoid height of 40 mm and width of 29 mm for males and height of 36.1 mm and width of 25.7 mm for females [57] as well as height of 31.7 ± 3.7 mm and width of 24.7 ± 3.5 mm for both sexes combined [58]. However, our data on glenoid size was smaller than the glenoid height of 45.7 mm in a USA study on 4 men and 4 women [59]. On the other hand, our results are larger than in men with a height of 37.5 mm and width of 27.8 mm, and in women, a height of 32.6 mm and width of 23.6 mm. The smaller data from this historical bone collection as compared to more recent data may support the assumption that this may not reflect the patients undergoing surgery today [26]. For a contemporary Mexican population, the need for better knowledge on sex dimorphism of glenoid size and the importance of population-specific discriminants for scapulae was highlighted for forensic scenes [44]. Further, a recent study postulated that larger sample sizes for ethnic groups should be explored. This study identified sex as the strongest independent predictor of glenoid size. Men exhibited a larger glenoid, however, patient height was found to be predictive only in patients of the same sex. The authors further observed variations in glenoid size and version also among ethnicities [58].

In the present study, on isolated scapulae a mean glenoid inclination angle of 5° in males and 4° in females were measured, which are rather similar to findings of 4° in male donors (range −7° - 15.8°), and 4.5° (range −1.5° - 15.3°) in female donors [26] and of 7.1° ± 1.7° in 4 men and 4 women [59]. In another study, a mean inclination angle of 12° (range −21° - 50°) was determined by postoperative CT-scanning of predominantly female patients, from which the authors concluded there was frequent malpositioning of the baseplate [6]. Nevertheless, the mean value of 13° for the inclination angle measured by CT was higher as compared to our findings in bone, and to the CT-data of 1° in male and 4° in female normal glenoids from another study, which reported no significant difference to osteoarthritic type B2 glenoids [51].

Using historical scapulae with a mean age of 25.6 years, Churchill and co-workers [26] measured mean glenoid version angles of 0.35° in black and 3.49° in white men, and 0.79° in black and 2.8° in white women. Recently, using CT scans, a mean version of 0.05 ± 9.05 was measured from which the authors proposed that males are expected to exhibit 8.4° more retroversion than females, and Hispanics demonstrate 6.4° more anteversion compared to African-Americans [58]. Retroversion of 4° - 8° has been described as normal, while higher retroversion angles predispose for dorsal shoulder luxation and glenoid loosening secondary to abnormal forces across the implant and the cement-bone interface [12, 30].

We attribute our own retroversion angles of −3.5° on bones (range −13.5°- 4.5°) and of −1° on CT scans (range −10° - 10°) to the pronouncedly higher age of the population we investigated. Our data were comparatively similar to findings of −4° (range − 18° - 5°) measured in a stable control group of a clinical study [14] by MRI according to Friedman [45] and of - 8.5° ± 5.2° by 3D-CT-reconstruction [19]. In a study comparing a new 2D measurement method, retroversion angle of −19° ± 3° were measured in the control group, whilst the method by Friedman [45] revealed a retroversion of −1° ± 6° [13]. We attribute the discrepancies between bone and CT-measurements in our study to the complex morphology of the scapula, which in a minority of cases was difficult to orientate due to pronounced deformations in 6 samples from 4 individuals aged 81–94 years. Furthermore, remnants of cartilage present on the extracted scapulae may account for these observed differences. Nevertheless, the difference between our morphological and radiological measurements was within a similar order of magnitude as reported for 2D- and 3D-CT measurements, with a range for the glenoid version angle of 0.1°–23°, and for the inclination angle of 0.2°–4.5° [12–15, 52, 60, 61].

To summarise, proper sizing and correct placement of prosthetic components are mandatory. 3D-imaging and patient specific instrumentation will have to be based on a profound knowledge of glenoid morphology [8, 61]. We hereby add a new systematic dataset regarding glenoid size, version and inclination angles and scapular distances to the literature. The glenoid angles measured by morphological and 3D-CT reflect the differences in elderly male and female patients undergoing total shoulder arthroplasty.

However, there are some limitations in this study: First of all, measurements by 3D-CT differed from those on the isolated scapulae, which may, as outlined above, be expected from published differences in the literature. Secondly, drillings were performed using a 2-screw system with a clear focus on the superior screw and the danger to the suprascapular nerve. Thirdly, central positioning of the baseplate was applied as used in previous work [17, 42], but differed for another study [19], which used inferior inclination of the baseplate. Nevertheless, to the best of our knowledge, this is one of the first studies to comprehensively present such a broad spectrum of morphological data in a mixed elderly population.

Conclusions

As also indicated in the literature, in some women and smaller individuals, smaller baseplates should be selected. The published safe zone of 20 mm is generally feasible also for superior screw placement. However, in small patients careful consideration is necessary that the distance between the glenoid and the scapular notch may be shorter than expected and be as little as 13 and 15 mm, respectively. While glenoid height and width correlated with each other in the present data set, no correlation between glenoid height or width with the length of the drilling canal towards the scapular notch was found. Preoperative CT-based treatment planning to determine version and inclination angles as well as the distance between the glenoid and the scapular notch is recommended.

Abbreviations

RTSA: Reverse total shoulder arthroplasty; TSA: Anatomical total shoulder arthroplasty

Acknowledgements

The authors are very grateful to Dr. Magdalena Vich and Heinz Sonderegger (photographs used in the figures), Institute of Anatomy, and Dr. Nikola Koepke, Institute of Evolutionary Medicine (IEM), University of Zürich for helpful, competent and friendly support.

Funding

The study was financially supported by the Mäxi Foundation (to F.-J.R.), the Swiss National Science Foundation (project No. 31003A-156299/1 to M.H.) and the Prof. Dr. med. Karl and Rena Theiler-Haag Foundation (to K.L.). The funding bodies had no role in the design of the study, collection, analysis or interpretation of the data, nor in writing the manuscript.

Authors' contributions

All authors have made substantial contributions to the study: HRB, EE, GH, and FQ initiated the study. HRB, EE, F-JR, MT and OU supervised study design and performance. FMB, HB, HRB, MB, EE, NF, DG, MH, KL, SM, NS, and STS collected, analysed and interpreted the data. I.F. provided technical support and created the drawings. EE, KL and SM discussed the data and drafted the manuscript. HRB, MM-G, G.H., MH, FQ, F-JR, STS and OU discussed the data and contributed to manuscript writing. All authors read and approved the final draft of the manuscript.

Competing interests

Hans-Rudolf Bloch was Medical Director of Lima Corporate SA, Italy, during the initiation and conduction of the study until December 2015. After that date, no commercial associations (e.g. consultancies, stock ownership, equity interest, patent/licensing arrangements, etc.) exist that might pose a conflict of interest in connection with the submitted article. Baseplate material for definition of the drilling holes was provided by Lima Corporate SA, Italy. The other authors certify that no commercial associations (e.g. consultancies, stock ownership, equity interest, patent/licensing arrangements, etc.) exist that might pose a conflict of interest in connection with the submitted article.

Consent for publication

Not applicable. This manuscript does not contain any individual persons data.

Author details

[1]Institute of Evolutionary Medicine (IEM), University of Zurich, Winterthurerstrasse 190, CH-8057 Zurich, Switzerland. [2]Division of Gross Anatomy, Institute of Anatomy, University of Zurich, Zurich, Switzerland. [3]Medical Radiology Institute, Schulthess Clinic, Zurich, Switzerland. [4]Medical Faculty, University of Zurich, Zurich, Switzerland. [5]Institute of Forensic Medicine, University of Zurich, Zurich, Switzerland. [6]Institute of Neuroradiology, University Hospital Magdeburg, Magdeburg, Germany. [7]Musculoskeletal Research Unit, Department of Biomedicine, University of Basel, Basel, Switzerland. [8]Shoulder Unit, Queen Alexandra Hospital,

Portsmouth, UK. [9]Shoulder Unit, Doncaster Royal Infirmary, Doncaster, UK. [10]Technical Orthopedics Unit, University Hospital Balgrist, Zurich, Switzerland. [11]Shoulder Surgery Unit, Ospedale Civico, Lugano, Switzerland.

References

1. Alentorn-Geli E, Samitier G, Torrens C, Wright TW. Reverse shoulder arthroplasty. Part 2: Systematic review of reoperations, revisions, problems, and complications. Int J Shoulder Surg. 2015;9(2):60–7.
2. Hawi N, Reinhold A, Suero EM, Liodakis E, Przyklenk S, Brandes J, Schmiedl A, Krettek C, Meller R. The anatomic basis for the arthroscopic Latarjet Procedure: A cadaveric study. Am J Sport Med. 2016;44(2):497–503.
3. Merkle TP, Beckmann N, Bruckner T, Zeifang F. Shoulder joint replacement can improve quality of life and outcome in patients with dysmelia: a case series. BMC Musculoskelet Disord. 2016;17:185-193.
4. Longo UG, Petrillo S, Berton A, Denaro V. Reverse total shoulder arthroplasty for the management of fractures of the proximal humerus: a systematic review. Musculoskelet Surg. 2016;100(2):83–91.
5. von Eisenhart-Rothe R, Muller-Gerbl M, Wiedemann E, Englmeier KH, Graichen H. Functional malcentering of the humeral head and asymmetric long-term stress on the glenoid: Potential reasons for glenoid loosening in total shoulder arthroplasty. J Shoulder Elb Surg. 2008;17(5):695–702.
6. Gregory TM, Sankey A, Augereau B, Vandenbussche E, Amis A, Emery R, Hansen U. Accuracy of glenoid component placement in total shoulder arthroplasty and its effect on clinical and radiological outcome in a retrospective, longitudinal, monocentric open study. Plos One. 2013;8(10): e75791.
7. Stephens BF, Hebert CT, Azar FM, Mihalko WM, Throckmorton TW. Optimal baseplate rotational alignment for locking-screw fixation in reverse total shoulder arthroplasty: a three-dimensional computer-aided design study. J Shoulder Elb Surg. 2015;24(9):1367–71.
8. Zumstein V, Kraljevic M, Hoechel S, Conzen A, Nowakowski AM, Muller-Gerbl M. The glenohumeral joint - a mismatching system? A morphological analysis of the cartilaginous and osseous curvature of the humeral head and the glenoid cavity. J Orthop Surg Res. 2014;9:34.
9. Chae SW, Kim SY, Lee H, Yon JR, Lee J, Han SH. Effect of baseplate size on primary glenoid stability and impingement-free range of motion in reverse shoulder arthroplasty. BMC Musculoskelet Disord. 2014;15:417.
10. Langohr GDG, Willing R, Medley JB, Athwal GS, Johnson JA. Contact mechanics of reverse total shoulder arthroplasty during abduction: the effect of neck-shaft angle, humeral cup depth, and glenosphere diameter. J Shoulder Elb Surg. 2016;25(4):589–97.
11. Lädermann A, Gueorguiev B, Charbonnier C, Stimec BV, Fasel JHD, Zderic I, Hagen J, Walch G. Scapular notching on kinematic simulated range of motion after Reverse Shoulder Arthroplasty is not the result of impingement in adduction. Medicine. 2015;94(38):e1615.
12. Hoenecke HR, Hermida JC, Flores-Hernandez C, D'Lima DD. Accuracy of CT-based measurements of glenoid version for total shoulder arthroplasty. J Shoulder Elb Surg. 2010;19(2):166–71.
13. Poon PC, Ting FSH. A 2-dimensional glenoid vault method for measuring glenoid version on computed tomography. J Shoulder Elb Surg. 2012;21(3): 329–35.
14. Privitera DM, Siegel EJ, Miller LR, Sinz NJ, Higgins LD. Glenoid version and its relationship to glenohumeral instability and labral tears. J Shoulder Elb Surg. 2016;25(7):1056–63.
15. Maurer A, Fucentese SF, Pfirrmann CWA, Wirth SH, Djahangiri A, Jost B, Gerber C. Assessment of glenoid inclination on routine clinical radiographs and computed tomography examinations of the shoulder. J Shoulder Elb Surg. 2012;21(8):1096–103.
16. Lädermann A, Stimec BV, Denard PJ, Cunningham G, Collin P, Fasel JHD. Injury to the axillary nerve after reverse shoulder arthroplasty: An anatomical study. Orthop Traumatol-Sur. 2014;100(1):105–8.
17. Molony DC, Gheiti AJC, Kennedy J, Green C, Schepens A, Mullett HJ. A cadaveric model for suprascapular nerve injury during glenoid component screw insertion in reverse-geometry shoulder arthroplasty. J Shoulder Elb Surg. 2011;20(8):1323–7.
18. Wang VM, Krishnan R, Ugwonali OFC, Flatow EL, Bigliani LU, Ateshian GA. Biomechanical evaluation of a novel glenoid design in total shoulder arthroplasty. J Shoulder Elb Surg. 2005;14(1):129s–40s.
19. DiStefano JG, Park AY, Nguyen TQD, Diederichs G, Buckley JM, Montgomery WH. Optimal screw placement for base plate fixation in reverse total shoulder arthroplasty. J Shoulder Elb Surg. 2011;20(3):467–76.
20. Farshad M, Grogli M, Catanzaro S, Gerber C. Revision of reversed total shoulder arthroplasty. Indications and outcome. BMC Musculoskelet Disord. 2012;13:160.
21. Shi LL, Freehill MT, Yannopoulos P, Warner JJ. Suprascapular nerve: is it important in cuff pathology? Adv Orthop. 2012;2012:516985.
22. McFarland EG, Huri G, Hyun YS, Petersen SA, Srikumaran U. Reverse total shoulder arthroplasty without bone-grafting for severe glenoid bone loss in patients with osteoarthritis and Intact rotator cuff. J Bone Joint Surg Am. 2016;98(21):1801–7.
23. Mizuno N, Denard PJ, Raiss P, Walch G. Reverse total shoulder arthroplasty for primary glenohumeral osteoarthritis in patients with a biconcave glenoid. J Bone Joint Surg Am. 2013;95(14):1297–304.
24. Anetzberger H, Maier M, Zysk S, Schulz C, Putz R. The architecture of the subacromial space in humans with full thickness supraspinatus tears. Z Orthop Grenzgeb. 2004;142(2):221–7.
25. Anetzberger H, Putz R. The scapula: Principles of construction and stress. Acta Anat. 1996;156(1):70–80.
26. Churchill RS, Brems JJ, Kotschi H. Glenoid size, inclination, and version: An anatomic study. J Shoulder Elb Surg. 2001;10(4):327–32.
27. Gumina S, Albino P, Giaracuni M, Vestri A, Ripani M, Postacchini F. The safe zone for avoiding suprascapular nerve injury during shoulder arthroscopy: an anatomical study on 500 dry scapulae. J Shoulder Elb Surg. 2011;20(8):1317–22.
28. Polguj M, Jedrzejewski KS, Topol M. Sexual dimorphism of the suprascapular notch - morphometric study. Arch Med Sci. 2013;9(1):177–83.
29. Polguj M, Majos A, Waszczykowski M, Fabiś J, Stefańczyk K, Podgórski M, Topol M. A computed tomography study on the correlation between the morphometry of the suprascapular notch and anthropometric measurements of the scapula. Folia Morphol. 2015;75(1):87–92.
30. Prescher A. Anatomical basics, variations, and degenerative changes of the shoulder joint and shoulder girdle. Eur J Radiol. 2000;35(2):88–102.
31. Codsi MJ, Bennetts C, Gordiev K, Boeck DM, Kwon Y, Brems J, Powell K, Iannotti JP. Normal glenoid vault anatomy and validation of a novel glenoid implant shape. J Shoulder Elb Surg. 2008;17(3):471–8.
32. Sangam MR, Sarada Devi SS, Krupadanam K, Anasuya K. A study on the morphology of the suprascapular notch and its distance from the glenoid cavity. J Clin Diagn Res. 2013;7(2):189–92.
33. Lädermann A, Denard PJ, Burkhart SS. Injury of the suprascapular nerve during Latarjet Procedure: An anatomic study. Arthroscopy. 2012;28(3):316–21.
34. Longo UG, Forriol F, Loppini M, Lanotte A, Salvatore G, Maffulli N, Denaro V. The safe zone for avoiding suprascapular nerve injury in bone block procedures for shoulder instability. A cadaveric study. Knee Surg Sport Tr A. 2015;23(5):1506–10.
35. Maquieira GJ, Gerber C, Schneeberger AG. Suprascapular nerve palsy after the Latarjet procedure. J Shoulder Elb Surg. 2007;16(2):e13–5.
36. Morgan RT, Henn RF, Paryavi E, Dreese J. Injury to the suprascapular nerve during superior labrum anterior and posterior repair: Is a rotator interval portal safer than an anterosuperior portal? Arthroscopy. 2014;30(11):1418–23.
37. Bigliani LU, Dalsey RM, McCann PD, April EW. An anatomical study of the suprascapular nerve. Arthroscopy. 1990;6(4):301–5.
38. Shishido H, Kikuchi S. Injury of the suprascapular nerve in shoulder surgery: An anatomic study. J Shoulder Elb Surg. 2001;10(4):372–6.
39. Tom JA, Mesfin A, Shah MP, Javandel M, Lee DJ, Cerynik DL, Amin NH. Anatomical considerations of the suprascapular nerve in rotator cuff repairs. Anat Res In. 2014;2014. doi:10.1155/2014/674179.
40. Longo UG, Loppini M, Rizzello G, Romeo G, Huijsmans PE, Denaro V. Glenoid and humeral head bone loss in traumatic anterior glenohumeral instability: a systematic review. Knee Surg Sports Traumatol Arthrosc. 2014; 22(2):392–414.
41. Codsi MJ, Bennetts C, Powell K, Iannotti JP. Locations for screw fixed beyond the glenoid vault for fixation of glenoid implants into the scapula: An anatomic study. J Shoulder Elb Surg. 2007;16(3):84s–9s.
42. Hart ND, Clark JC, Wade Krause FR, Kissenberth MJ, Bragg WE, Hawkins RJ. Glenoid screw position in the Encore Reverse Shoulder Prosthesis: an anatomic dissection study of screw relationship to surrounding structures. J Shoulder Elb Surg. 2013;22(6):814–20.
43. Athwal GS, MacDermid JC, Reddy KM, Marsh JP, Faber KJ, Drosdowech D. Does bony increased-offset reverse shoulder arthroplasty decrease scapular notching? J Shoulder Elb Surg. 2015;24(3):468–73.
44. Hudson A, Peckmann TR, Logar CJ, Meek S. Sex determination in a

contemporary Mexican population using the scapula. J Forensic Leg Med. 2016;37:91–6.
45. Friedman RJ, Hawthorne KB, Genez BM. The use of computerized-tomography in the measurement of glenoid version. J Bone Joint Surg Am. 1992; 74A(7):1032–7.
46. Schramek GGR, Stoevesandt D, Reising A, Kielstein JT, Hiss M, Kielstein H. Imaging in anatomy: a comparison of imaging techniques in embalmed human cadavers. BMC Med Educ. 2013;13(1):1.
47. Martin R, Saller K. Lehrbuch der Anthropologie in systematischer Darstellung mit besonderer Berücksichtigung der anthropologischen Methoden. G. Stuttgart: Fischer; 1957.
48. Lima. SMR Surgical technique. Villanova di San Daniele del Friuli, Italy: Lima Corporate; 2012.
49. Burkhard M, Mathews S, Link K, Franke I, Harper G, Quereshi F, Bloch H, Ullrich O, Eppler E, Ruhli F. The human glenoid morphology - a comparative cadaver based study. Am J Phys Anthropol. 2015;156:95–6.
50. Mathews S, Burkhard M, Link K, Franke I, Harper G, Quereshi F, Bloch HR, Ullrich O, Ruhli F, Eppler E. Assessing bone and soft tissue morphology of the scapula region: a cadaver dissection-based study to improve uncemented glenoid metalback fixation. Faseb J. 2014;28(1).
51. Knowles NK, Ferreira LM, Athwal GS. Premorbid retroversion is significantly greater in type B2 glenoids. J Shoulder Elb Surg. 2016;25(7):1064–8.
52. Bryce CD, Davison AC, Lewis GS, Wang L, Flemming DJ, Armstrong AD. Two-dimensional glenoid version measurements vary with coronal and sagittal scapular rotation. J Bone Joint Surg Am. 2010;92(3):692–9.
53. Nyffeler RW, Jost B, Pfirrmann CWA, Gerber C. Measurement of glenoid version: Conventional radiographs versus computed tomography scans. J Shoulder Elb Surg. 2003;12(5):493–6.
54. Ekin A, Magden O, Icke C. Anatomy and relationship of the suprascapular nerve. Int Congr Ser. 1995;1085:379–84.
55. Sinkeet SR, Awori KO, Odula PO, Ogeng'o JA, Mwachaka PM. The suprascapular notch: its morphology and distance from the glenoid cavity in a Kenyan population. Folia Morphol. 2010;69(4):241–5.
56. Athwal GS, Faber KJ. Outcomes of reverse shoulder arthroplasty using a mini 25-mm glenoid baseplate. Int Orthop. 2016;40(1):109–13.
57. Polguj M, Jedrzejewski KS, Podgorski M, Topol M. Correlation between morphometry of the suprascapular notch and anthropometric measurements of the scapula. Folia Morphol. 2011;70(2):109–15.
58. Piponov HI, Savin D, Shah N, Esposito D, Schwartz B, Moretti V, Goldberg B. Glenoid version and size: does gender, ethnicity, or body size play a role? Int Orthop. 2016;40(11):2347-53.
59. Wong AS, Gallo L, Kuhn JE, Carpenter JE, Hughes RE. The effect of glenoid inclination on superior humeral head migration. J Shoulder Elb Surg. 2003; 12(4):360–4.
60. Van Haver A, Heylen S, Vuylsteke K, Declercq G, Verborgt O. Reliability analysis of glenoid component inclination measurements on postoperative radiographs and computed tomography-based 3D models in total and reversed shoulder arthroplasty patients. J Shoulder Elb Surg. 2016;25(4):632–40.
61. Dallalana RJ, McMahon RA, East B, Geraghty L. Accuracy of patient-specific instrumentation in anatomic and reverse total shoulder arthroplasty. Int J Shoulder Surg. 2016;10(2):59–66.

6

Identifying complications requiring re-operation following primary hip or knee arthroplasty

Bill Reynolds[1], Nick Maister[2], Stephen D. Gill[1,3,4*], Shaun Waring[2], Peter Schoch[1], Sally Beattie[3], Andrew Thomson[2] and Richard S. Page[2,3,4]

Abstract

Background: The number of hip and knee arthroplasties completed is expected to double over the next decade. In public hospitals, regular post-arthroplasty orthopaedic review has commonly occurred for the duration of a patient's life, which requires substantial outpatient resources. However, there is limited evidence regarding the utility of these reviews for identifying complications. The current study investigated when and where complications requiring re-operation were identified following primary hip or knee arthroplasty.

Methods: The medical records of all patients requiring re-operation for complications following primary hip arthroplasty ($n = 48$, 2004 to 2015) or knee primary arthroplasty ($n = 50$, 1998 to 2015) at a large regional health service were evaluated. Data were extracted by one of four investigators using a standardised electronic data extraction tool. Variables of interest included the health setting where the complication was initially identified, how long following the original operation the complication was identified and whether the complication was symptomatic.

Results: Routine post-arthroplasty orthopaedic appointments identified 15 (15.3%) complications requiring re-operation; all were identified in the first-year post-surgery. For each complication identified in the first-year post-surgery, approximately 1000 orthopaedic outpatient appointments were required. After the first year, all complications were identified in Emergency Departments ($n = 30$, 30.6%), General Practice ($n = 24$, 24.5%) or non-routine orthopaedic outpatient appointments ($n = 19$, 19.4%). All patients with complications reported symptoms.

Conclusions: Routine post-arthroplasty review appointments were an inefficient mechanism for identifying complications requiring re-operation more than one year following surgery. Public health services should consider assessing and redesigning post-arthroplasty review services to reduce the burden on patients and the demand for outpatient appointments.

Keywords: Arthroplasty, Complications, Revision surgery, Hip, Knee

* Correspondence: stephen.gill2@deakin.edu.au
[1]Physiotherapy Department, Barwon Health, Geelong, VIC 3220, Australia
[3]Barwon Centre for Orthopaedic Research and Education (B-CORE), St John of God Hospital and Barwon Health, Geelong, VIC 3220, Australia
Full list of author information is available at the end of the article

Background

The number of referrals to public orthopaedic outpatient services are increasing, and waiting times for appointments often exceed recommended targets [1, 2]. Review appointments following hip or knee arthroplasty constitute a large number of appointments. For example, our health service completed approximately 1600 routine hip or knee post-arthroplasty review appointments in 2015 [3]; a figure predicted to increase as the number of hip and knee replacements performed per annum is expected to double in the next decade [4].

The primary purpose of post-arthroplasty review appointments is to identify post-operative complications, such as aseptic prosthetic loosening, that might lead to catastrophic failure if untreated. The frequency of post-arthroplasty review varies between surgeons [5–8]. The Arthroplasty Society of Australia Position Statement indicated that routine reviews following uncomplicated primary arthroplasty in low risk patients and prostheses should take place 2–6 months post implantation, and then at 1–2 years, 5 years and then biennially thereafter [4]. Considering only arthroplasties that occurred in Australian public hospitals in 2016, [9] this review schedule requires approximately 64,000 outpatient appointments in 2017-8 to review the 32,000 primary hip and knee arthroplasties that occurred in 2016; additional appointments would be required to review patients who are 5 years or more following surgery. However, there is little empirical evidence to indicate how often post-arthroplasty review appointments should occur or whether they are necessary at all [2, 5, 10]. The review schedule creates a high burden and cost to patients, families, health services and arthroplasty surgeons. Surgeons cannot regularly review all joint replacement patients without compromising their ability to manage increasing numbers of new patients [4]. Regular review of asymptomatic patients might also contribute to high non-attendance rates amongst this cohort of patients [5, 11].

The current study investigated whether routine orthopaedic outpatient appointments after primary hip or knee arthroplasty were responsible for identifying post-operative complications. Specifically, we aimed to determine 1) the healthcare setting where complications requiring re-operation were initially identified 2) how long after surgery the complications were identified, 3) the type of complication/s identified and 4) the symptomatic and radiological indicators of complications.

Methods

Setting

The study was conducted at [removed for anonymous review] (UHG), a 432-bed regional teaching hospital in [removed for anonymous review] that is the only publicly funded hospital in the region. The UHG Orthopaedic Unit currently comprises 8 lower limb arthroplasty surgeons that performed 292 primary hip arthroplasties and 154 primary knee arthroplasties in 2015 [3]. At the time of the study, post-operative *routine* reviews were conducted at the hospital in each surgeon's weekly outpatient clinic. Patients could be seen post-operatively by the surgeon, orthopaedic registrar or a supervised junior doctor at 6 weeks, 3 months and 12 months, then at 5 and 8 years, and then every two years thereafter. Hip hemiarthroplasties were reviewed in the same manner, provided patients were community ambulant preceding surgery. More frequent *non-routine* reviews occurred at the surgeon's discretion if there were concerns of increased risk of complications, for example, for prostheses with known higher revision rates. The decision to organise non-routine reviews could be made at any time, including immediately following surgery.

Study design

We planned to retrospectively analyse 100 consecutive primary hip or knee arthroplasties that required re-operation. All hip re-operations that occurred at UHG between 2004 and 2015 ($n = 49$) and all knee re-operations that occurred at UHG between 1998 and 2015 ($n = 51$) were screened for eligibility (see Fig. 1). Including 100 consecutive re-operations was a pragmatic decision based on our ability to identify arthroplasties requiring re-operation (described below) and the resources available to complete the review. Two patients were subsequently excluded from the final data set (see Fig. 1).

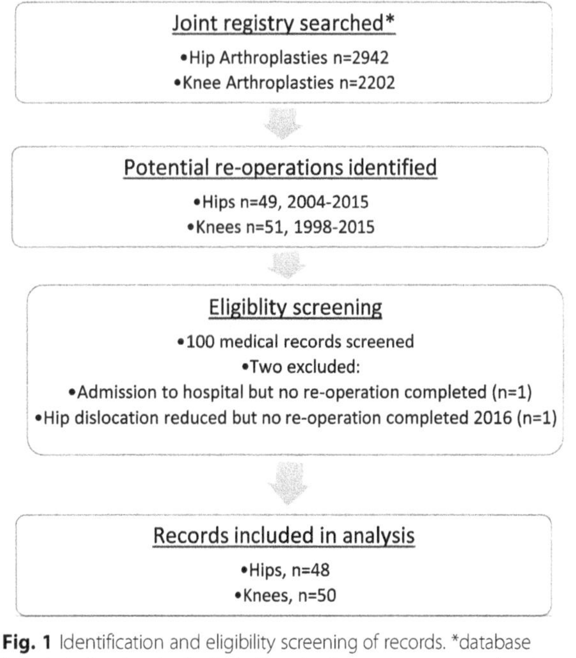

Fig. 1 Identification and eligibility screening of records. *database included all arthroplasties including elective, post-trauma, total and partial replacements and re-operations between 1 Jan 1998 to 30 Sept 2015 for knees and between 1 Jan 2004 to 30 Sept 2015 for hips

Participants

Eligible participants had undergone primary hip or knee joint arthroplasty at UHG followed by re-operation at UHG. Arthroplasty included total or partial replacement including resurfacing, and a variety of prosthesis types were used at the discretion of each surgeon over the study period. Re-operation included major revision (replacement of components fixed to bone), minor revision (replacement of components not fixed to bone) or washout. Patients with joint dislocation were included only if they subsequently required revision surgery (e.g. patients whose hip dislocations were reduced and had no further orthopaedic intervention were excluded). Patients who underwent multiple revisions had only their first revision included in the analysis.

Data collection, collation and analysis

Data were extracted from the organisation's joint replacement registry, which prospectively collects pre-operative and post-operative demographic and outcome data for all people undergoing hip or knee arthroplasty at UHG [12]. Registry data was collected according to the organisation's routine post-arthroplasty review schedule. Approximately 14% of primary hip arthroplasties and 14% of primary knee arthroplasties have been lost to follow-up since 2004 and 1998 respectively [3]. People requiring re-operation following hip or knee arthroplasty were identified from the joint replacement registry.

The medical records of eligible patients were inspected by one of four members of the research team (BR, NM, SW, PS). Each member analysed 25 cases which were arbitrarily assigned by the primary author (BR). Data extractors were trained by the primary author to collect data in a standardised manner using an electronic data collection template located in the REDCap data management system, hosted at our health service [13]. A senior orthopaedic surgeon (RP or AT) adjudicated to reach consensus if uncertainty existed regarding the classification of information.

Patient demographic data included age, sex and the American Society of Anesthesiologists (ASA) Score [14]. The healthcare setting where the complication was initially identified was classified as either orthopaedic outpatients (routine or non-routine review), inpatients (acute or subacute during the immediate post-operative period), General Practice (GP), Emergency Departments (ED), or other community setting.

Complications were classified as symptomatic, if symptoms were present preceding the re-operation. Radiological indicators were collected from the radiologist's report and doctor's notes in the patient's hospital medical record. How long after the primary operation the complication was identified was categorised as: less than one year, 1-5 years, 6-10 years and more than 10 years.

Data were analysed using descriptive statistics. The chi-square statistic was used to determine if the proportion of people requiring re-operation that were identified at routine orthopaedic outpatient review appointments was different from the proportion of people identified elsewhere. Metal on metal hip resurfacing arthroplasty ($n = 9$) was reported separately due to previously reported high complication rates and unique monitoring requirements [4].

Results

Participant characteristics

Of the 48 hip arthroplasty patients, 36 were elective and 12 were post proximal femur fracture of whom 10 received hemi-arthroplasty. The group's mean age at the time of re-operation was 70.0 years (SD 14.6), 29 (60.4%) were female and the mean ASA score was 2.3 (SD 0.8, 15 patient's ASA score was irretrievable). Primary hip arthroplasties were completed 6.6 years (average) prior to re-operation (range 15 days to 26.5 years).

Of the 50 knee elective arthroplasty patients, nine received a unilateral knee replacement. The group's mean age at the time of re-operation was 73.0 years (SD 8.6), 26 (52.0%) were female and the mean ASA score was 2.5 (SD 0.6, 12 patient's ASA score was irretrievable). Primary knee arthroplasties were completed 4.9 years (average) prior to re-operation (range 7 days to 19.0 years).

Re-operations completed

Eighty-two re-operations (83.7%) were revisions: 51 (52.0%) were major revisions including both sides of the joint; 28 (28.6%) were major revisions including one side of the joint; and 3 (3.1%) were minor revisions. Fourteen (14.3%) re-operations were washouts, of which 11 subsequently had revision arthroplasty. One patient (1.0%) had an open reduction and internal fixation for periprosthetic fracture and the prosthesis was not replaced. One patient (1.0%) had arthroscopic release and joint manipulation for arthrofibrosis.

The approximate cumulative re-operation rate at the hospital (as of 30 September 2015) was 1.0% for primary hip arthroplasties completed between 2004 and 2015 and 1.7% for primary knee arthroplasties completed between 1998-2015.

Health setting where complication was initially identified

A significantly larger proportion of people requiring re-operation were identified outside of routine orthopaedic outpatient appointments (84.7%) than at routine appointments (15.3%) ($p < .01$) (see Table 1). Of the people identified at routine orthopaedic review appointments, all were identified in the first-year post-surgery ($n = 15$, 15.3%). Complications were most frequently identified in

Table 1 Health service where complication was initially identified

	Routine orthopaedic outpatient review		Non-routine orthopaedic outpatient review	ED[a]	GP	Inpatient[b]
	≤ 1 year	> 1 year				
Hip ($n = 39$)	6 (15.4%)	0	5 (12.8%)	14 (35.9%)	8 (20.5%)	6 (15.4%)
Metal on metal ($n = 9$)	0	0	8 (88.9%)	1 (11.1%)	0	0
Knee ($n = 50$)	9 (18.0%)	0	6 (12.0%)	15 (30.0%)	16 (32.0%)	4 (8.0%)
Total	15 (15.3%)	0	19 (19.4%)	30 (30.6%)	24 (24.5%)	10 (10.2%)

No complications were identified in 'other community settings'
[a]Emergency Department attached to study hospital, except $n = 2$ that were identified by other EDs and referred to the study hospital;
[b]hospital or rehabilitation during the immediate post-operative period (range 2-19 days)

EDs ($n = 30$, 30.6%.), GP ($n = 24$, 24.5%) and non-routine orthopaedic outpatient reviews ($n = 19$, 19.4%).

Between 2004 and 2015, approximately 8500 routine 6-week, 12-week and 1-year post hip-arthroplasty review appointments were scheduled [3]. Between 1998 and 2015, approximately 6500 routine 6-week, 12-week and 1-year post knee-arthroplasty review appointments were scheduled [3]. These appointments identified 15 complications, an approximate yield of 1 complication for every 1000 scheduled appointments.

Duration following primary arthroplasty that complications were identified

Forty-four (44.9%) patients with complications requiring re-operation were identified in the first year following arthroplasty, which increased to 69 (70.4%) by the end of the 5th year (see Table 2).

Types of complications

Aseptic loosening was the most common complication which affected 37 (37.8%) patients, followed by infection (19.4%), fracture (15.3%) and dislocation/instability (13.3%) (see Table 3).

Symptoms and radiological features of complications

All patients reported joint related pain prior to re-operation, and some patients reported reduced mobility ($n = 35$, 35.7%), joint locking/clicking/stiffness/giving way ($n = 20$, 20.4%) or erythema/swelling/discharge near the joint ($n = 19$, 19.4%). Osteolysis or prosthetic loosening was the most commonly reported x-ray finding ($n = 36$, 36.7%) (see Table 4). No x-ray abnormality was reported for 30 (30.6%) patients.

Table 2 Duration following primary arthroplasty when complication was identified (years)

	≤1 year	> 1 ≤ 6 years	6 ≤ 11 years	> 11 years
Hip ($n = 39$)	19 (48.7%)	4 (10.3%)	8 (20.5%)	8 (20.5%)
Hip metal on metal ($n = 9$)	4 (44.4%)	4 (44.4%)	1 (11.1%)	0
Knee ($n = 50$)	21 (42%)	17 (34%)	9 (18%)	3 (6%)
Total	44 (44.9%)	25 (25.5%)	18 (18.4%)	11 (11.2%)

Note: % = (number of re-operations for time period)/(number of re-operations for that arthroplasty type)

Discussion

Post-arthroplasty review is recommended to occur at regular intervals to identify complications [7, 8, 10, 16]. In the current study, routine post-arthroplasty outpatient appointments were an inefficient mechanism for identifying complications that required re-operation, identifying only 15.3% of complications, all in the first-year post-surgery; 1000 routine appointments were required for every complication identified in the first year following arthroplasty. Given the increasing numbers of people requiring joint replacement, routine post-arthroplasty outpatient appointments, particularly beyond 12 months post-surgery, may place unnecessary demand on public health services and alternative models of care should be considered.

Symptoms, rather than radiographic changes were the primary trigger for re-operation; all participants were symptomatic, and 30.6% had normal x-rays. Consistent with our results, Silverwood et al. [17] found that all 183 patients requiring revision total hip arthroplasties were symptomatic, and Hacking et al [18] found 96.4% of 110 total hip arthroplasties were symptomatic [5, 19]. Radiological signs of implant failure can precede symptoms [7], but these patients are commonly kept under observation until symptoms develop, at which point surgery occurs [2]. Because patients self-initiate professional assessment of their symptoms, usually via GP or an ED, following which referral to orthopaedics can be made, regular review of routine post-arthroplasty patients appears duplicative. General practitioners' and ED staff's first-point-of-care role for arthroplasty patients requires they have adequate training, knowledge and skills to assess for complications. Efficient communication and referral pathways to orthopaedic care is also required, such as proposed by HealthPathways [20].

Consistent with recommendations, [4] the results of the current study indicate that surgeon discretion might still be necessary when scheduling review appointments; 19.4% of complications were detected at non-routine

Table 3 Types of complications

	Aseptic loosening	Infection	Fracture	Dislocation	Progressive joint disease	Defective prosthesis	Mal-alignment	Other
Hip ($n = 39$)	11 (28.2%)	6 (15.4%)	10 (25.6%)	8 (20.5%)	4[a] (10.3%)	1[c] (2.6%)	0	0
Hip metal on metal ($n = 9$)	3 (33.3%)	0	1 (11.1%)	0 (0%)	0	4[d] (44.4%)	0	1[f](11.1%)
Knee ($n = 50$)	25 (50.0%)	13 (26.0%)	4 (8.0%)	2 (4.0%)	4[b] (8.0%)	1[e] (2.0%)	2 (4.0%)	4[g] (8.0%)
Total	39 (39.8%)	19 (19.4%)	15 (15.3%)	10 (10.2%)	8 (8.2%)	6 (6.1%)	2 (2.0%)	5 (5.1%)

Note: more than one diagnosis possible (five patients had two diagnoses); % is proportion of patients with complication for that arthroplasty type. [a]Acetabular disease post hemiarthroplasty; [b]Patello-femoral disease ($n = 2$) or tibio-femoral disease ($n = 2$) post unilateral replacement; [c]Articular Surface Replacement (ASR) acetabular system [15]; [d]ASR resurfacing system [15]; [e]failure of zimmer rotating hinge; [f]pain without radiological abnormality; [g]arthrofibrosis ($n = 1$), loose body ($n = 1$), synovitis without infection ($n = 1$), instability (tibiofemoral subluxation) ($n = 1$)

review appointments. It is unknown however, whether these patients would have been identified in community settings in a timely fashion if non-routine orthopaedic review had not occurred.

Our health service redesigned its post-arthroplasty review service in response to the current investigation. Low risk patients are reviewed in-person at 6 and 12 weeks post primary arthroplasty and then surveyed via mail-out questionnaire at 1, 5 and 8 years post-operatively and then biennially thereafter. The questionnaire used in our remote review system screens for possible complications, expecting that most patients with complications will be symptomatic. Patients with suspected complications are reviewed by the patient's surgeon. Surgeons can schedule in-person reviews at any time if they are concerned about possible complications, including from higher risk prostheses. Elsewhere, studies indicate that remote post-arthroplasty review compared to in-person review produces lower financial costs to patients, shorter review times, less travel time, less burden on carers, fewer unscheduled outpatient visits and high levels of patient satisfaction; all without missing complications [21–23]. Modelling indicates substantial cost savings and increased quality-adjusted life years from remote models of care [24, 25].

Our remote review system for routine low-risk post-arthroplasty patients is expected to substantially reduce the number of outpatient appointments occurring at our health service. Modelling indicates that in the first year alone, approximately 450 12-month post-operative review appointments will be avoided. An additional 1000 in-person review appointments will be avoided for patients undergoing five-year or longer post-operative review. Reducing the number of post-arthroplasty review appointments will improve the orthopaedic unit's capacity to see new patients, without requiring additional resources. Adopting this model of care in all Australian public hospitals could reduce the number of scheduled 12-month post-operative review appointments by up to 32,000 in 2017; additional reductions would occur for patients being reviewed at 5 years or beyond.

Consumer-centered care requires that patient preferences are incorporated into all stages of healthcare decision-making including service re-design [26]. Patient preferences regarding post-arthroplasty review are largely unknown and require investigation. Baxter et al. [27] found that 76 of 105 hip or knee arthroplasty patient wanted long-term follow-up, and Sharareh et al [23] found that 59% of patients preferred remote web-based post-arthroplasty review compared to in-clinic review.

Providing remote care requires organisational resources to survey patients; however, we expect a net benefit in favour of reduced organisation costs, consistent with predictions by others [24]. Employing allied staff to provide remote care might be controversial for some surgeons, [19] but preliminary evidence suggests that allied staff, such as physiotherapists can safely and effectively complete post-arthroplasty reviews [28, 29]. Our new service model is in its infancy; its evaluation, including cost-effectiveness and safety is necessary and ongoing.

Table 4 X-ray findings

	No visible abnormality	Loosening/ osteolysis	Fracture	Mal-alignment	Polyethylene wear	Effusion	Progressive joint disease
Hip ($n = 39$)	9 (23.1%)	12 (30.8%)	9 (23.1%)	14 (35.9%)	4 (10.3%)	NA	3 (7.7%)
Hip metal on metal ($n = 9$)	5 (55.6%)	3 (33.3%)	1 (11.1%)	2 (2.2%)	NA	NA	0
Knee ($n = 50$)	16 (32.0%)	21 (42.0%)	4 (8.0%)	9 (18.0%)	3 (6.0%)	7 (14%)	4 (8.0%)
Total	30 (30.6%)	36 (36.7%)	14 (14.3%)	25 (25.5%)	7 (7.1%)	7 (7.1%)	7 (7.1%)

Note: x-ray findings according to radiologist's report and outpatient notes. More than one x-ray finding possible. % is proportion of patients with finding for that arthroplasty type

Limitations of the current study

The current study identified complications requiring re-operation from an established regional joint replacement registry which relies on surgeons and staff registering re-operations. Although extensive efforts are made by the orthopaedic research unit to identify all re-operations, it is possible that not all were captured in the database used by the current study. Re-operations might have occurred at other health services that were not included in our database. Our retrospective analysis could only collect information recorded in medical histories, which might be incomplete or inaccurate. We only included patients with complications requiring re-operations following primary arthroplasty; the pathways and outcomes for patients with complications not requiring re-operation remain unknown. The results of the current study might not be generalisable to other health services with different populations, prosthesis types, complication rates or follow-up procedures.

Conclusion

Hip and knee arthroplasties have low rates of post-operative complications and most review appointments are uneventful with no change in clinical management [21] . The current study is the first to our knowledge to report the healthcare setting where complications requiring re-operation are initially detected. Our results indicate that routine post-arthroplasty review appointments are an inefficient mechanism for identifying complications requiring re-operation. Health services should assess their own services and consider alternate models of post-arthroplasty review to meet patient expectations and help manage current and future demand for orthopaedic outpatient services.

Abbreviations

ASA: American Society of Anesthesiologists; ED: Emergency Department; GP: General Practitce; OA: Osteoarthritis; UHG: University Hospital Geelong

Acknowledgements

Mr Richard Angliss Mr David Bainbridge Mr David Bowyer Mr Glenn Boyce Mr Graeme Brown Mrs Amanada Cowland Mr Nathan Donovan Mr Kevin Eng Mr Chatar Goyal Mrs Pam Kennedy Mr Ben Miller Mr John Skelley Mr Andrew Wilkinson Mr Simon Williams.

Funding

The Victorian Department of Health and Human Services provided funding for the project as part of a state-wide implementation of Advanced Practice Physiotherapy led Post Arthroplasty Review (PAR) Services.

Authors' contributions

BR: Study design, data collection, data analysis, literature review, manuscript writing NM: Data collection, data analysis, literature review, manuscript writing. SDG: Study design, data analysis, literature review, manuscript writing. SW: Data collection, data analysis, manuscript writing. PS: Data collection, manuscript writing. SB: Data collection, study design, manuscript writing. AT: Study design, data analysis, manuscript writing. RSP: Study design, process design, data analysis, literature review, manuscript writing. All authors read and approved the final manuscript.

Consent for publication

Not applicable.

Competing interests

RSP and AT receive institutional educational support from De Puy Synthes, New Brunswick, New Jersey, United States. BR, NM, SDG, SW, PS and SB have no competing interests.

Author details

[1]Physiotherapy Department, Barwon Health, Geelong, VIC 3220, Australia. [2]Orthopaedic Department, Barwon Health, Geelong, Victoria 3220, Australia. [3]Barwon Centre for Orthopaedic Research and Education (B-CORE), St John of God Hospital and Barwon Health, Geelong, VIC 3220, Australia. [4]School of Medicine, Deakin University, Waurn Ponds, VIC 3220, Australia.

References

1. Schoch PA, Adair L. Successfully reforming orthopaedic outpatients. Aust Health Rev. 2012;36(2):233–7.
2. Kingsbury SR, Dube B, Thomas CM, Conaghan PG, Stone MH. Is a questionnaire and radiograph-based follow-up model for patients with primary hip and knee arthroplasty a viable alternative to traditional regular outpatient follow-up clinic? Bone Joint J. 2016;98-B(2):201–8.
3. Barwon Centre for Orthopaedic Research & Education (B-CORE). Joint Replacement Registry. Geelong: B-CORE; 2017.
4. Australian Orthopaedic Association. Position statement on the follow-up of hip and knee arthroplasty. In: Arthroplasty Society of Australia; 2016.
5. Choi JK, Geller JA, Patrick DA Jr, Wang W, Macaulay W. How are those "lost to follow-up" patients really doing? A compliance comparison in arthroplasty patients. World J Orthop. 2015;6(1):150–5.
6. Veysi VT, Jones S, Stone MH, Limb D. Out-patient follow-up after total hip replacement in one health region. J R Coll Surg Edinb. 1998;43(2):95–6.
7. Teeny SM, York SC, Mesko JW, Rea RE. Long-term follow-up care recommendations after total hip and knee arthroplasty: results of the American Association of hip and Knee Surgeons' member survey. J Arthroplast. 2003;18(8):954–62.
8. British Orthopaedic Association and British Association for Surgery of the Knee. Knee replacement: a guide to good practice. London: British Orthopaedic Association and British Association for Surgery of the Knee; 1999.
9. Australian Orthopaedic Association National Joint Replacement Registry (AOANJRR). Hip, knee & shoulder arthroplasty: 2017 annual report. Adelaide: AOA; 2017.
10. Broughton N, Collopy D, Solomon M. Arthroplasty Society of Australia Position Statement of follow-up of joint replacement patients. In: Arthroplasty Society of Australia; 2016.
11. Clohisy JC, Kamath GV, Byrd GD, Steger-May K, Wright RW. Patient compliance with clinical follow-up after total joint arthroplasty. J Bone Joint Surg Am. 2008;90(9):1848–54.
12. Page RS, Beattie S, Williams S, Gill SD. Clinical quality registries: local registries complement national registries. An example from joint arthroplasty. ANZ J Surg. 2018; in press
13. Harris PA, Taylor R, Thielke R, Payne J, Gonzalez N, Conde JG. Research electronic data capture (REDCap)–a metadata-driven methodology and workflow process for providing translational research informatics support. J Biomed Inform. 2009;42(2):377–81.
14. Owens WD, Felts JA, Spitznagel EL Jr. ASA physical status classifications: a study of consistency of ratings. Anesthesiology. 1978;49(4):239–43.
15. de Steiger RN, Hang JR, Miller LN, Graves SE, Davidson DC. Five-year results of the ASR XL acetabular system and the ASR hip resurfacing system: an analysis from the Australian Orthopaedic Association National Joint Replacement Registry. J Bone Joint Surg Am. 2011;93(24):2287–93.
16. British Orthopaedic Association. Primary total hip replacement: a guide to good practice. London: British Orthopaedic Association; 2012.
17. Silverwood R, Lawton R, Barnett K, Finlayson D: Is long-term follow-up after

uncomplicated primary total hip arthroplasty necessary? Orthopaedic Proceedings. 2012;94B(supp XXXIX):176.

18. Hacking C, Weinrauch P, Whitehouse SL, Crawford RW, Donnelly WJ. Is there a need for routine follow-up after primary total hip arthroplasty? ANZ J Surg. 2010;80(10):737–40.
19. Haddad FS, Ashby E, Konangamparambath S. Should follow-up of patients with arthroplasties be carried out by general practitioners? J Bone Joint Surg Br. 2007;89(9):1133–4.
20. Robinson S, Varhol R, Bell C, Quirk F, Durrington L. HealthPathways: creating a pathway for health systems reform. Aust Health Rev. 2015;39(1):9–11.
21. Marsh JD, Bryant DM, MacDonald SJ, Naudie DD, McCalden RW, Howard JL, Bourne RB, McAuley JP. Feasibility, effectiveness and costs associated with a web-based follow-up assessment following total joint arthroplasty. J Arthroplast. 2014;29(9):1723–8.
22. Wood G, Naudie D, MacDonald S, McCalden R, Bourne R. An electronic clinic for arthroplasty follow-up: a pilot study. Can J Surg. 2011;54(6):381–6.
23. Sharareh B, Schwarzkopf R. Effectiveness of telemedical applications in postoperative follow-up after total joint arthroplasty. J Arthroplast. 2014; 29(5):918–22. e1
24. Bitsaki M, Koutras G, Heep H, Koutras C. Cost-effective mobile-based healthcare system for managing Total joint arthroplasty follow-up. Healthc Inform Res. 2017;23(1):67–73.
25. Bolz KM, Crawford RW, Donnelly B, Whitehouse SL, Graves N. The cost-effectiveness of routine follow-up after primary total hip arthroplasty. J Arthroplast. 2010;25(2):191–6.
26. Australian Commission on Safety and Quality in Health Care (ACSQHC). National safety and quality health service standards. Sydney: ACSQHC; 2012.
27. Baxter JA, Courtman NH. Patient perception of follow-up review after hip and knee arthroplasty. The Bulletin of the Royal College of Surgeons of England. 2015;97(1):E5–8.
28. Large KE, Page CJ, Brock K, Dowsey MM, Choong PF. Physiotherapy-led arthroplasty review clinic: a preliminary outcomes analysis. Aust Health Rev. 2014;38(5):510–6.
29. Waring S, Reynolds B, Schoch P, Thomson A, Williams S, Page R. Improved access orthopaedic joint replacement review clinic. ANZ J Surg. 2015; 85(Suppl. 1):81–8.

7

Variation in Prosthetic Joint Infection and treatment strategies during 4.5 years of follow-up after primary joint arthroplasty using administrative data of 41397 patients across Australian, European and United States hospitals

Perla J. Marang-van de Mheen[1*], Ellie Bragan Turner[2], Susan Liew[3], Nora Mutalima[4,5], Ton Tran[4], Sten Rasmussen[6,7], Rob G. H. H. Nelissen[8] and Andrew Gordon[9]

Abstract

Background: To identify best practices and quality improvement initiatives, we aimed to assess whether the incidence of Periprosthetic Joint Infection (PJI) and treatment strategies differed across patients treated in Australian, European and United States (US) hospitals.

Methods: Routinely collected administrative data for 41397 patients undergoing a primary total hip or knee arthroplasty between July 2007-December 2010 across 22 hospitals were included. Patients were followed for 2 years looking for PJI occurrence, defined as early (within 4 weeks) and late PJI, and surgical treatment during 2.5 years after PJI diagnosis. Logistic and Poisson regression models were used to test for differences in PJI occurrence and treatment strategies across the three geographical regions, adjusted for age, sex, joint and Elixhauser comorbidity groups.

Results: PJI occurrence varied from 1.4% in European to 1.7% in Australian patients, which were significantly higher than US patients after adjustment for patient characteristics (OR 1.24 [1.01–1.52] and 1.40 [1.03–1.91] respectively). Early PJIs varied between 0.3% in European to 0.6% in Australian patients, but adjusted rates were similar. Revision following PJI was significantly lower in Australian than in US patients (OR 0.46 [0.25–0.86]) as were the total number of revisions (RR 0.51 [0.36–0.71]) and number of surgical procedures (RR 0.60 [0.44–0.81]) used to treat PJI.

Conclusion: The overall PJI rate was significantly higher in Australian patients, but fewer procedures were needed to treat these PJIs. Future research should reveal whether this reflects PJIs caught earlier or less severe when diagnosed, and whether this is associated with the longer length of stay after primary arthroplasty in Australian hospitals.

Keywords: Periprosthetic Joint Infection, International variation, Total joint replacement, Treatment strategies

* Correspondence: p.j.marang@lumc.nl
[1]Department of Medical Decision Making, Leiden University Medical Center, J10-S, PO Box 9600, 2300 RC Leiden, The Netherlands
Full list of author information is available at the end of the article

Background

Worldwide about two million total hip (THA) and total knee arthroplasties (TKA) are performed annually, with the majority in the United States and Europe [1, 2]. The number of arthroplasties is expected to increase considerably over the next decades, [3, 4] due to the ageing population, an increasing prevalence of obesity, and the demand and expectation of these procedures in increasingly younger patients [5]. This increased burden on our healthcare systems will have considerable societal and economic consequences [6].

Although these procedures are very effective in reducing pain and improving functionality of patients, complications do occur and have shown to vary between hospitals [7]. Periprosthetic Joint Infection (PJI) following primary THA or TKA is one of the most devastating complications, with rates typically around 1–2% and slightly higher for TKA than THA [7–10]. The occurrence of PJI has huge impact on the patient, such as an increased rate of mortality and/or readmission to hospital [11] with the resulting experience of a PJI being a major trauma for which patients would like psychological support [12]. Projections indicate a three-fold increase of PJIs by the year 2030 [3, 13]. However, PJI rates may vary, not only between hospitals but also between health care systems, and with respect to treatment strategies used. By studying these variations, we may be able to identify best practices and thus directions for quality improvement. Furthermore, with the expected growth in THA and TKA procedures to be performed in the coming decades, the rise in antimicrobial resistance of organisms and the increased complexity of patients being cared for, the number of PJIs is likely to increase accordingly along with significant costs to treat PJI [11, 14].

The aim of the present study is firstly to assess whether PJI occurrence differs across patients treated in hospitals from different geographical regions (Australia, Europe and United States (US)), and secondly to examine whether treatment strategies for PJI differ between these patient groups.

Methods

Patients

Patient data from the Global Comparators Project were used, in which hospitals from various countries all over the world share their experiences and compare their outcomes using routinely collected administrative admission data. As previously described, diagnoses and procedures were combined into groups and comorbidities were defined within this Project, which were matched across countries to reconcile the different coding systems being used [15]. For the present study, all patients who underwent a primary THA or TKA in the period July 2007-December 2010 were selected; data were available for patients from 22 hospitals across six countries (Australia, Belgium, Denmark, Netherlands, United Kingdom (UK), and the US). We distinguished three geographical regions: Australia (four hospitals), Europe (11 hospitals) and United States (seven hospitals). The names of individual hospitals contributing data are listed in the Additional file 1: Table A. Patients receiving a primary THA or TKA with a primary diagnosis of cancer in the same admission, that is any C-code (ICD-10) or codes between 104 and 2097 (ICD-9), were excluded.

Definitions

All patients with a procedure code for a primary THA or TKA were followed over a 2-year period for the occurrence of a PJI during subsequent admissions. The following codes were used to define a PJI, as the primary or secondary diagnosis of an admission: 996.66 (ICD-9, for the Netherlands 996.6), T84.5 or T84.7 (ICD-10 and ICD-AM). These represent billable medical codes that can be used to indicate a diagnosis on a reimbursement claim. Only those PJIs that occurred within 2 years after the initial admission for the primary THA or TKA were included. We distinguished between early PJI (occurring within 4 weeks) and late PJI (after 4 weeks) based on clinical relevance, as treatments are likely to differ between these two groups.

The primary and secondary procedure codes of all admissions in these patients were then examined for any codes indicating a surgical treatment of the PJI, in a period of 2.5 years after PJI diagnosis. Additional file 1: Table B shows the codes used to identify the various possible treatments in the different coding systems. For the analysis, the placement of an antibiotic spacer was aggregated with revision or resection arthroplasty, as some coding systems were not able to distinguish between these groups and even more, these procedures are used in various combinations in clinical practice (i.e. the antibiotic spacer is put in when the prosthesis is removed).

In addition, the following case-mix variables were collected: age 70+ versus <70, gender and all 32 Elixhauser comorbidity groups (yes/no variable) as identified from the secondary diagnoses data.

Statistical analysis

The mean PJI occurrence among patients treated in hospitals from the three regions with 95% confidence intervals was calculated first. This was done separately for primary THA or TKA, and separately for early and late PJI occurrence as defined above. Testing was then undertaken for differences in PJI occurrence between the three regions after adjustment for case-mix, using stepwise backwards logistic regression analysis. The following factors were included as possible confounding variables: age group, sex, Elixhauser comorbidity groups, TKA versus THA, and region. Region however, was mandatory for the model and so was not eliminated as part of the stepwise backwards analysis. An Elixhauser comorbidity group was only included if at least 10 patients with that comorbidity had also experienced a PJI, to prevent unstable estimates and improve model fit.

Model fit was examined using both the C-statistic and the Nagelkerke R-squared. The same analysis was done for early PJI occurrence.

To assess whether treatment for PJI differed between patients from hospitals in different regions, we looked at the differences in the surgical procedure following the PJI. First we looked at revision following PJI using backwards logistic regression analysis within patients with a PJI diagnosis, with the same variables included as above and revision/resection (yes/no) as the dependent variable. Region was a mandatory factor in the model. However, revision surgery (i.e. one-stage revision) or resection arthroplasty surgery (i.e. removal of implant) as the first surgical procedure may indicate a more aggressive approach, compared with irrigation and debridement as the first procedure and so was subject to further sensitivity analysis with a further condition being that revision/resection (yes/no) was performed as the first surgical procedure as the dependent variable. The same independent variables as above were included and region was again a mandatory factor in the model. The same analysis was done with irrigation and debridement (yes/no) as the first surgical procedure.

But even if the first surgical procedure is more aggressive, this may still be a more effective course of action if it means that the patient undergoes fewer procedures. Therefore, the total number of surgical procedures used to treat PJI across patients from hospitals in the three regions was also examined. This was done using Poisson regression analysis, with region mandated in the model and using the same case-mix variables mentioned above. The same analysis was done for the total number of revisions/resections, to assess whether a less invasive initial approach might still result in more invasive procedures being necessary.

In all analyses, a p-value < 0.05 was considered to be statistically significant.

Results

Data from 22 hospitals across the three geographical regions were included, covering 41397 primary procedures (Table 1). Patient characteristics varied between regions and in particular the percentage of patients with any comorbidities being much higher in the US. The length of stay in the US was much lower in the admission when the primary arthroplasty took place (on average 9 days shorter than Australia).

Crude PJI rates were highest in Australian patients (1.7%) and lowest in Europe (1.4%). Figure 1 shows that the higher PJI rate in Australian patients was mainly in early PJIs occurring within 4 weeks, but that late PJI rates were similar. After adjustment for differences in patient characteristics, the likelihood of a PJI diagnosis was significantly higher in both Australian and European patients compared to the US (Table 2). Table 2 also shows that the likelihood of a PJI was significantly increased for male patients with various types of comorbidities undergoing TKA. PJI was less likely to be diagnosed in elderly patients (70+ years of age) independent from any comorbidity, which probably reflects a healthy selection of elderly patients without comorbidity undergoing THA or TKA or alternatively, these patients receive antibiotic suppression therapy to prevent PJI because they are too frail to undergo revision surgery. Looking only at early PJI, rates were similar as the US after adjustment for patient characteristics (OR 1.46 [0.86–2.47] for Australia and 0.98 [0.67–1.42] for Europe).

Table 3 shows that after adjustment for differences in patient characteristics, chances of a revision as treatment following PJI diagnosis are significantly lower in Australian patients (54% lower). Figure 2 shows that treatment strategies seem to differ across regions with irrigation and debridement more often used as first treatment following PJI diagnosis in Australia and revision more often as first treatment in the US. After adjustment for differences in patient characteristics, chances of a revision as first treatment following PJI diagnosis was significantly lower in Australia (OR 0.50 [0.28–0.92]) and similar in Europe (OR 0.71 [0.48–1.06]) compared to the US. Differences in irrigation and debridement as first treatment were not statistically different after adjustment for patient characteristics (data not shown). Looking at the number of procedures, both the

Table 1 Patient characteristics, PJI rate and treatment across 3 regions

	Australia	Europe	US	Total
Hospitals				
Number of hospitals	4	11	7	22
Arthroplasties				
Number of arthroplasties	3705	26993	10699	41397
% Hip	47%	50%	46%	49%
Patient characteristics at primary arthroplasty				
Average age	68.4	68.2	62.3	66.7
Median age	70	69	63	68
% Females	62%	61%	60%	61%
% with 1 or more comorbidities	42%	56%	80%	61%
Average number of comorbidities	0.8	0.9	1.7	1.1
Median number of comorbidities	0	1	2	1
Length of stay (LOS) of primary arthroplasty admission				
Average LOS in arthroplasty spell	12.4	7.7	3.3	7.0
Median LOS in arthroplasty spell	7	6	3	5
% patients in upper quartile LOS	46%	33%	2%	26%
Prosthetic joint infections (PJI)				
PJI rate within 2 years	1.7%	1.4%	1.5%	1.4%
Treatment of prosthetic joint infection within 2.5 years				
Average number of procedures	0.9	1.3	1.6	1.4
Median number of procedures	1	1	1	1

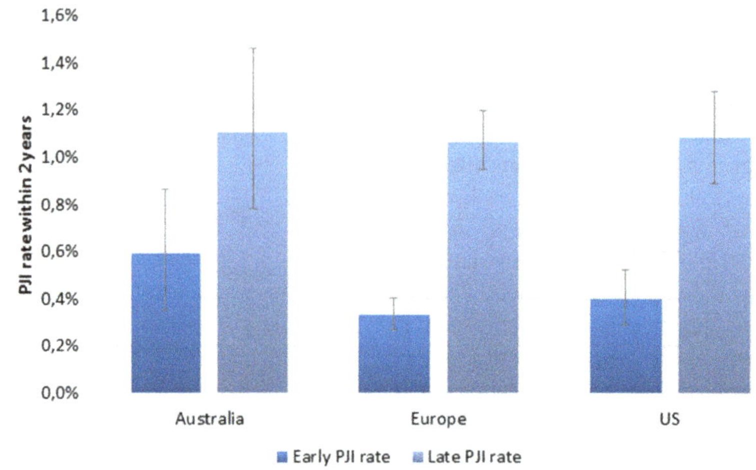

Fig. 1 Crude early Periprosthetic Joint Infection (PJI) rate (<4 weeks) versus late PJI rate (<2 years) across 3 regions

number of revisions and the total number of surgical procedures following PJI diagnosis are significantly lower in Australia after adjustment for differences in patient characteristics (Fig. 3). Europe also has significantly fewer revisions following PJI diagnosis compared to the US, but the total number of surgical procedures does not differ significantly.

Discussion

The present study has shown that PJI after primary THA and TKA is diagnosed more frequently in Australian and European patients than in US patients, but that occurrence of early PJI within 4 weeks is similar. The PJI rate was significantly higher in patients with various types of comorbidities as well as after knee arthroplasty. Treatment strategies following PJI were also different across these three regions, with revisions being less frequently used as first treatment in Australia as well as fewer revisions and a lower total number of surgical procedures. Europe also had fewer revisions following PJI diagnosis but the same total number of surgical procedures as the US. The hypothesis that would fit these findings is that PJIs in Australia are caught earlier or are less severe when diagnosed resulting in fewer surgical procedures being necessary, which should be further investigated.

Limitations of our study include the use of administratively collected data which may overestimate or underestimate the presence of comorbidities and complications, with differences across hospitals and health care systems due to different coding practices. In the present study the average number of reported comorbidities in patients was clearly higher for US patients, most likely due to the financial incentives associated with coding [16], which may

Table 2 Influence of patient characteristics and region on Periprosthetic Joint Infection (PJI) rate

Variable	Odds Ratio [95% CI]
Age > =70 years	**0.75 [0.63-0.89]**
Sex (Males versus Females)	**1.38 [1.17–1.63]**
Comorbidities	
Cardiac arrhythmias (yes/no)	1.32 [0.99–1.74]
Congestive heart failure (yes/no)	1.58 [0.98–2.53]
Rheumatoid arthritis, collagen or vascular disease (yes/no)	**1.96 [1.39–2.75]**
Diabetes uncomplicated (yes/no)	**1.28 [1.00–1.64]**
Coagulopathy (yes/no)	**2.28 [1.29–4.03]**
Fluid and electrolyte disorders (yes/no)	**1.63 [1.15–2.30]**
Depression (yes/no)	**2.04 [1.46–2.86]**
Joint (knee versus hip)	**1.52 [1.28–1.79]**
Region	
Australia versus US	**1.40 [1.03–1.91]**
Europe versus US	**1.24 [1.01–1.52]**

Significant differences are indicated in bold; Model fit: C statistic = 0,61 Nagelkerke R^2 = 0,018

Table 3 Influence of patient characteristics and region on having a revision as surgical treatment following Periprosthetic Joint Infection (PJI)

Variable	Odds Ratio [95% CI]
Age > =70 years	**0.62 [0.43–0.87]**
Comorbidities	
Obesity (yes/no)	0.63 [0.36–1.12]
Fluid and electrolyte disorders (yes/no)	**0.43 [0.22–0.86]**
Region	
Australia versus US	**0.46 [0.25–0.86]**
Europe versus US	0.77 [0.51–1.16]

Significant differences are indicated in bold; Model fit: C statistic = 0,62 Nagelkerke R^2 = 0,053

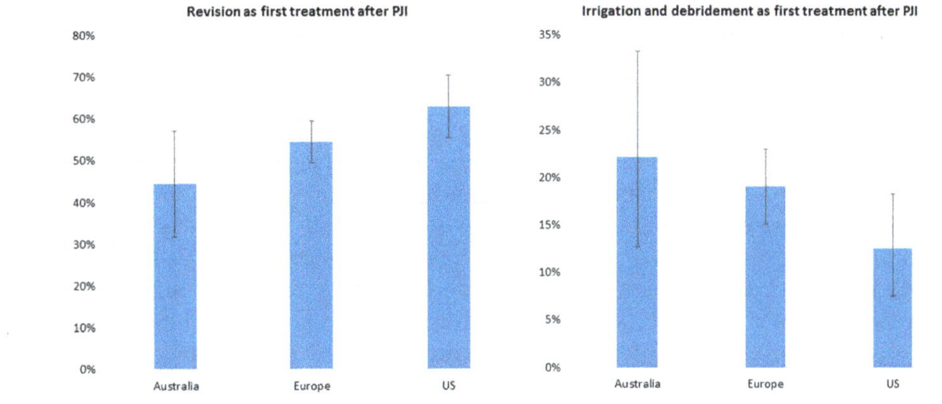

Fig. 2 Crude rates of first treatment of Periprosthetic Joint Infection (PJI) across 3 regions

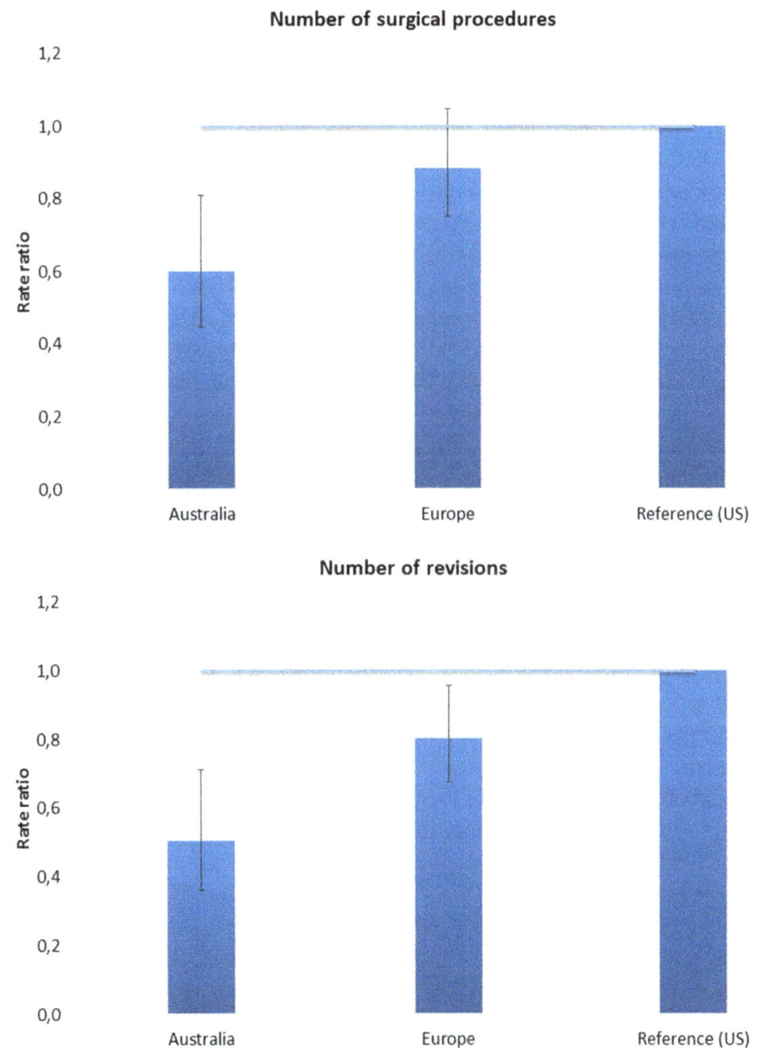

Fig. 3 Difference between regions in number of surgical procedures and number of revisions for Periprosthetic Joint Infection (PJI), adjusted for differences in patient characteristics

result in PJI rates in the US being underestimated after adjustment for these reported comorbidities. However, reimbursement of health services in Australia also depends on clinical coding [17], but did not result in a higher number of reported comorbidities, so that it does not seem likely that this will explain the results entirely. Another issue is the ability to correctly identify PJI from administrative data. Lange et al have recently shown an 85% positive predictive value for periprosthetic hip joint infection using administrative discharge registers from Denmark, which slightly increased to 86% when combined with an infection-specific surgical procedure code [18]. Bozic et al also argued that diagnoses like PJI are less influenced by coding practices and found 99% agreement after medical record validation [7]. Related to this, variation in the definition of PJI across centres could have influenced our findings. However, given the use of clinical admission data with ICD9 or ICD10 coding, only those PJIs serious enough to warrant readmission will have been included, and less subject to variation in applied definitions. Finally, bias in procedures to treat PJI is far less likely but nevertheless there was still variation in surgical treatment strategy amongst the three health care systems, with fewer procedures required to treat PJI in Australia. When checking all the data for incomplete follow-up time after PJI diagnosis (i.e. less than 2.5 years), it was found that 4% of the PJIs in Europe had incomplete follow-up, 0% in the US and 0% in Australia. As these percentages are very low, it is not likely to affect the results to a great extent. If anything, this means that the number of revisions following PJI might have been underestimated in Europe, so that the difference with the US may be smaller in reality, but it cannot explain the difference between Australia and the US. The number of primary arthroplasties per patient was also checked, to investigate the possibility that another "primary arthroplasty" may have been coded for when in reality a revision is performed. However, numbers of more than two primary arthroplasties in a patient were extremely low, particularly in the US (0.04%, versus 0.05% in Australia and 0.07% in Europe) so this also is not likely to have influenced our results. Finally we checked the extent to which PJIs were diagnosed in the same admission as the primary arthroplasty, whereas only PJIs in subsequent admissions were counted in the primary analysis. As expected, rates were low (0.5% for Australia, 0.3% for Europe and 0.1% for US) so that the difference in PJI between patients from different regions might even have been underestimated.

It is important to note that the study findings are only based on a limited number of hospitals within the countries and regions examined. As each centre was a large academic medical unit, outcomes between centres included in our study will be fairly comparable with respect to their patient population, but may differ from other units in the selected countries. Therefore it is possible that observed differences in this study are only found among complex patients typically treated in academic centres but are not representative for patients treated in other hospitals in these regions. Still, the overall PJI rate of 1.4% within 2 years after the primary arthroplasty and 0.4% of early PJIs within 4 weeks fits well in the reported range of PJI in previous studies, when differences in duration of follow-up between studies are taken into account [7, 8, 10]. Another reason for discrepancies with previously reported rates is that some studies only include PJIs with a related procedure [7, 8]. Excluding PJI with an unrelated procedure in the present study, would result in similar PJI rates around 1% as reported in those studies. Furthermore, the factors identified to increase the likelihood of a PJI such as coagulopathy and rheumatoid arthritis as well as being higher after primary TKA, are consistent with previous reports [9, 19, 20].

Conclusions and implications

What the present study has shown for the first time is that both PJI diagnosis and the associated treatment strategy seem to differ across patients treated in different health care systems. Discussions among collaborating hospitals did not suggest any difference in preoperative infection prophylaxis strategy but no patient level data were available to substantiate this. Combining the significantly higher PJI rate in Australia with the less aggressive treatment strategy of revisions being less often the first treatment following PJI and fewer surgical procedures, results in the hypothesis of less severe PJIs when diagnosed or PJIs caught earlier. This may be associated with the considerable longer length of stay in Australian hospitals, which may indicate (early signs of) the PJI or alternatively, being more of a 'standard duration' in this health care system but thereby enabling identification of the PJI compared with US hospitals discharging patients early so early PJIs may not be identified. This is supported by the difference in PJI rates diagnosed in the same admission as the primary arthroplasty. Diagnosing the PJI earlier is also likely to affect the treatment strategy, that is requiring either less aggressive or fewer procedures to be treated adequately. Another explanation may be an active surveillance system being present as for instance the Victorian Healthcare Associated Infection Surveillance System (VICNISS) reporting a significant reduction of surgical site infections over time including a reduction in deep surgical site infections [21]. However, similar surveillance systems are also present in the United States and in Europe (e.g. the CDC and the ECDC), so that it does not seem likely that this would explain the observed difference between regions. Finally, the higher number of revisions and surgical procedures being performed in the US may be due to the time of presentation or the patients' clinical status at the time of presentation, but another thing to consider is that it may not just be clinical practice but also an effect of remuneration for procedures across the different health care systems, given for instance the higher fees for hip replacements in the US than in Australia and European countries [22].

An important question is whether the initial longer length of stay for THA and TKA in Australia, in fact is a cost-effective approach if it results in complications like PJI being caught earlier and fewer readmissions and treatments being required. Multiplying the initial longer length of stay in Australia compared to the US from Table 1, with the bed day costs of about £400 [23] and divided by the difference in number of revisions, this would amount to £410.241 health care costs per prevented revision in Australia. For Europe, health care costs would be £363.866 higher. These costs are likely to be overestimated as only hospital bed days were included in this study and patients in the US routinely go to rehabilitation centres after leaving the hospital. Assuming the same total length of stay in the US as in Europe, would still amount to £213.366 per prevented revision in Australia. These costs exceed the average costs for revision surgery of £25.974. [23, 24] Including societal costs by assuming that 50% of patients would be absent from work for 8 weeks because of the revision, amounting to £1.400 per week, costs in Australia and Europe were still considerably (£378.667 and £332.292 respectively) higher than the costs for revision surgery. Assuming a threshold of £30.000 per Quality Adjusted Life Years (QALY) for a cost-effective intervention, this would mean that 12,6 QALY's have to be gained by preventing revisions, for the Australian strategy to be cost-effective compared to the US (11,1 QALY's for Europe). This is highly unlikely, given that even under assumptions of temporary health loss of 50% during 6 months and 20% permanent health loss for 10% of the patients, this would only amount to about 1 QALY gained. Our results thus have important implications for future directions in clinical practice, but also strongly illustrate the value of international collaboratives allowing us to compare outcomes, learn from each other, and enable improvements in quality of care.

Acknowledgements

The study was carried out on behalf of the ORTHO GOAL Dr Foster Global Comparators (GC) Project, Dr Foster/Telstra Health in association with the Dr Foster Unit at Imperial College London. The ORTHO GOAL currently consists of the following participants: Andrew Gordon (Sheffield Teaching Hospitals NHS Trust) Jarkko Leskinen (Teng Hospital District of Helsinki Uusimaa), Nora Mutalima (Monash Health), Ove Talsnes (Sykehuset Innlandet HF), Perla Marang-van de Mheen (Leiden University Medical Center), Peter Thompson (University Hospitals Coventry & Warwickshire NHS Trust), Rob Nelissen (Leiden University Medical Center), Sten Rasmussen (Aalborg University Hospital), Susan Liew (Alfred Health), Ton Tran (Monash Health)
We would like to thank Bethan Mackay (Dr Foster), Neil Casey (Dr Foster), Dany Gammall (Dr Foster) and Erik Hansen (University of California) for their contributions to the early stages of this project.

Funding

None.

Authors' contributions

AG had the original idea, AG EBT & PMvdM designed the study, EBT recoded and harmonised all datasets for analysis, EBT & PMvdM conducted the analysis, PMvdM, EBT, SL, NM, TT, SR, RN, AG participated in interpreting the results, PMvdM wrote the first draft of the manuscript, all authors have approved the final version of the manuscript. PMvdM acts as guarantor of the study and affirms that the manuscript is an honest, accurate, and transparent account of the study being reported, and that no important aspects of the study have been omitted.

Competing interests

The authors declare that they have no competing interests.

Consent for publication

Not applicable.

Author details

[1]Department of Medical Decision Making, Leiden University Medical Center, J10-S, PO Box 9600, 2300 RC Leiden, The Netherlands. [2]Dr Foster Ltd, London, UK. [3]Department of Orthopaedic Surgery, Alfred Hospital, Melbourne, Australia. [4]Department of Orthopaedic Surgery, Monash Health, Dandenong, Australia. [5]Department of Surgery, Monash University, Dandenong, Australia. [6]Orthopaedic Surgery Research Unit, Aalborg University Hospital, Aalborg, Denmark. [7]Department of Clinical Medicine, Aalborg University, Aalborg, Denmark. [8]Department of Orthopaedic Surgery, Leiden University Medical Center, Leiden, The Netherlands. [9]Department of Orthopaedic Surgery, Sheffield Teaching Hospitals NHS trust, Sheffield, UK.

References

1. Kremers HM, Larson DR, Crowson CR, et al. Prevalence of total hip and knee replacement in the United States. J Bone Joint Surg. 2015;97:1386–97.
2. OECD. Hip and Knee replacement. In: Health at a Glance: Europe 2012. Paris: OECD publishing; 2012. pp. 86–7.
3. Kurtz S, Ong K, Lau E, Mowat F, Halpern M. Projections of primary and revision hip and knee arthroplasty in the United States from 2005 to 2030. J Bone Joint Surg. 2007;89:780–5.
4. Kurtz SM, Ong KL, Lau E, et al. International survey or primary and revision total knee replacement. Int Orthop. 2011;35:1783–9.
5. Kurtz SM, Lau E, Ong K, Zhao K, Kelly M, Bozic KJ. Future young patient demand for primary and revision joint replacement: national projections from 2010–2030. Clin Orthop Relat Res. 2009;467:2606–12.
6. Kurtz SM, Ong KL, Lau E, Bozic KJ. Impact of the economic downturn on total joint replacement demand in the United States: update projections to 2021. J Bone Joint Surg. 2014;96:724–30.
7. Bozic KJ, Grosso LM, Lin Z, et al. Variation in hospital-level risk-standardized complication rates following elective primary total hip and knee arthroplasty. J Bone Joint Surg Am. 2014;96:640–7.
8. Gundtoft PH, Overgaard S, Schønheyder HC, et al. The "true" incidence of surgically treated deep prosthetic joint infection after 32,896 primary total hip arthroplasties: a prospective cohort study. Acta Orthop. 2015;86:326–34.
9. Pulido L, Ghanem E, Joshi A, Purtill JJ, Parvizi J. Periprosthetic joint infection. The incidence, timing and predisposing factors. Clin Orthop Relat Res. 2008; 466:1710–5.
10. Tsaras G, Osmon DR, Mabry T, et al. Incidence, secular trends and outcomes of prosthetic joint infection (PJI): a population-based study, Olmsted county, Minnesota, 1969–2007. Infect Control Hosp Epidemiol. 2012;33:1207–12.
11. Kirkland KB, Briggs JP, Trivette SL, Wilkinson WE, Sexton DJ. The impact of surgical-site infections in the 1990s: attributable mortality, excess length of hospitalization and extra costs. Infect Control Hosp Epidemiol. 1999;20:725–30.
12. Moore AJ, Blom AW, Whitehouse MR, Gooberman-Hill R. Deep prosthetic joint infection: a qualitative study of the impact on patients and their experiences of revision surgery. BMJ Open. 2015;5:e009495.
13. Dale H, Fenstad AM, Hallan G, et al. Increasing risk of prosthetic joint infection after total hip arthroplasty. Acta Orthop. 2012;83:449–58.
14. Yi SH, Baggs J, Culler SD, Berrios-Torres SI, Jerrigan JA. Medicare reimbursement attributable to periprosthetic joint infection following primary hip and knee arthroplasty. J Arthroplasty. 2015;30:931–8.

15. Bottle A, Middleton S, Kalkman CJ, Livingston EH, Aylin P. Global comparators project: international comparison of hospital outcomes using administrative data. Health Serv Res. 2013;48:2081–100.
16. O'Malley KJ, Cook KF, Price MD, Raiford Wildes K, Hurdle JF, Ashton CM. Measuring diagnoses: ICD code accuracy. Health Serv Res. 2005;40:1620–39.
17. Cheng P, Gilchrist A, Robinson KM, Paul L. The risk and consequences of clinical miscoding due to inadequate medical documentation: a case study of the impact on health services funding. HIM J. 2009;38:35–46.
18. Lange J, Pedersen AB, Troelsen A, Søballe K. Do hip prosthesis related infection codes in administrative discharge registers correctly classify periprosthetic hip joint infection? Hip Int. 2015;25:568–73.
19. Zhu I, Zhang F, Chen W, Liu S, Zhang Q, Zhang Y. Risk factors for periprosthetic joint infection after total joint arthroplasty: a systematic review and meta-analysis. J Hosp Infect. 2015;89:82–9.
20. Schrama JC, Fenstad AM, Dale H, et al. Increased risk of revision for infection in rheumatoid arthritis patients with total hip replacements. Acta Orthop. 2015;86:469–76.
21. Worth LJ, Bull AL, Brett J, Richards MJ. Diminishing surgical site infections in Australia: time trends in infection rates, pathogens and antimicrobial resistance using a comprehensive Victorian surveillance program, 2002–2013. Infect Control Hosp Epidemiol. 2015;36:409–16.
22. Squires DA. Explaining high health care spending in the United States: an international comparison of supply, utilization, prices and quality. Commonwealth Fund publication 1595;10:1–13. Available at: http://www.commonwealthfund.org/~/media/files/publications/issue-brief/2012/may/1595_squires_explaining_high_hlt_care_spending_intl_brief.pdf. Accessed 16 May 2017.
23. Vanhegan IS, Malik AK, Jayakumar P, Ul Islam S, Haddad FS. A financial analysis of revision hip arthroplasty. The economic burden in relation to the national tariff. J Bone Joint Surg. 2012;94B:619–23.
24. Kallala RF, Vanhegan IS, Ibrahim MS, Sarmah S, Haddad FS. Financial analysis of revision knee surgery based on NHS tariffs and hospital costs. Does it pay to provide a revision service? Bone Joint J. 2015;97B:197–201.

8

Ankle joint distraction arthroplasty for severe ankle arthritis

Yang Xu[1,2†], Yuan Zhu[1†] and Xiang-yang Xu[1*]

Abstract

Background: Ankle distraction arthroplasty is one option for the treatment of severe ankle arthritis in young patients. The outcomes and factors predicting success in distraction arthroplasty are poorly understood.

Methods: From January 2011 to May 2015, 16 patients who had undergone ankle distraction arthroplasty for ankle arthritis were operated, including six males and ten females. All patients were available for analysis. The main outcome measurements included joint space on weight bearing radiographs, AOFAS-AH scores (American Orthopaedic Foot & Ankle Society ankle-hindfoot score), VAS scores and SF-36 scores.

Results: All 16 patients were followed for a mean follow-up of 40.9 ± 14.7 months (range, 17–67 months). Fourteen of the 16 patients still had their native ankle joints. One patient had undergone ankle arthrodesis 1 year after the operation and one patient had converted to spontaneous ankle fusion at the 3 years follow-up postoperative. The VAS score improved from 5.9 ± 0.8 to 3.7 ± 2.2 ($p = 0.0028$). The mean AOFAS-AH score improved from 41.9 ± 7.2 preoperatively to 68.1 ± 20.0 postoperatively ($p = 0.001$). The mean SF-36 score improved from 43.1 ± 7.6 preoperatively to 62.7 ± 18.8 postoperatively ($p = 0.002$). A weight-bearing ankle space larger than 3 mm at 1 year following distraction is a positive predictive factor.

Conclusions: In this study, the treatment of ankle motion distraction for end stage ankle arthritis showed benefit in 9/16 (56.25%) patients at 41 months. It is a promising method for young patients with severe ankle arthritis.

Keywords: Ankle joint, Distraction, Arthroplasty

Background

Ankle joint distraction arthroplasty is a promising treatment method for ankle arthritis but the outcomes of distraction arthroplasty are poorly understood. It is an effective treatment for young patients with end-stage ankle arthritis, providing the benefits of pain reduction and functional improvement. In addition to ankle osteoarthritis, young patients with rheumatoid arthritis of the ankle joint also achieved good results [1]. The purpose of ankle distraction is to allow for intermittent intra-articular fluid pressures, the relief of mechanical stress on the cartilage and sustained, diminished subchondral sclerosis following the procedure [2, 3]. All of the mechanisms mentioned above are of benefit for cartilage repair and the reduction of cartilage damage. However, the current literature lacks good studies on distraction arthroplasty [4].

On the basis of the available clinical evidence, we conducted this study and hypothesized that ankle motion distraction would alleviate symptoms, improve ankle function and delay the time to ankle arthroplasty or arthrodesis while maintaining the joint space for a long period of time.

Methods

Approval for this retrospective study was obtained from our hospital's ethics committee.

The inclusion criteria for patients included the following: (1) symptomatic isolated, unilateral severe ankle osteoarthritis; (2) younger than 60 years old; (3) painful ankle arthritis with more than 1 year of conservative treatment including ankle debridement and medication.

The exclusion criteria included the following: (1) acute or chronic infection; (2) older than 60 years old; (3) poor general health condition; (4) patients who had ankle

* Correspondence: xu664531@hotmail.com
[†]Equal contributors
[1]Department of Orthopedics, Shanghai Ruijin Hospital, Shanghai Jiaotong University School of Medicine, Shanghai 200025, China
Full list of author information is available at the end of the article

surgery like supramalleolar osteotomy during ankle distraction or during follow-up. Because we were not sure whether or not the outcomes were due to ankle distraction.

All the patients were followed and none dropped out. Since we decided to analyze the outcomes of ankle distraction, all patients were required to come to our clinic during the last 3 months before submission of this paper. We got 15 patients' X-rays and latest information during this period. The other patient was operated 6 years ago. The last X-ray of her was 4 years postoperative. But we still keep contact with her via telephone.

Preoperative preparation

All patients were evaluated and their complete histories were obtained. Preoperative routine weight bearing radiographs were performed, including anteroposterior, mortise and lateral views of the ankle joint. The hindfoot alignment view was also made to help in the evaluation of hindfoot alignment. The hindfoot alignment view we used was recommended by Saltzman and el-Khoury [5]. CT and MRI scans were obtained before the surgery and at the follow-up visits to evaluate the condition of the ankle joint cartilage and subchondral bone.

Before the surgery, the patients were examined and circumferential external fixators were constructed based on the size and length of each patient's leg and foot. All VAS scores, AOFAS-AH scores (American Orthopaedic Foot & Ankle Society ankle-hindfoot score) and SF-36 scores were collected preoperatively as customary at our center. The VAS score was used to evaluate the degree of pain. The AOFAS-AH score and SF-36 score were used to evaluate ankle function.

Surgical technique

The patient was placed supine on the operating table. First, a complete cheilectomy was performed to clear the osseous impingement. We did adequate resection of anterior tibial osteophytes to make sure that when dorsiflexing the ankle joint, there was no impingement. Intraoperative lateral fluoroscopic images were used to assess the resection. All visual osteophytes around ankle joint were completely resected. Osteophytes around the ankle joint were removed through an anterior open incision or a lateral or posterior incision, if necessary.

The external fixator was applied in a standard fashion. The external fixator included two tibial rings and one podalic ring. The whole external fixator was constructed and sterilized before the surgery. A K-wire was inserted into the axis of the ankle motion from the tip of the medial malleolus to the tip of the lateral malleolus temporarily and the external fixation frame was installed to make sure that the axis of the ankle motion was consistent with the axis of the external fixation frame motion. This was the most important step. The frame was fixed with K-wires or half pins if necessary. Each tibial ring was fixed with two crossed K-wires. If the patient had osteoporosis, half pins were utilized to help stabilize the external fixator. Foot fixation included four 2.0 mm tensioned K-wires. Two crossed K-wires were inserted through the calcaneum, and two K-wires were drilled through the metatarsals and midfoot to fix the forefoot and midfoot. C-arm fluoroscopy was used to ensure ideal wire placement. After all wires and pins were placed correctly, the temporary K-wire inserted into the axis of ankle motion was removed (Fig. 1).

Postoperative management

Distraction by 1 mm per day was performed after surgery and was assessed by radiography. Full weight bearing was permitted 2 weeks postoperatively. We required the patients walk with the fixators 2 weeks postoperatively, and the motion exercises were performed from the 2nd week to the 12th week. After the surgery, every patient underwent routine pinhole nursing every day. The distractor was removed 3 months after surgery. Each patient was required to come to the outpatient department every year to evaluate the function of the ankle and to take radiographs. Unfortunately, not every patient complied with this demand to visit every year. The postoperative VAS, AOFAS-AH and SF-36 scores analyzed in this study were the latest information collected by telephone or outpatient visit.

Statistical methods

The significance level was set at $\alpha = 0.05$. All data analyses were performed with SAS software version 8.1 (SAS Institute, Inc, Cary, NC). The results were presented as the mean and standard deviation. The paired Student's *t*-test was used to compare the preoperative and postoperative radiographic measurements and ankle function scores.

Results

From January 2011 to May 2015, 126 patients were screened and 17 patients entered into this study. One patient had supramalleolar osteotomy during ankle joint distraction and was excluded. In this case, the patients had a history of severe Pilon fracture and had severe posttraumatic ankle varus deformity and ankle arthritis. So we did a supramalleolar osteotomy to realign the ankle alignment. The remaining 16 patients (6 males and 10 females) who had undergone ankle distraction arthroplasty met the criteria. Table 1 shows the patient's detailed information. The average patient age at surgery was 30.3 ± 14.3 years old (range, 14 to 60 years). Among these, 13 patients had a history of ankle fracture or Pilon fracture. One patient had a history of an old talus fracture.

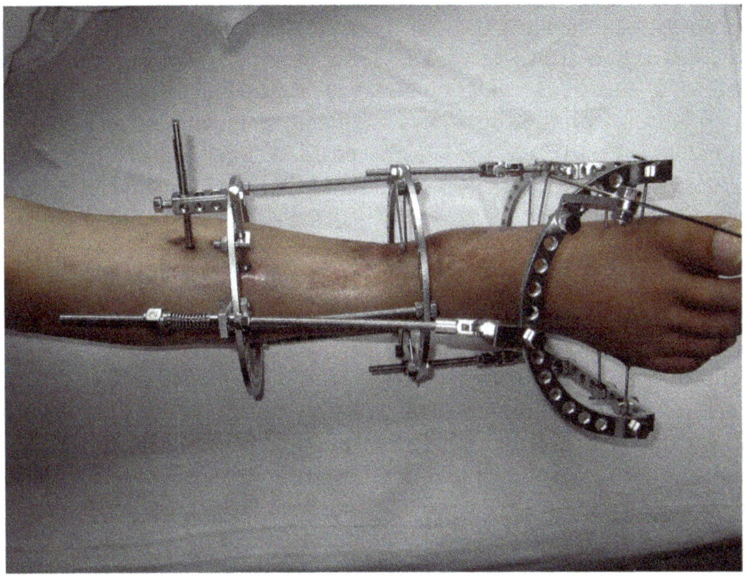

Fig. 1 Photograph of ankle distractor

One patient had a history of ankle sprain 10 years prior to the study, and the other one had no prior history of ankle injury. One patient also underwent the fibula reduction with distraction at the same time. Debridement and removal of osteophytes were performed in 6 patients. The Achilles tendons of two patients were lengthened at the time of operation with percutaneous Hoke method. The mean follow-up time was 40.9 ± 14.7 months (range, 17 to 67 months) (Table 1).

During the follow-up, one patient had talonavicular joint arthritis 3 years after the operation, but the patient was very satisfied with the ankle joint function although the ankle joint motion was comparatively less than normal. One patient had calcaneal osteotomy due to hindfoot valgus alignment. Five patients had their ankle space return to the same as or narrower than their preoperative joint space. One patient's ankle joint converted to spontaneous fusion at the 3-year follow-up, and this

Table 1 Outcomes of ankle distraction for ankle arthritis

Patient no.	Left/Right	History	Time of follow-up (month)	VAS preop	AOFAS preop	SF-36 preop	VAS postop	AOFAS postop	SF-36 postop	Clinical outcome
1	L	ankle fracture	17	6	36	33.53	3	78	57.74	good
2	R	ankle fracture	24	6	42	44.36	1	81	77.61	good
3	L	ankle fracture	44	7	29	66.22	2	88	78.02	good
4	R	-	66	6	39	42.05	6	39	41.94	fair
5	R	ankle fracture	63	5	48	41.12	6	46	41.31	fair
6	L	ankle fracture	36	7	51	50.35	5	58	67.44	good
7	L	ankle sprain	29	5	36	39.97	5	41	41.36	fair
8	R	ankle fracture	67	6	42	43.34	4	60	59.72	good
9	R	ankle fracture	32	5	31	37.09	0	100	89.64	excellent
10	L	ankle fracture	50	6	51	42.41	6	57	50.13	fair
11	R	talus fracture	37	-	-	-	-	-	-	failed
12	R	ankle fracture	32	7	44	43.01	7	56	43.9	fair
13	L	ankle fracture	32	7	52	40.78	2	90	87.55	excellent
14	L	ankle fracture	39	5	44	42.84	4	68	51.28	good
15	R	pilon fracture	37	-	-	-	-	-	-	failed
16	L	ankle fracture	49	5	42	48.72	1	91	90.06	excellent

patient had pain relief. One of the patients with severe Pilon fracture ultimately transferred to ankle arthrodesis in 2015, 2 years after ankle distraction arthroplasty. The other 9 patients remained at a normal or wider joint space at the latest follow-up and had positive outcomes. A total of 14 patients had native ankle joints at the latest follow-up. Table 2 shows that the mean VAS score improved from 5.9 ± 0.8, preoperatively, to 3.7 ± 2.2, postoperatively ($p = 0.0028$). The mean AOFAS-AH score improved from 41.9 ± 7.2, preoperatively, to 68.1 ± 20.0, postoperatively ($p = 0.001$). The mean SF-36 score improved from 43.1 ± 7.6, preoperatively, to 62.7 ± 18.8, postoperatively ($p = 0.002$) (Table 2). In this study, 3 patients rated their outcomes as "excellent", and a "good" outcome was observed in 6 patients. Five patients rated their results as "fair" because of the consistent discomfort. On the other hand, 2 distraction surgeries failed, with one patient undergoing ankle arthrodesis and another with the spontaneous fusion of the ankle joint. Only two patients had pin-site infection. In this study, the use of ankle motion distraction for the treatment of severe ankle arthritis showed benefit in 9/16 patients at 41 months. The mean preoperative ankle space was 1.9 mm (range, 1.6 to 2.4 mm), the mean ankle space during distraction was 6.2 (range, 5 to 8.83 mm), and the mean ankle space of last follow-up was 4.1 mm (range, 2.2 to 5.48 mm). We noticed that patients with ankle space larger than 3 mm tended to achieve better outcomes. A weight-bearing ankle space larger than 3 mm at 1 year following distraction is a positive predictive factor.

The average preoperative and postoperative ankle dorsiflexion ranges were 6.5° (range, 0 to 12°) and 8° (range, 0 to 15°) ($p > 0.05$). The average preoperative and postoperative ankle plantarflexion ranges were 33.2° (range, 20° to 45°) and 36° (range, 20° to 50°) ($p < 0.05$). The average preoperative and postoperative ankle motion ranges were 39.7° (range, 20° to 55°) and 44° (range, 25° to 60°) ($p < 0.05$).

Fisher's Exact Test was used to analyze whether gender was one of the prognostic factors. And the *P* value was larger than 0.05, which showed gender had no effect on prognosis (Fig. 2a) (b).

Discussion

Posttraumatic arthritis is the most common form of ankle arthritis. Ankle fractures can cause altered biomechanics and structural changes even with adequate open reduction and internal fixation [3]. Ligamentous injury is another important cause of posttraumatic ankle arthritis.

Table 2 Functional outcomes after ankle distraction

	Preop	Postop	*P* value
VAS	5.9 ± 0.8	3.7 ± 2.2	0.0028
AOFAS-AH	41.9 ± 7.2	68.1 ± 20.0	0.001
SF-36	43.1 ± 7.6	62.7 ± 18.8	0.002

The goals of treatment for ankle osteoarthritis are reducing pain and restoring as much ankle function as possible [6]. Conservative treatments for early stage ankle arthritis include lifestyle adaption, oral medicine such as NSAIDS. Joint preservation surgical treatments include ankle debridement, osteotomy and joint distraction. Joint sacrificing treatments include arthrodesis and joint replacement. Ankle distraction, arthrodesis and replacement are indicated for end-stage ankle osteoarthritis. Arthrodesis has the potential risk of adjacent joint arthritis, continuous pain, nonunion and decreased function [7–10]. Ankle replacement is associated with the risk of device-related infection and major revision surgery [11, 12]. For ankle arthritis, supramalleolar osteotomy is indicated for early ankle arthritis with partially preserved ankle joint surface, ankle frontal alignment deformities and retaining the motion of the ankle [13–15]. Ankle arthritis with subsequent subtalar arthritis is a good indication of tibiotalocalcaneal arthrodesis [16].

However, for relatively young cases, ankle distraction may be a better choice. The mechanisms of ankle distraction may attribute to the relief of mechanical stress on the cartilage, the formation of intermittent fluid pressure that is beneficial to the nutrition of cartilage and decreasing subcohondral sclerosis [2].

Van valburg et al. recommended that distraction should be carried out over a distance of 5 mm on weight-bearing X-rays [17]. Fragomen et al. came to the conclusion through cadaveric experiments that a 5.8 mm distraction gap on X-ray was needed under weight-bearing conditions, while a 7.0 mm distraction gap on X-ray was needed under non-weight-bearing conditions [18]. Few studies emphasize the ankle space change after ankle distraction. In our study, we noticed that there was a reduction of ankle space after taking off the external fixation. However, if the ankle space could maintain a normal or larger than normal space 1 year postoperatively, the joint space may continue to stay in this condition long term.

The fixator used in the distraction arthroplasty can be fixed or mobilizable. In our study, all patients' fixators were mobilizable. In a prospective randomized controlled trial, Saltzman et al. reported that outcomes after motion distraction were significantly better than those using fixed distraction [19]. Moreover, in their subsequent study, Nguyen et al. reported that AOS scores at 2 years after distraction and age at the time of surgery were the most important predictive factors of ankle survival. They thought that those with an AOS score smaller than 42 and older patients tended to achieve better outcomes [20]. They questioned whether motion distraction was superior to fixed distraction because of

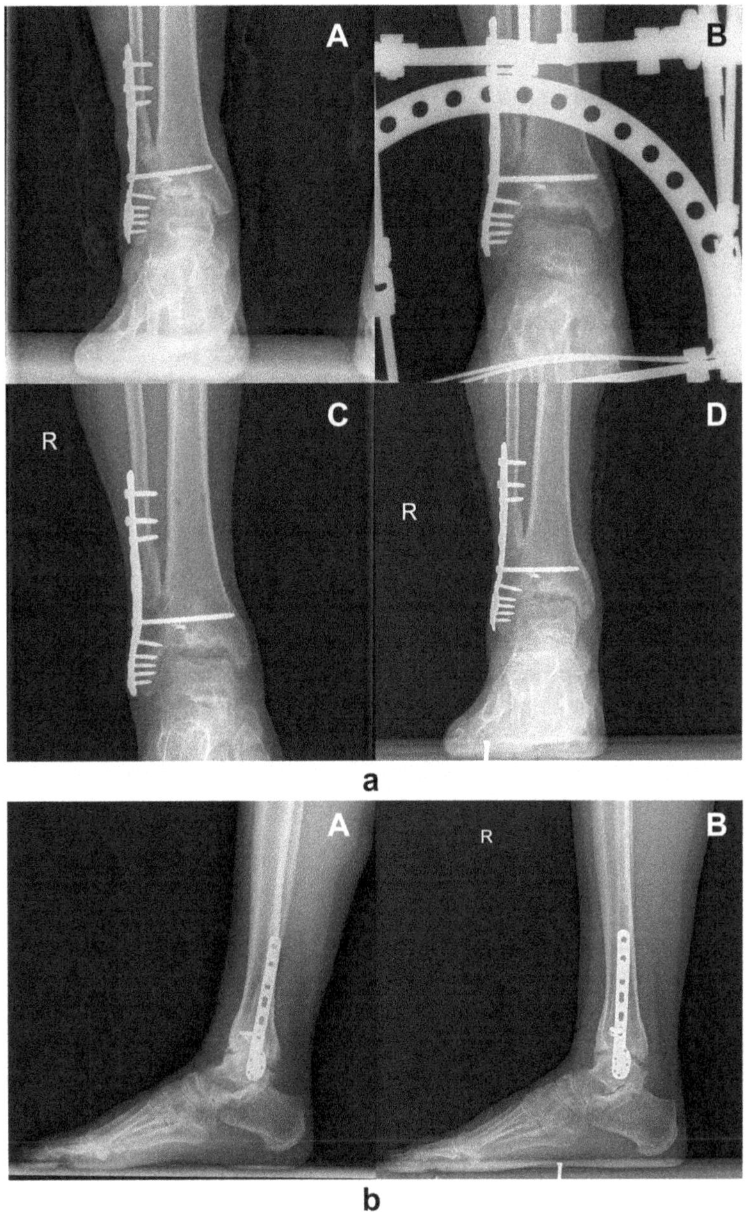

Fig. 2 **a** radiographs of a female with severe ankle arthritis. *a* preoperative ankle joint. *b* ankle joint during ankle distraction. *c* ankle joint after removal of external fixation. *d* 1 year postoperative. **b** lateral radiographs of a female with severe ankle arthritis. *a* lateral view of the same patient before operation. *b* lateral view of the same patient at 1 year after operation

the limited number of patients and the fixed group regaining motion over time. However, in their studies, there was no description of the distraction distance before and after the operation and no mention of joint space improvement. Marijnissen et al. found that the female gender is a predictor of failure of distraction arthroplasty [21]. Female patients had a higher likelihood of failure than male patients, which is a finding similar to that found in hip distraction. In our study, we found that it is the postoperative ankle space that is the most important predictive factor. If the ankle space remained larger than 3 mm at the 1-year postoperative follow-up under the weight-bearing situation, the outcomes tend to be better than those with an ankle space smaller than 3 mm. The weight-baring ankle spaces of those who achieved pain relief or clinical symptoms improvement were larger than 3 mm.

In this study, six patients had preceding arthroscopic debridement or debridement with open incision. In previous studies, ankle distraction had a statistically significant better result than debridement, and it was demonstrated that the improvement in the clinical outcome after ankle distraction was not due to debridement [2, 22].

The most common complication of distraction is pin-site infection. Others like osteomyelitis, deep vein thrombosis and K-wire breakage were reported [23]. In our study only two patients had pin-site infection, which was resolved by oral antibiotics and routinely dressing change.

There are several limitations of this study. First, it was a retrospective study of a case series, and there was no control group. Thus, we were not sure whether there was a placebo effect. Six patients underwent ankle joint debridement and osteophyte excision, and one of the patients also underwent a reduction of the fibula. We were not sure how much these additional procedures could have influenced the outcomes, although a previous study has demonstrated that the clinical outcome improvement is not due to debridement [2]. The articular surface of severe ankle arthritis patients is blurred, which makes it hard to measure the joint space. Although we tried to measure the space as many times as possible, it may not represent the real ankle space. Thus, the ankle space during long-term visits may not represent the real average. Since we noticed an ankle fusion during follow-up, the possibility of spontaneous ankle fusion should not be neglected even though the patient experienced pain relief.

Conclusion

In this study, the treatment of ankle motion distraction for severe ankle arthritis showed benefit in 9/16 (56.25%) patients at 41 months. It is a promising method for young patients with severe ankle arthritis.

Abbreviations

AOFAS-AH: American Orthopaedic Foot & Ankle Society ankle-hindfoot; AOS: Ankle Osteoarthritis scale; SF-36: Short form-36; VAS: Visual analogue scale

Acknowledgements

The authors gratefully acknowledge all collaborating researchers in collecting information during this study. We would also like to thank the subjects whose participation made this investigation possible.

Funding

This research did not receive any specific grant from funding agencies in the public, commercial, or not-for-profit sectors.

Authors' contributions

YX: literature research, experimental studies, statistical analysis and manuscript preparation. YZ: experimental studies and manuscript editing. X-YX concepts and study design, experimental studies. All authors read and approved the final manuscript.

Competing interests

The authors declare that they have no competing interests.

Consent for publication

Not applicable.

Author details

[1]Department of Orthopedics, Shanghai Ruijin Hospital, Shanghai Jiaotong University School of Medicine, Shanghai 200025, China. [2]Shanghai Institute of Traumatology and Orthopedics, Shanghai, China.

References

1. Nakasa T, Adachi N, Kato T, Ochi M. Distraction arthroplasty with arthroscopic microfracture in a patient with rheumatoid arthritis of the ankle joint. J Foot Ankle Surg. 2015;54(2):280–4.
2. Marijnissen AC, van Roermund PM, van Melkebeek J, Lafeber FP. Clinical benefit of joint distraction in the treatment of ankle osteoarthritis. Foot Ankle Clin. 2003;8(2):335–46.
3. Martin RL, Stewart GW, Conti SF. Posttraumatic ankle arthritis: an update on conservative and surgical management. J Orthop Sports Phys Ther. 2007;37(5):253–9.
4. Smith NC, Beaman D, Rozbruch SR, Glazebrook MA. Evidence-based indications for distraction ankle arthroplasty. Foot Ankle Int. 2012;33(8):632–6.
5. Saltzman CL, el-Khoury GY. The hindfoot alignment view. Foot Ankle Int. 1995;16(9):572–6.
6. Grunfeld R, Aydogan U, Juliano P. Ankle arthritis: review of diagnosis and operative management. Med Clin North Am. 2014;98(2):267–89.
7. Buchner M, Sabo D. Ankle fusion attributable to posttraumatic arthrosis: a long-term followup of 48 patients. Clin Orthop Relat Res. 2003;406:155–64.
8. Muir DC, Amendola A, Saltzman CL. Long-term outcome of ankle arthrodesis. Foot Ankle Clin. 2002;7(4):703–8.
9. Hendrickx RP, Stufkens SA, de Bruijn EE, Sierevelt IN, van Dijk CN, Kerkhoffs GM. Medium- to long-term outcome of ankle arthrodesis. Foot Ankle Int. 2011;32(10):940–7.
10. Coester LM, Saltzman CL, Leupold J, Pontarelli W. Long-term results following ankle arthrodesis for post-traumatic arthritis. J Bone Joint Surg Am. 2001;83-A(2):219–28.
11. SooHoo NF, Zingmond DS, Ko CY. Comparison of reoperation rates following ankle arthrodesis and total ankle arthroplasty. J Bone Joint Surg Am. 2007;89(10):2143–9.
12. Matsumoto T, Yasunaga H, Matsui H, Fushimi K, Izawa N, Yasui T, et al. Time trends and risk factors for perioperative complications in total ankle arthroplasty: retrospective analysis using a national database in Japan. BMC Musculoskelet Disord. 2016;17(1):450.
13. Tanaka Y. The concept of ankle joint preserving surgery: why does supramalleolar osteotomy work and how to decide when to do an osteotomy or joint replacement. Foot Ankle Clin. 2012;17(4):545–53.
14. Barg A, Pagenstert GI, Horisberger M, Paul J, Gloyer M, Henninger HB, et al. Supramalleolar osteotomies for degenerative joint disease of the ankle joint: indication, technique and results. Int Orthop. 2013;37(9):1683–95.
15. Colin F, Gaudot F, Odri G, Judet T. Supramalleolar osteotomy: techniques, indications and outcomes in a series of 83 cases. Orthop Traumatol Surg Res. 2014;100(4):413–8.
16. Fang Z, Claassen L, Windhagen H, Daniilidis K, Stukenborg-Colsman C, Waizy H. Tibiotalocalcaneal arthrodesis using a retrograde intramedullary nail with a valgus curve. Orthop Surg. 2015;7(2):125–31.
17. van Valburg AA, van Roermund PM, Lammens J, van Melkebeek J, Verbout AJ, Lafeber EP, et al. Can Ilizarov joint distraction delay the need for an arthrodesis of the ankle? A preliminary report. J Bone Joint Surg Br. 1995;77(5):720–5.
18. Fragomen AT, McCoy TH, Meyers KN, Rozbruch SR. Minimum distraction gap: how much ankle joint space is enough in ankle distraction arthroplasty? HSS J. 2014;10(1):6–12.
19. Saltzman CL, Hillis SL, Stolley MP, Anderson DD, Amendola A. Motion versus fixed distraction of the joint in the treatment of ankle osteoarthritis: a prospective randomized controlled trial. J Bone Joint Surg Am. 2012;94(11):961–70.
20. Nguyen MP, Pedersen DR, Gao Y, Saltzman CL, Amendola A. Intermediate-term follow-up after ankle distraction for treatment of end-stage osteoarthritis. J Bone Joint Surg Am. 2015;97(7):590–6.
21. Marijnissen AC, Hoekstra MC, Pre BC, van Roermund PM, van Melkebeek J, Amendola A, et al. Patient characteristics as predictors of clinical outcome of distraction in treatment of severe ankle osteoarthritis. J Orthop Res. 2014;32(1):96–101.

9

Topical zoledronic acid decreases micromotion induced bone resorption in a sheep arthroplasty model

Thomas Jakobsen[1,2*], Søren Kold[1,2], Juan Shiguetomi-Medina[1], Jorgen Baas[1], Kjeld Soballe[1] and Ole Rahbek[1]

Abstract

Background: Initial micromotion of a total hip replacement is associated with aseptic loosening. The use of bisphosphonates could be one way to reduce peri-implant bone resorption induced by micromotion. Bisphosphonates compounds are inhibitors of bone resorption. The aim of this study was to investigate whether local treatment with bisphosphonate would reduce bone resorption and fibrous tissue around an experimental implant subjected to micromotion.

Methods: One micromotion implant were inserted into each medial femoral condyle in ten sheep. During each gait cycle the implant axially piston 0.5 mm. During surgery one of the femoral condyles were locally treated with 0.8 mg zoledronate. The other condyle served as control. Observation period was 12 weeks.

Results: Histological evaluation showed a fibrous capsule around both the control and bisphosphonate implants. Histomorphometrical analysis showed that 97% of the surface on both control and bisphosphonate implants were covered by fibrous tissue. However, the bisphosphonate was able to preserve bone in a 1 mm zone around the implants.

Conclusion: This study indicates that local treatment with bisphosphonate cannot prevent the formation of a fibrous capsule around an implant subjected to micromotion, but bisphosphonate is able to reduce resorption of peri-prosthetic bone.

Keywords: Bisphosphonate, Osseointegration, Implant, Animal, Arthroplasty

Background

Initial stable implant fixation is important for long-term survival of total joint replacements [1, 2]. Radiostereometrical studies indicate that early migration is a associated with later revision [1–3]. Treatment strategies that optimize initial implant fixation and prevents early implant migration could have the potential to reduce risks of later revision.

Failure of initial implant osseointegration will result in early implant migration and bone resorption [4]. Early implant migration is associated with reduced resistance to withstand implant movement induced by external load [5]. Continues implant migration is associated with implant failure [3]. Early bone resorption can be initiated by an unstable implant generating micro-movement or fluid pressure [6–8]. We have previously shown that implant micromotion without the presence of wear debris can generate a fibrous membrane and cause bone resorption [9]. In vivo studies suggest that instability induced bone resorption works through similar molecular mechanisms as particle induced bone resorption [10, 11]. Aseptic loosening of an implant involves several steps. One of the first steps could be bone resorption due to micro-movement of the implant. The resorption bone is replaced with fibrous tissue. Wear debris will subsequently migrate from the joint articulation along the fibrous tissue to the bone to implant interface and aggravate the process [12, 13]. Longevity of the implant might potentially be increased if micro-

* Correspondence: Thomas.Jakobsen@ki.au.dk
[1]Orthopaedic Research Laboratory, Department of Orthopaedics, Aarhus University Hospital, Norrebrogade 44, Building 1A, DK-8000 Aarhus, Denmark
[2]Department of Orthopaedics, Aalborg University Hospital, Aalborg, Denmark

movement of the implant were not allowed to induce bone resorption.

One way to reduce micromotion induced bone resorption and fibrous membrane formation could be with the use of bisphosphonates. These compounds binds strongly to bone, inhibit osteoclastic activity, and reduce bone resorption [14]. Systemic bisphosphonate treatment has previously in an experimental model of osteolysis been able to reduce bone resorption [15]. We have previously shown that local treatment with bisphosphonate can increase new bone formation, preserve lamellar bone and allograft, and increase biomechanical implant fixation in an experimental joint replacement model [9]. In a clinical study, local treatment with bisphosphonate was shown to reduce acetabular component migration measured by radiostereometrical analysis [16]. The same effect has been observed in the study investigating local ibandronate treatment in total knee arthroplasties [17]. Others have shown the local or systemic treatment with bisphosphonates can reduce but not prevent osteolytic bone resorption and formation of fibrous tissue in a rat model of prosthetic loosening [18, 19]. Our group has previously shown in a large animal model that systemic alendronate can reduce bone resorption around unstable implants but not prevent it [20]. A stronger stimulus might be needed. Only way to obtain a stronger stimulus could be with topical administration of a third generation bisphosphonate. The aim of this study was to investigate in a sheep arthroplasty model whether topical treatment with bisphosphonate would reduce bone resorption and fibrous tissue.

We tested the hypothesis that local zoledronate treatment would reduce bone resorption and fibrous tissue formation around implants subjected to micromotion.

Methods

Study design

We used 10 skeletally mature Danish Landrace sheep with a mean weight of 40 kg (range, 35–50 kg). The sheep were obtained though our Institutional farm (Påskehøjgaardcentret, 8380 Trige, Denmark) affiliated with our Research facility. Our Institutional Animal Care and Use Committee approved the study. Institutional guidelines for the treatment and care of experimental animals were followed.

In this study, we used a paired design with intervention and control group in the same sheep. We have previously shown that the used model of micromotion is able to induce bone resorption [9]. In each sheep, we inserted one loaded micromotion device (Fig. 1) into each of the medial femoral condyles. Zoledronate was administered locally in one of the knees. Saline was used as control in the contralateral knee. The zoledronate and control implants were systematically alternated between left and right knee. Our observation period was 12 weeks.

Our sample size calculation was based on a previous study [9]. We assumed the standard deviation of the relative change to be 50%. Two-sided α and β were set to 5% and 20%, respectively. We added two extra animals to the calculated sample size of eight to counteract if implants from one or two animals were lost for subsequent analysis.

Implants

We used 20 custom-made micromotion implant devices (Fig. 1). Our micromotion device has previously been described in detail [9, 21]. In short, the micromotion device allows a polymethylmethacrylate (PMMA) implant to piston 0.5 mm with respect to the bone during each step the animal takes. The micromotion creates shear forces in the bone to implant interface. The implants in this study were made sterile by gamma irradiation (25–50 kGy for 16 h, Codan Steritex, Espergaerde, Denmark).

Surgery

With the sheep under general anesthesia, we used our standard anteromedial surgical approach to the knee [9, 21, 22]. Our micromotion device was inserted into the weight-bearing portion of the medial femoral condyle. The procedure has been described in detail in our previously study [9]. During each surgery, we tested and assured that the micromotion device would piston during each gait cycle.

Before the PMMA implant was mounted onto the anchor screw, we soaked the bone cavity for 60 s with either saline as control or 1 mL saline containing 0.8 mg zoledronate (Aclasta, Novartis Healthcare A/S, Copenhagen, Denmark) as intervention. After soaking the bone for 60 s, the cavity was rinsed with saline and excess zoledronate or saline together with blood coming from the marrow cavity was sucked away. In this study, all sheep were weight bearing on the operated leg within 5 days of surgery. After the 12 weeks observation period the sheep were euthanized with an overdose of hypersaturated barbiturate and the bones were collected for preparation and analyses. At harvest, all pistons were movable.

Specimen preparation

Bone specimens were stored at −20 °C immediately. We cut each specimen perpendicular to the long axis of the implant using a water-cooled bad saw (Exact Apparatebau, Nordenstedt, Germany) (Fig. 2). The specimens was fixed in 70% ethanol and used for later analysis. Preparation and subsequent evaluation were blinded.

Histology and Histomorphometry

All bone-implant specimen were dehydrated in ethanol (70%–96%) containing basic fuchsin, and embedded in Epoxy (EPOFIX, Struers, Copenhagen, Denmark). Four

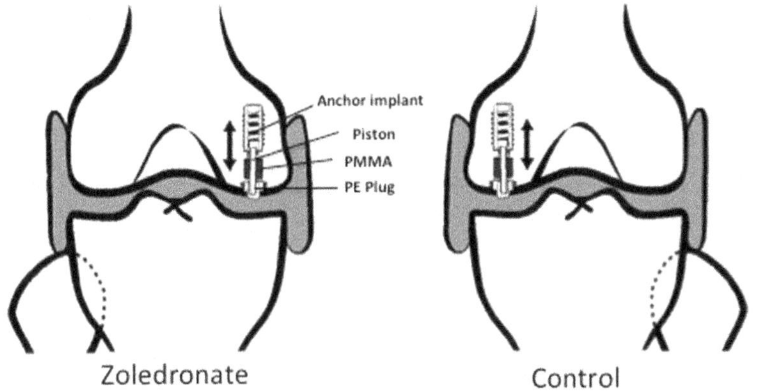

Fig. 1 Schematic drawing showing implant position in the medial femoral condyle. Reproduced with permission from copyright holder/author

25-μm thick sections were cut with a hard tissue microtome (KDG-95, MeProTech, Heerhugowaard, The Netherlands) around the center part of each implant [23]. The sections were cut with a distance of 400 μm. Before making the sections, the implant was randomly rotated around its long axis. The sections were cut parallel to this axis. These techniques provide reliable results with negligible bias [24]. Before the sections were mounted on glass, we surface stained them with 2% light-green (BDH Laboratory Supplies, Poole, England).

We used a stereological software program (newCAST, Visiopharm A/S, Horsholm, Denmark) for the histomorphometrical analysis. Volume fractions of bone were estimated by point counting [25] in a zone from the implant surface and 1 mm into the surrounding bone. Fractions of bone in contact with the implant surface were estimated using sine-weighted lines [26].

Statistical analysis

Intercooled Stata 9.0 (Stata Inc., College Station, TX, USA) were used for statistical analysis. Statistical analyses were done on ratios between paired data, which were not normally distributed. All variables were log-transformed and Student's paired t-test was performed on absolute differences between normally distributed log-transformed paired data. An absolute difference between the logarithms of a pair of data equals the logarithm of the ratio within the pair [27].

Results

Surgery

One sheep died during surgery and was excluded. The remaining 9 sheep completed the 12-weeks observation period. No clinical signs of infection were present at time of euthanization.

Histology

The most striking difference between the control and zoledronate implants was the presence of a 200–300 μm thick fibrous membrane around the control implants (Fig. 3). A fibrous membrane was also present around the zoledronate implants, but the membrane was thinner with an approximately thickness of 50 μm. The fibrous membrane in both the control and zoledronate group consisted of dense paralleled fibers. No qualitative morphological difference was found between the two groups

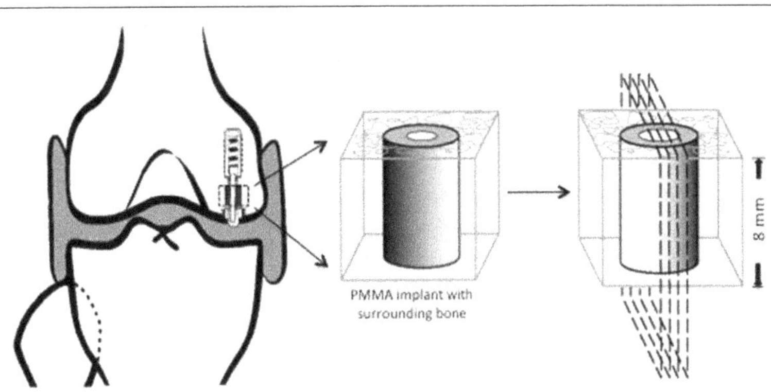

Fig. 2 Schematic diagram showing the specimen preparation. Each bone-implant specimen is embedded and cut into four slides for histomorphometrical analysis. Reproduced with permission from copyright holder/author

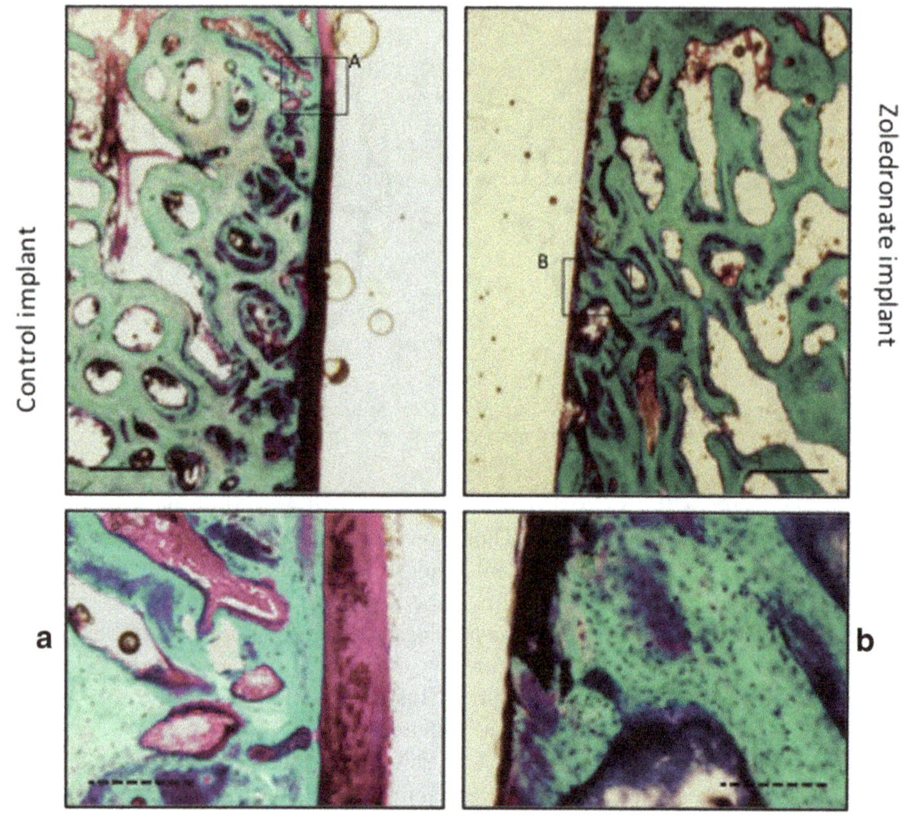

Fig. 3 Representative photomicrographs of samples from the same animal. The samples were stained with basic fuchsin and counterstained with 2% light green. Note the thick fibrous membrane around the control implant compared to the zoledronate implant. Solid bar = 1 mm. Dotted bar = 0.3 mm

when looking at the bone in the peri-implant zone. The bone consisted mainly of lamellae with spindle-shaped osteocytes in between. Sparse amount of osteoclasts were observed in both groups. No retained bone debris was observed in any of the groups.

Histomorphometrical analysis

The local zoledronate treatment preserved 14% (p = 0.02) more total bone around the implants in a 1 mm zone in the zoledronate group compared to the control group (Fig. 4). We found a total peri-implant bone volume fraction of 57% (95% CI: 46% - 67%) in the control group and 66% (95% CI: 53% - 78%) in the zoledronate group. No statistically significant changes were found when comparing bone volume fractions for woven (p = 0.08) or lamellar (p = 0.32) bone (Fig. 3). In the zoledronate group, 16% (95% CI: 2% - 29%) of 1 mm peri-implant zone was made of fibrous tissue compared to 23% (95% CI: 14% - 33%) in the control group (p = 0.22).

The implant surfaces in the both the zoledronate and control group were virtually covered by fibrous tissue. The surface fraction for fibrous tissue was 97% (95% CI: 94%- 100%) in the zoledronate group compared to 97% (95% CI: 94% - 99%) in the control group (p = 0.65). We found no significant differences in the surface-fractions of woven, lamellar, and total bone (p = 0.76, p = 0.42, p = 0.71).

Discussion

The purpose of this study was to investigate whether topical treatment with zoledronate could prevent bone resorption and fibrous tissue formation in our large animal model of micromotion induced bone resorption. We found that zoledronate did not prevent formation of a fibrous membrane, but was able to reduce bone resorption and thickness of the fibrous membrane.

The used model is intended to imitate the bone to cement interface of a total hip replacement. We have previously demonstrated that our experimental model are able to induce peri-implant bone resorption and therefore also suitable to test local adjuvant therapies against bone resorption [9]. The paired design allowed us to eliminate the biological difference between individuals.

Our study is limited by an observation period of 12 weeks and only nine animals completed the study.

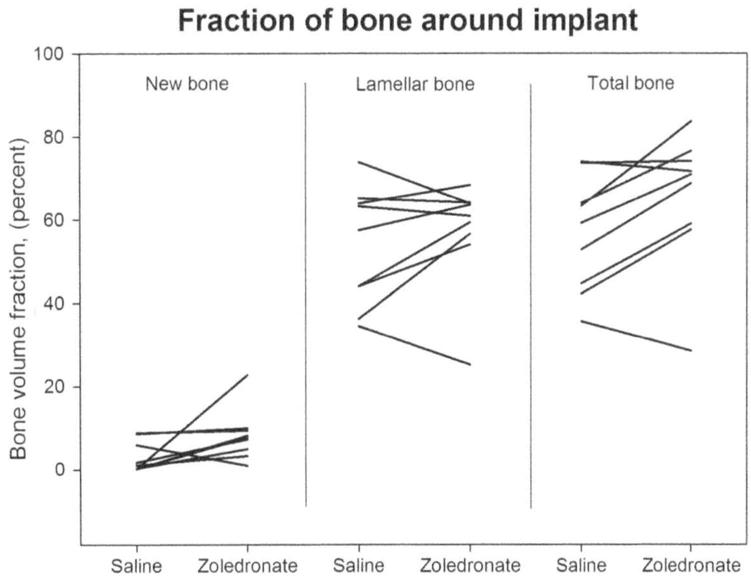

Fig. 4 Tissue-volume fractions in a 0–1 mm zone around implants. Paired data connected by line

Non-significant differences should therefore be interpreted with caution.

Zoledronate is a potent inhibitor of bone resorption [28]. We have previously shown that local treatment with zoledronate can inhibit resorption of allograft and increase fixation of both primary and revision implants [29, 30]. In this study, we show that local treatment with zoledronate can reduce resorption of bone in a 1 mm peri-implant zone around an implant subjected to controlled micromotion.

Our model of micromotion has a piston that allows a 0.5 mm movement of the implant during each loading. The model was designed to imitate a cemented femoral implant subjected to micromotion. The amplitude of movement of our implant is above the accepted threshold of 0.15 mm studies and suggested by Van der Voort based on RSA and thereby comparable to clinical implants with a high risk of as aseptic loosening [31]. Furthermore, the loading conditions of both clinical femoral implants and our experimental implants are comparable; both implants transfers load by shear forces though the bone-cement imterface. In our model, movement will occur at the implant-to-bone interface during each gait cycle and thereby create high shear forces and strain between the implant and tissue in contact with the implant. According to studies by and Carter and Giori, the amplitude of strain dictates which tissue can be formed [32, 33]. A high strain will induce bone resorption and formation of fibrous tissue. We found that local zoledronate treatment were able to partly counteract the strain/micromotion induced bone resorption and preserve 14% more total bone compared to our control.

An interesting histological finding is the difference in thickness of the fibrous membrane between the zoledronate and control groups. We know from previous studies from our group that micromotion is able to induce formation of a fibrous membrane [9, 34]. In this study we observed that local zoledronate treatment histologically reduced the thickness of the membrane. It could be that shear forces and stain at the tissue-to-implant interface are to high to by counteracted by zoledronate. Further away form the implant surface, strain and shear forces diminishes and zoledronate are able to partly preserve bone. We know from previous studies that increased amount of bone and decreased amount of fibrous tissue in correlated to increased implant stability [22]. The difference in fibrous layer thickness should therefore have the potential to make the zoledronate implants more mechanically stable.

It has previously been shown that systemic alendronate is able to inhibit bone resorption in a canine osteolytic hip arthroplasty model [15]. An animal study using a rodent model has shown that systemic treatment with alendronate or clodronate can reduce instability-induced bone resorption, but high doses are needed [19]. One likely explanation for the preserved bone volume density found in this study is the inhibitory effect of zoledronate on bone resorption. Previous studies have shown that preservation of lamellar bone often leads to increased formation of new bone [35–37]. The increased new bone formation is explained by increased osteoconductive properties of the preserved lamellar bone. In this study, we are not able to show a statistically significant increase in peri-implant formation of new bone (8% in zoledronate group vs. 3% in control group, $p = 0.08$). One possible explanation could be a to short observation period for new bone formation to occur. The effect on bone formation and resorption has been shown to be different over time [37]. A longer observation period might have shown a more pronounced effect of zoledronate on both bone formation and resorption.

Local treatment with zoledronate was not able to prevent formation of peri-implant fibrous tissue. However, zoledronate was able to reduce the thickness of the peri-implant fibrous membrane. This is in agreement with results from another study where local alendronate treatment reduced formation of soft tissue, but did not prevent its formation [19]. It is also in agreement with a clinical study were local ibandronate treatment reduced occurrences of radiolucent lines around acetabular cups lines, but not prevented them [16]. Based on our previous study were systemic alendronate reduced bone resorption around an unstable implant, we expected that a stronger anti-resorptive stimulus could be obtained with local zoledronate. We therefore expected that local zoledronate could prevent bone resorption and formation of fibrous tissue. It may be that implant micromotion is a too strong stimulus for even local zoledronate being able to completely prevent bone resorption. Another explanation could be that the single dose of zoledronate acts only as a defense again bone-resorption for a limited amount of time. Zoledronate, released from bone by osteoclastic resorption, could be slowly washed away from the implant-bone interface. By time the concentration will be too low to inhibit the continuous strong bone resorptive stimulus from micromotion.

In clinical practice, soaking the bone bed before implantation is a simple procedure. We know from a previous studies that the effect on implant osseointegration of local bisphosphonate is dose-dependent [29, 38]. Bisphosphonate bound to bone will only exert its effect on the osteoclast during bone resorption and intracellular internalization [39]. However, any cell, including bone-forming cells, can internalize unbound bisphosphonate. Removal of unbound bisphosphonate by irrigating the bone bed after soaking it with bisphosphonate is therefore of importance.

Conclusion

In conclusion, this study indicates that local treatment with zoledronate can reduce micromotion induced bone resorption, but not prevent it. Studies investigating the effect of different zoledronate doses and observation periods are needed.

Abbreviations

PE: polyethylene; PMMA: polymethylmethacrylate; RSA: Radiostereometric Analysis

Acknowledgements

The authors wish to thank Jane Pauli, Orthopaedic research Laboratory, Aarhus University Hospital, for technical expertise. The authors declare to have no professional or financial conflict of interest.

Authors'contributions

TJ, SK, JB, KS, and OR: Designed the study. TJ, SK, JB, and OR: performed the surgery. TJ and JSM: specimen preparation and histomorphometry. TJ, and JB: push-out test. TJ: Statistical analysis. TJ, SK, JSM, JB, KS, and OR: Interpretation of data. TJ wrote the first draft of the manuscript. SK, JSM, JB, KS, and OR: critically revision of manuscript. All authors read and approved the final manuscript.

Funding

This study was unconditionally funded by The Danish Ministry of Higher Education and Science.

Consent for publication

Not applicable.

Competing interests

The authors declare that they have no competing interests.

References

1. Kärrholm J, Borssén B, Löwenhielm G, Snorrason F. Does early micromotion matter? 4-7 year stereoradiographic follow-up of 84 cemented prostheses. J Bone Jt Surg - Br Vol. 1994;76:912–7.
2. Ryd L, Albrektsson E, Carlsson L, Dansgaard F, Herberts P, Regnér L, et al. Roentgen of knee of mechanical analysis loosening as a predictor continues. J Bone Jt Surg - Br Vol. 1995;77:377–83.
3. Nieuwenhuijse MJ, Valstar ER, Kaptein BL, Nelissen RGHH. Good diagnostic performance of early migration as a predictor of late aseptic loosening of acetabular cups: results from ten years of follow-up with Roentgen stereophotogrammetric analysis (RSA). J Bone Joint Surg Am. 2012;94:874–80.
4. Ollivere B, Wimhurst JA, Clark IM, Donell ST. Current concepts in osteolysis. J Bone Joint Surg Br. 2012;94:10–5.
5. Hilding MB, Yuan X, Ryd L. The stability of three different cementless tibial components. A randomized radiostereometric study in 45 knee arthroplasty patients. Acta Orthop Scand. 1995;66:21–7.
6. Aspenberg P, Herbertsson P. Periprosthetic bone resorption. J Bone Jt Surg Br. 1996;78:641–6.
7. Skripitz R, Aspenberg P. Pressure-induced periprosthetic osteolysis: a rat model. J Orthop Res. 2000;18:481–4.
8. Aspenberg P, Van der Vis H. Migration, particles, and fluid pressure. A discussion of causes of prosthetic loosening. Clin Orthop Relat Res. 1998:75–80.
9. Jakobsen T, Kold S, Baas J, Søballe K, Rahbek O. Sheep hip Arthroplasty model of failed implant Osseointegration. Open Orthop J. 2015;9:525–9.
10. Amirhosseini M, Andersson G, Aspenberg P, Fahlgren A. Mechanical instability and titanium particles induce similar transcriptomic changes in a rat model for periprosthetic osteolysis and aseptic loosening. Bone Reports. 2017;7:17–25.
11. Amirhosseini M, Madsen RV, Escott KJ, Bostrom M, Ross FP, Fahlgren A. GSK-3β inhibition suppresses instability-induced Osteolysis by a dual action on osteoblast and osteoclast differentiation. J Cell Physiol. 2017;
12. Goodman S, Gibon E, Yao Z. The basic science of Periprosthetic Osteolysis. Instr Course Lect. 2001:201–6.
13. Jacobs JJ, Roebuck KA, Archibeck M, Hallab NJ, Glant TT. Osteolysis: basic science. Clin Orthop Relat Res 2001:71–77.
14. Fleisch H. Development of bisphosphonates. Breast Cancer Res. 2002;4:30–4.
15. Shanbhag AS, Hasselman CT, Rubash HE. The John Charnley award. Inhibition of wear debris mediated osteolysis in a canine total hip arthroplasty model. Clin Orthop Relat Res. 1997:33–43.
16. Schilcher J, Palm L, Ivarsson I, Aspenberg P. Local bisphosphonate reduces migration and formation of radiolucent lines adjacent to cemented acetabular components. Bone Jt J. 2017;99:317–24.
17. Hilding M, Aspenberg P. Local peroperative treatment with a bisphosphonate improves the fixation of total knee prostheses: a

randomized, double-blind radiostereometric study of 50 patients. Acta Orthop. 2007;78:795–9.
18. Astrand J, Skripitz R, Skoglund B, Aspenberg PA. Rat model for testing pharmacologic treatments of pressure-related bone loss. Clin Orthop Relat Res. 2003:296–305.
19. Astrand J, Aspenberg P. Reduction of instability-induced bone resorption using bisphosphonates. Acta Orthop. 2002;73:24–30.
20. Søballe K, Chen X, Jensen TB, Kidder L, Bechtold JE. Alendronate treatment in the revision setting, with and without controlled implant motion: an experimental study in dogs. Acta Orthop. 2007;78:800–7.
21. Bechtold JE, Kubic V, Søballe KA. Controlled experimental model of revision implants. Acta Orthop Scand. 2001;72:642–9.
22. Jakobsen T, Kold S, Bechtold JE, Elmengaard B, Søballe K. Effect of topical alendronate treatment on fixation of implants inserted with bone compaction. Clin Orthop Relat Res. 2006;444:229–34.
23. Overgaard S, Søballe K, Jørgen H, Gundersen G. Efficiency of systematic sampling in histomorphometric bone research illustrated by hydroxyapatite-coated implants: optimizing the stereological vertical-section design. J Orthop Res. 2000;18:313–21.
24. Baas J. Adjuvant therapies of bone graft around non-cemented experimental orthopaedic implants. Acta Orthop. 2008;79:2–43.
25. Gundersen HJ, Bagger P, Bendtsen TF, Evans SM, Korbo L, Marcussen N, et al. The new stereological tools: disector, fractionator, nucleator and point sampled intercepts and their use in pathological research and diagnosis. APMIS. 1988;96:857–81.
26. Baddeley AJ, Gundersen HJ, Cruz-Orive LM. Estimation of surface area from vertical sections. J Microsc. 1986;142:259–76.
27. Bland JM, Altman DG. Statistics notes: the use of transformation when comparing two means. BMJ 1996;312:1153–1153.
28. Gatti D, Adami S. New bisphosphonates in the treatment of bone diseases. Drugs Aging. 1999;15:285–96.
29. Jakobsen T, Baas J, Bechtold JE, Elmengaard B, Søballe K. The effect of soaking allograft in bisphosphonate: a pilot dose-response study. Clin Orthop Relat Res. 2010;468:867–74.
30. Sørensen M, Barckman J, Bechtold JE, Soballe K, Baas J. Preclinical evaluation of Zoledronate to maintain bone allograft and improve implant fixation in. J Bone Jt Surg - Am Vol. 2013:1862–8.
31. van der Voort P, Pijls BG, Nieuwenhuijse MJ, Jasper J, Fiocco M, Plevier JWM, et al. Early subsidence of shape-closed hip arthroplasty stems is associated with late revision. A systematic review and meta-analysis of 24 RSA studies and 56 survival studies. Acta Orthop. 2015;86:575–85.
32. Giori NJ, Ryd L, Carter DR. Mechanical influences on tissue differentiation at bone-cement interfaces. J Arthroplast. 1995;10:514–22.
33. Carter DR, Fyhrie DP, Whalen RT. Trabecular bone density and loading history: regulation of connective tissue biology by mechanical energy. J Biomech. 1987;20:785–94.
34. Bechtold JE, Mouzin O, Kidder L, Part II. Implementation with loaded titanium implants and bone graft. Acta Orthop Scand. 2001;72:650–6.
35. Baas J, Elmengaard B, Jensen TB, Jakobsen T, Andersen NT, Soballe K. The effect of pretreating morselized allograft bone with rhBMP-2 and/or pamidronate on the fixation of porous Ti and HA-coated implants. Biomaterials. 2008;29:2915–22.
36. Jakobsen T, Kold S, Bechtold JE, Elmengaard B, Søballe K. Local alendronate increases fixation of implants inserted with bone compaction: 12-week canine study. J Orthop Res. 2007;25:432–41.
37. Kettenberger U, Ston J, Thein E, Procter P, Pioletti DP. Does locally delivered Zoledronate influence peri-implant bone formation? - Spatio-temporal monitoring of bone remodeling in vivo. Biomaterials. 2014;35:9995–10006.
38. Jakobsen T, Baas J, Bechtold JE, Elmengaard B, Søballe K. Soaking morselized allograft in bisphosphonate can impair implant fixation. Clin Orthop Relat Res. 2007;463:195–201.
39. Russell RGG. Bisphosphonates: mode of action and pharmacology. Pediatrics. 2007;119(Suppl):S150–62.

10

Patient Endorsement of the Outcome Measures in Rheumatology (OMERACT) Total Joint Replacement (TJR) clinical trial draft core domain set

Jasvinder A. Singh[1,2*], Michelle Dowsey[3] and Peter F. Choong[3]

Abstract

Background: A patient- and surgeon-Delphi-derived Outcome Measures in Rheumatology (OMERACT) draft core domain set for total joint arthroplasty (TJR) trials was recently developed. Our objective was to obtain further patient stakeholder endorsement of draft core domain set for TJR clinical trials.

Methods: We surveyed two patient groups: (1) OMERACT patient partners; and (2) patients who had undergone hip or knee TJR. Patients received an introductory email with explanations about the core domain set and instructions to rate the core domains, i.e., important aspects, of OMERACT TJR clinical trial draft core domain set. Rating was on a nominal scale, where 1–3 indicated a domain of limited importance, 4–6 an important, but not critical domain, and 7–9 a critical domain. We used Mann–Whitney test (a non-parametric test) to compare the distribution of ratings between the two groups.

Results: Thirty one survey participants from the OMERACT patient partner group and 118 knee/hip TJR patients responded with response rates of 66 and 80%, respectively. Majority of the survey respondents were female, 87 vs. 53%, and were 55 years or older, 57 vs. 94%. Median (interquartile range [IQR]) scores for six core domains by OMERACT and knee/hip TJR patient groups were, respectively: pain, 8 [8, 9] and 9 [8, 9]; function, 9 [8, 9] and 9 [8, 9]; patient satisfaction, 8 [8, 9] and 8 [7, 9]; revision surgery, 7 [7, 8] and 7 [5, 9]; adverse events, 8 [7, 9] and 8 [6, 9]; and death, 9 [6, 9] and 9 [4, 9]. No statistically significant differences in rating were noted for any of the six core domains between the two groups ($p \geq 0.31$). Among the additional domains, ratings for patient participation did not differ by group ($p = 0.98$), but ratings for cost were significantly different ($p = 0.005$). Patients provided qualitative feedback regarding core domains, and did not propose any modifications to the draft core domain set.

Conclusions: Two separate patient stakeholder groups endorsed the OMERACT TJR draft core domain set for TJR trials.

Background

Total Joint Replacement (TJR) is a very successful and cost effective surgical treatment for refractory end-stage arthritis in patients who report pain and/or functional limitation. Majority of the patients report impressive improvements in pain and function with this surgery [1, 2], while a small proportion have an unsatisfactory outcome from TJR [3, 4], including persistent pain and functional limitation [5–10]. Although hip and knee TJR are the most common joints replaced currently, we realize that TJR for other joints is also becoming more common in the recent years [11–15]. While the rapid advances in implant design and surgical techniques have occurred for TJR, TJR trial reporting has not kept pace with this quick evolution. Development of valid outcome measures, universal adoption and harmonization continues to be a big challenge. As a result, patients and surgeons have not been able to effectively capitalize on the large and growing body of data for cross study comparisons. Moreover, the heterogeneity in outcome measures used in TJR trials [16] prevents meta-analysis and literature

* Correspondence: Jasvinder.md@gmail.com
[1]University of Alabama at Birmingham, 510 20th Street S, Faculty Office Tower 805B, Birmingham, AL 35294, USA
[2]Birmingham Veterans Affairs Medical Center, 700 19th St S, Birmingham, AL 35233, USA
Full list of author information is available at the end of the article

synthesis and this is compounded by the limited validity of several of the outcome instruments being used [17]. Recent studies confirmed that these challenges continue in knee TJR trials [18, 19]. In 2006, our group recognized the need for consensus and harmonization of reporting of TJR trials [20]. We have built capacity and capability by undertaking several systematic reviews and building collaborations, which have continued over the last decade. This has led to the formation of an international Working group (WG) on TJR clinical trial outcomes that is now an orthopedist-patient-rheumatologist-methodologist multi-stakeholder collaborative [21].

Using the Outcomes Measures in Rheumatology (OMERACT) filter for developing core measurement sets, we developed a multi-stakeholder endorsed TJR trial draft core domain set, based on systematic literature reviews, followed by input from patients and surgeons using a Delphi process [21] and mailed surveys. The OMERACT TJR draft core domain set (for any joint) included the following: Pain, function, patient satisfaction, revision, adverse events, and death [21]. The OMERACT TJR trial draft core domain set was developed based on systematic literature reviews, several multi-stakeholder discussions at OMERACT and various orthopedic meetings that included leaders in arthroplasty registries, trials and outcome science, Delphi surveys and a face-to-face discussion of each potential core domains with patients, orthopedic surgeons, methodologist, physical and occupational therapists and rheumatologists, details provided elsewhere [21]. This outcome draft core domain set is consistent with previous systematic reviews of patient outcomes after TJR and qualitative studies of patient perspective of TJR outcomes [3, 16, 22–24]. In a subsequent consensus-building exercise, we achieved a complete consensus for this draft TJR core domain set with two independent groups of orthopaedic surgeons, who endorsed all six core domains [25].

As part of our long-term objective to develop and implement a TJR core measurement set, the aim of the current study was to obtain further endorsement of the OMERACT TJR trial draft core domain set, for any TJR for any joint, as defined previously [21]. We aimed to survey new patient groups, who are representative internationally, and are independent of the patient group that helped us develop the original draft core domain set. Another objective was to identify whether these independent patient surveys find evidence for modifying our preliminary OMERACT TJR trial core. This study describes the process of obtaining further endorsement of the OMERACT TJR trial draft core domain set for any joint from a wider patient audience.

Methods

We surveyed two groups of patients. The first group included the OMERACT patient research partner (PRPs), a group of patients with rheumatic diseases (predominantly arthritis, but also including patients with immune conditions) who had attended one of the biannual OMERACT meetings including the 2016 OMERACT meeting at Whistler, Canada ($n = 47$). The second group was a cohort of patients who had undergone hip or knee replacement at St. Vincent's Private Hospital (SVPH), Melbourne, Australia between January 2013 and December 2014 ($n = 147$). This cohort was identified through the St. Vincent's Melbourne Arthroplasty Registry (SMART), approved by the Human ethics committee at St. Vincent's Hospital, Australia (HREC-A 100/14; there is no published protocol). We recruited patients after knee or hip TJR, since our goal was to develop a core domain set for TJR trials, and therefore recruiting pre-operative patients does not address our main question.

We developed and pre-tested a survey questionnaire, which was reviewed by several colleagues with previous TJR attending the OMERACT meeting, study team members as well as patients in the SMART registry. Subsequently, it was iteratively modified, based on the feedback, including clarification of the questions and simplification of the cover letter, the background and the purpose of the questionnaire. The survey queried patient characteristics and the importance of each domain of the OMERACT TJR trial draft core domain set, including the six core areas/domains (pain, function [ability to function in society, work; work productivity, employability; disability; work disability], patient satisfaction [satisfaction with the outcome, satisfaction with the procedure], revision surgery, adverse event and death) and two optional areas/domains (patient participation in life/social activities, cost).

Patients rated each core domain on a 1–9 scale, developed by the GRADE group, used by us for rating outcomes in previous studies of development of treatment guideline [26, 27] and our previous studies ranking disease core domains [25, 28]: 1–3 indicated a domain of limited importance, 4–6 an important, but not critical domain, and 7–9 a critically important domain. Surveys were emailed to both groups of patients. In addition, a hard copy was mailed to patients from the SVPH cohort without email addresses ($n = 23$). Patients completed these annonymized surveys using Survey Monkey link sent to their emails or a mailed copy. Those not responding received two reminders at least 1-week apart.

We defined the purpose of patient surveys in our previous paper, which was to assess whether patients could achieve consensus on the current core domain set for TJR trials, seek patient endorsement of the core domain set and in case of any suggestions for modification/s, the reasons for change in core domains [21]. We defined the consensus as follows. If both groups of patients would rate each core domain between 7–9, i.e., critical, this would constitute complete consensus. If both patient groups rated a majority of the six core domains, but not all, as critical, we would consider this as incomplete consensus. In case of incomplete consensus, we would have further discussion with patients and we would plan to modify the draft TJR trial core domain set for any joint. If the patient groups achieved complete consensus on core domains, given the previous complete consensus by orthopaedic surgeons [25], the draft TJR core domain set would be considered endorsed by both patients and orthopaedic surgeons at this stage. We calculated summary statistics including proportions and medians (interquartile range), as applicable, separately for the OMERACT PRP and the SVPH patient cohorts. We used a non-parametric test, Mann–Whitney to compare the distribution of ratings between the two groups and considered a p-value <0.05 to be statistically significant.

Results

Survey response rates were good to excellent, 66% for OMERACT PRPs and 80%, for SVPH patients. The two cohorts differed in gender, age and diagnosis (Table 1). Compared to the SVPH cohort, OMERACT PRP group had greater proportions of females, 87 vs. 53%, those with a diagnosis of RA, 4 vs. 54%, and was younger (Table 1). 85% of OMERACT and 97% of SVPH patients had a diagnosis of arthritis. A key difference was that 27% of OMERACT and 100% of the SVPH cohort had had a joint replacement.

Despite these differences, both cohorts rated OMERACT TJR clinical trials core domains similarly (Table 2). On a 1 to 9 scale, all six-core domains were rated as critical domains (score 7–9); the additional domains of cost and participation were scored important to critical (scores 6–8) (Table 2). None of the core domain set ratings differed significantly between the two groups (Table 2). For additional domains, participation ratings were not statistically significantly different by group but rating for cost as an additional domain was statistically significantly higher for the SVPH Cohort compared to the OMERACT patient cohort ($p = 0.005$; Table 2).

We received additional free text comments, which provided insight into defining these core domains further and suggestions as to which instruments we should consider for the next step in the development of the TJR clinical trial core measurement set (Additional file 1). Additional areas brought up for consideration included several that are either included as core domain or are closely related to it: [1] life of an implant (same as the core domain, revision); [2] Recovery and rehabilitation (similar to pain, function or functional ability, satisfaction); [3] Independence (similar to function or functional ability).

Table 1 Participant characteristics of the two patient cohorts

	OMERACT Patient research partner (PRP) Cohort survey ($N = 47$)	Total Joint Replacement SVPH Cohort ($N = 147$)
# Survey participants	$N = 31$ (66%)	$N = 118^a$ (80%)
% Male[b]	4 (13%)	50 (47%)
Age category[b]		
18-24	0	0
25-34	1 (3%)	0
35-44	3 (10%)	1 (1%)
45-54	9 (30%)	5 (5%)
55-64	11 (37%)	26 (25%)
65-74	6 (20%)	36 (34%)
≥75	0	37 (35%)
Missing	2 (7%)	2
Had a joint replacement	13 (42%)	107 (100%)
Type of arthritis		
Osteoarthritis	2 (7%)	93 (87%)
Rheumatoid arthritis	15 (54%)	4 (4%)
Other inflammatory arthritis	7 (26%)	7 (6%)
Joint aches/pains, no arthritis diagnosed or no joint aches/pains	4 (15%)	3 (3%)

[a]Of the 147 patients who received the survey (email, $n = 124$; mailed survey, $n = 23$), 118 responded (email, $n = 109$; mailed survey, $n = 9$), of which 107 were usable (email, $n = 99$; mailed survey, $n = 9$). Therefore, most proportions are out of 107 (73% valid surveys)

[b]Missing responses for variables for OMERACT PRPs vs. TJR SVPH cohorts: sex: 0 vs. 2; age, 0 vs. 2

Discussion

This study describes patient consensus and endorsement of the OMERACT TJR trial draft core domain set, which was first developed and endorsed with multi-stakeholder input in 2014, including patients and surgeons, after completing several systematic reviews that helped identify potential core domain set [21]. As described in our previous study, the current study completes step 5, i.e., patient endorsement of the preliminary OMERACT TJR trial core domain set, such that we now have an OMERACT TJR trial draft core domain set. We specified a priori that patients and surgeons were our two key stakeholders [21]. Therefore, the completion of this patient survey that followed surgeon survey [25], which was published in the interim, provided us with consensus we were aiming for TJR trial core domain set. Both surgeons and patients have achieved consensus on TJR trial core domain set consisting of six core domains, and no modification is needed, based on the results of these two studies. Several findings in this study merit further discussion.

Table 2 Patient Consensus on OMERACT TJR Clinical Trial Core Areas/Domains

	OMERACT PRP ($n = 31$) Median [IQR]	SVPH Cohort ($n = 118$[a]) Median [IQR]	p-value (Mann–Whitney test)
Core Domains to be reported in every TJR clinical trial			
Joint Pain	8 [8, 9]	9 [8, 9]	0.75
Function or functional ability (ability to function in society, work; work productivity, employability; disability; work disability)	9 [8, 9]	9 [8, 9]	0.31
Patient Satisfaction (satisfaction with the outcome, satisfaction with the procedure)	8 [8, 9]	8 [7, 9]	0.86
Revision surgery (including reoperation)	7 [7, 8]	7 [5, 9]	0.97
Adverse events (total and specific)	8 [7, 9]	8 [6, 9]	0.84
Death	9 [6, 9]	9 [4, 9]	0.70
Additional domains for consideration for reporting in TJR clinical trials			
Patient Participation	8 [6.5, 8]	7 [6, 9]	0.98
Cost	6 [5, 7]	7 [6, 8]	0.005

[a]118 responded, of which 107 had valid, analyzable responses

A key aspect of core domain development is its endorsement by a wider group of stakeholders. The OMERACT process uses cutting-edge methodological science and rigor and is a data-driven and consensus-based development of outcome instruments for clinical trials. The OMERACT filter 2.0 provides a well-described framework for the development of core domain and core measurement sets [29]. Although this process of developing a multi-stakeholder group and developing the core domain set has taken a long time since we started a decade ago, we have followed the OMERACT methodology rigorously [21]. We believe that this rigor will ultimately help with a wider acceptance and uptake of the TJR trial core domain set. We have now developed core domain set for TJR trials based on the OMERACT filter 2.0 [29, 30].

Our current study shows that two groups of patients endorsed the OMERACT TJR trial preliminary core domain set, rating all six domains as critical. Despite differences in patient characteristics, the ratings by two cohorts were similar, which is a testament to a rigorous process that we have used to develop this draft core domain set. This draft TJR trial core domain set has now been endorsed by several independent groups of patients and orthopaedic surgeons, two key stakeholders.

The methodology for core domain set development for TJR trials was a standard method of defining every domain that is core to the condition, i.e., there is no prioritization [29–31]. Therefore, the patient survey elicited responses whether each of the core/additional domains was core to TJR outcome or not at its own merit, without asking them to prioritize the domains. The last two steps in this process are dissemination and a wider endorsement of the core domain set by orthopedic surgeons, and the development, validation and endorsement of a TJR trial core measurement set by a multi-stakeholder group, and possible co-branding of this OMERACT TJR trial draft core domain set and core measurement set by interested orthopedic societies.

This study shows that a few patients identified additional potential domains, including recovery and rehabilitation. It may be debated whether these are already represented by the core domains currently included i.e. pain, function or functional ability and patient satisfaction. The definitions for function [ability to function in society, work; work productivity, employability; disability; work disability] and satisfaction [[satisfaction with the outcome, satisfaction with the procedure] and domain of pain indicated to us that recovery and rehabilitation are processes that are intertwined with these core domains and perhaps already captured to some extent with these domains. However, in order to ensure appropriate rigor and inclusiveness, further discussions are required with wide stakeholder input, regarding whether these should be optional domains or be on research agenda.

We noted that real-world concerns were also brought up by a few participants related to TJR that are not relevant for TJR clinical trial reporting. Examples include access to and wait times for TJR, which are related to health care access and are country and setting-specific contextual factors, likely relevant for observational studies and/or public policy discussions. These are important policy concerns, but not relevant to TJR clinical trial core domain selection.

Our study has several limitations. Survey response rates were 66 and 80%, but we do not have non-responder characteristics to understand how non-response influenced our findings. However, the high response rate should give readers more confidence in these findings. To strengthen our conclusions, we attempted to get a wide perspective by polling representative groups, including patients who had undergone knee/hip TJR. We surveyed only adults and focused on knee or hip TJR trials. These findings cannot be generalized to TJR that involve other joints. Study strengths included the assessment of the validity of core domain sets in two patient populations, an international representativeness of sample, robustness of findings despite patient characteristic differences in survey participants, and a high response rate.

Conclusions

In conclusion, two patient groups in separate surveys have now endorsed the OMERACT TJR trial draft core domain set. The OMERACT TJR draft core domain set was previously developed with multi-stakeholder input, including patients and surgeons. All current core and additional domains were endorsed as they are, without any modification. With a parallel consensus from orthopaedic surgeons showing consensus for the 6 domains (In a different study of the same core domains), both patients have achieved consensus on TJR trial draft core domain set consisting of six core domains, and based on the results of these two studies, no modification is needed. We also obtained important feedback regarding these domains, which will be instrumental in our next steps of instrument selection for each of the core domains. The planning is currently underway to seek a wider dissemination to and/or endorsement by general membership of arthroplasty surgeon societies and/or OMERACT. If the draft core domain set is also endorsed by a wider orthopedic society membership, we will proceed with the development of first consensus-based data-driven TJR trial core measurement set.

Abbreviations

OMERACT: Outcome Measures in Rheumatology; PRPs: Patient research partner; SMART: St. Vincent's Melbourne Arthroplasty Registry; SVPH: St. Vincent's Private Hospital; TJR: Total Joint Replacement; WG: Working Group

Acknowledgements

A/Prof Dowsey holds a National Health & Medical Research Council Career Development Fellowship (APP1122526). We thank the patients for participating in this study.

Funding

No funding support was obtained for this study.

Authors' contributions

JAS designed the study, developed study protocol, and survey, collected data, reviewed analyses and wrote the first draft of the paper. MD reviewed the protocol, helped with data collection and reviewed analyses. PC reviewed the protocol and reviewed analyses. All authors revised the manuscript, read and approved the final manuscript.

Author's information

JAS and PC are the co-chairs of the OMERACT Working Group assessing the outcome measures in arthroplasty. JAS has served as expert/lead on task forces for the specialty societies and the US FDA.

"The views expressed in this article are those of the authors and do not necessarily reflect the position or policy of the Department of Veterans Affairs or the United States government."

Competing interests

JAS is a member of the Editorial Board of BMC Musculoskeletal Disorders. JAS has received research grants from Takeda and Savient and consultant fees from Savient, Takeda, Regeneron and Allergan. JAS is a member of the executive committee of OMERACT, an organization that develops outcome measures in rheumatology and receives arms-length funding from 36 companies; a member of the American College of Rheumatology's Guidelines Subcommittee of the Quality of Care Committee; and a member of the Veterans Affairs Rheumatology Field Advisory Committee. Michael Dohm receives no direct funding and has no financial conflicts. He is a member of the American Joint Replacement Registry (AJRR) and Chairman of the Data Elements Committee as well as an associate member of the International Society of Arthroplasty Registers (ISAR), is a member of the evidence based practice committee for AAHKS and Chairman of the AAOS Outcome Special Interest Group. PC has received consultancy fees from DePuy, Zimmer and Stryker as part of surgeon design or research teams. PC's and MD's institution has received research grant funding from Allergan, DePuy and Medacta.

Consent for publication

Not applicable.

Author details

[1]University of Alabama at Birmingham, 510 20th Street S, Faculty Office Tower 805B, Birmingham, AL 35294, USA. [2]Birmingham Veterans Affairs Medical Center, 700 19th St S, Birmingham, AL 35233, USA. [3]Department of Surgery, University of Melbourne, St. Vincent's Hospital, Melbourne, Australia.

References

1. Ethgen O, Bruyere O, Richy F, Dardennes C, Reginster JY. Health-related quality of life in total hip and total knee arthroplasty. A qualitative and systematic review of the literature. J Bone Joint Surg Am. 2004;86-A(5):963–74.
2. Singh JA. Epidemiology of knee and hip arthroplasty: a systematic review. Open Orthop J. 2011;5:80–5.
3. Bourne RB, Chesworth BM, Davis AM, Mahomed NN, Charron KD. Patient satisfaction after total knee arthroplasty: who is satisfied and who is not? Clin Orthop Relat Res. 2010;468(1):57–63.
4. Scott CE, Howie CR, MacDonald D, Biant LC. Predicting dissatisfaction following total knee replacement: a prospective study of 1217 patients. J Bone Joint Surg (Br). 2010;92(9):1253–8.
5. Singh JA, Lewallen DG. Better functional and similar pain outcomes in osteoarthritis compared to rheumatoid arthritis after primary total knee arthroplasty: a cohort study. Arthritis Care Res. 2013;65(12):1936–41.
6. Singh JA, Lewallen DG. Medical and psychological comorbidity predicts poor pain outcomes after total knee arthroplasty. Rheumatology (Oxford). 2013;52(5):916–23.
7. Singh JA, Gabriel SE, Lewallen DG. Higher body mass index is not associated with worse pain outcomes after primary or revision total knee arthroplasty. J Arthroplasty. 2011;26(3):366–74. e1.
8. Singh JA, Lewallen D. Age, gender, obesity, and depression are associated with patient-related pain and function outcome after revision total hip arthroplasty. Clin Rheumatol. 2009;28(12):1419–30.
9. Brander V, Gondek S, Martin E, Stulberg SD. Pain and depression influence outcome 5 years after knee replacement surgery. Clin Orthop Relat Res. 2007;464:21–6.
10. Brander VA, Stulberg SD, Adams AD, Harden RN, Bruehl S, Stanos SP, et al. Predicting total knee replacement pain: a prospective, observational study. Clin Orthop Relat Res. 2003;416:27–36.
11. Singh JA, Ramachandran R. Time trends in total ankle arthroplasty in the USA: a study of the National Inpatient Sample. Clin Rheumatol. 2016;35(1):239–45.

12. Singh JA, Ramachandran R. Sex differences in characteristics, utilization, and outcomes of patient undergoing total elbow arthroplasty: a study of the US nationwide inpatient sample. Clin Rheumatol. 2016;35(3):723–31.
13. Singh JA, Ramachandran R. Age-related differences in the use of total shoulder arthroplasty over time: use and outcomes. Bone Joint J. 2015;97-B(10):1385–9.
14. Jain NB, Higgins LD, Guller U, Pietrobon R, Katz JN. Trends in the epidemiology of total shoulder arthroplasty in the United States from 1990–2000. Arthritis Rheum. 2006;55(4):591–7.
15. Gay DM, Lyman S, Do H, Hotchkiss RN, Marx RG, Daluiski A. Indications and reoperation rates for total elbow arthroplasty: an analysis of trends in New York State. J Bone Joint Surg Am. 2012;94(2):110–7.
16. Riddle DL, Stratford PW, Bowman DH. Findings of extensive variation in the types of outcome measures used in hip and knee replacement clinical trials: a systematic review. Arthritis Rheum. 2008;59(6):876–83.
17. Singh J, Sloan JA, Johanson NA. Challenges with health-related quality of life assessment in arthroplasty patients: problems and solutions. J Am Acad Orthop Surg. 2010;18(2):72–82.
18. Gagnier JJ, Mullins M, Huang H, Marinac-Dabic D, Ghambaryan A, Eloff B, et al. A Systematic Review of Measurement Properties of Patient-Reported Outcome Measures Used in Patients Undergoing Total Knee Arthroplasty. J Arthroplasty. 2017.
19. Lange T, Rataj E, Kopkow C, Lützner J, Günther K-P, Schmitt J. Outcome Assessment in Total Knee Arthroplasty: A Systematic Review and Critical Appraisal. J Arthroplasty. 2017;32(2):653–65.e1.
20. Riddle DL, Stratford PW, Singh JA, Strand CV. Variation in outcome measures in hip and knee arthroplasty clinical trials: a proposed approach to achieving consensus. J Rheumatol. 2009;36(9):2050–6.
21. Singh JA, Dohm M, Sprowson AP, Wall PD, Richards BL, Gossec L, et al. Outcome Domains and Measures in Total Joint Replacement Clinical Trials: Can We Harmonize Them? An OMERACT Collaborative Initiative. J Rheumatol. 2015;42:2496-502.
22. Mancuso CA, Sculco TP, Wickiewicz TL, Jones EC, Robbins L, Warren RF, et al. Patients' expectations of knee surgery. J Bone Joint Surg Am. 2001;83-A(7):1005–12.
23. Santaguida PL, Hawker GA, Hudak PL, Glazier R, Mahomed NN, Kreder HJ, et al. Patient characteristics affecting the prognosis of total hip and knee joint arthroplasty: a systematic review. Can J Surg. 2008;51(6):428–36.
24. Baker PN, van der Meulen JH, Lewsey J, Gregg PJ. The role of pain and function in determining patient satisfaction after total knee replacement. Data from the National Joint Registry for England and Wales. J Bone Joint Surg (Br). 2007;89(7):893–900.
25. Singh JA, Dohm M, Choong PF. Consensus on draft OMERACT core domains for clinical trials of Total Joint Replacement outcome by orthopaedic surgeons: a report from the International consensus on outcome measures in TJR trials (I-COMiTT) group. BMC Musculoskelet Disord. 2017;18(1):45.
26. Singh JA, Saag KG, Bridges Jr SL, Akl EA, Bannuru RR, Sullivan MC, et al. 2015 American College of Rheumatology Guideline for the Treatment of Rheumatoid Arthritis. Arthritis Rheumatol. 2016;68(1):1–26.
27. Singh JA, Furst DE, Bharat A, Curtis JR, Kavanaugh AF, Kremer JM, et al. 2012 update of the 2008 American College of Rheumatology recommendations for the use of disease-modifying antirheumatic drugs and biologic agents in the treatment of rheumatoid arthritis. Arthritis Care Res. 2012;64(5):625–39.
28. Singh JA, Dohm M. Towards Consensus on the Reporting of Core Outcome Domains in Total Joint Replacement Clinical Trials: The Derivation of the Preliminary Core Outcome Domain Set. J Arthritis. 2016;5:6.
29. Boers M, Kirwan JR, Wells G, Beaton D, Gossec L, d'Agostino MA, et al. Developing core outcome measurement sets for clinical trials: OMERACT filter 2.0. J Clin Epidemiol. 2014;67(7):745–53.
30. Boers M, Kirwan JR, Gossec L, Conaghan PG, D'Agostino MA, Bingham 3rd CO, et al. How to choose core outcome measurement sets for clinical trials: OMERACT 11 approves filter 2.0. J Rheumatol. 2014;41(5):1025–30.
31. Boers M, Brooks P, Strand CV, Tugwell P. The OMERACT filter for Outcome Measures in Rheumatology. J Rheumatol. 1998;25(2):198–9.

11

Clinical and radiographic outcome of dynamic cervical implant (DCI) arthroplasty for degenerative cervical disc disease: a minimal five-year follow-up

Lin-nan Wang, Bo-wen Hu, Lei Wang[*†], Yue-ming Song[*†], Xi Yang, Li-min Liu and Hao Liu

Abstract

Background: To evaluate the mid- to long-term clinical and radiographic outcomes of anterior cervical discectomy and dynamic cervical implant (DCI) arthroplasty for degenerative cervical disc disease.

Methods: From April 2010 to October 2010, 38 patients with single- or double-level cervical disc herniation underwent anterior cervical discectomy and DCI arthroplasty. The clinical results and radiographic outcomes of these 38 patients (42 levels) were retrospectively evaluated. The clinical results included the visual analogue scale, Japanese Orthopaedic Association score, Neck Disability Index score, 36-item short form health survey questionnaire, and incidences of complications and neurological deterioration. Radiographic results including cervical alignment, intervertebral height, cervical range of motion (ROM), ROM of the functional spinal unit, adjacent intervertebral ROM, migration, subsidence, and heterotopic ossification (HO) were assessed on plain radiography, three-dimensional computed tomography, and magnetic resonance imaging.

Results: The mean follow-up period was 72.3 months (range 68–78 months). During follow-up, all patients showed significant improvements in the visual analogue scale score, Japanese Orthopaedic Association score, Neck Disability Index score, 36-item short form health survey physical component summary score and mental component summary score. The ROM of the functional spinal unit was partly reduced. The DCI migrated forward in 10 of 42 (23.8%) cases, and HO was detected in 24 of the 42 (57.1%) DCI segments. Subsidence was observed in 14 of 42 (33.3%) DCI segments. Two patients experienced symptom recurrence, and were treated conservatively.

Conclusions: The clinical efficacy of DCI arthroplasty was maintained during mid- to long-term follow-up. HO formation is a common phenomenon, leading to a substantial decrease in ROM at the index level and recurrence of neurological symptoms. The incidence of implant subsidence and migration is relatively high, leaving a potential risk of symptoms at the index level and adjacent segment degeneration. We consider that the first choice for patients with degenerative cervical disc disease should still be total disc replacement or anterior cervical discectomy and fusion, rather than DCI arthroplasty.

Keywords: Dynamic cervical implant, Degenerative cervical disc disease, Heterotopic ossification, Anterior migration, Subsidence

* Correspondence: wang_lei13245@163.com; prof_songyueming@163.com
†Equal contributors
Department of Orthopedics, West China Hospital, Sichuan University, 37 Guoxue Rd, Chengdu 610041, China

Background

The standard anterior surgical procedure for degenerative cervical disc disease is currently anterior cervical discectomy and fusion (ACDF). ACDF achieves a satisfactory clinical outcome and fusion rate; however, it also increases the motion and intradiscal pressure of the adjacent segments [1, 2], resulting in adjacent segment degeneration (ASD) [3, 4]. This complication led to the search for motion-preserving alternative procedures that could provide sufficient stability and simultaneously decrease the rate of ASD [5–7]. The most common non-fusion technique is total disc replacement (TDR). Several randomized controlled trials have reported that TDR has equivalent or superior clinical outcomes and a lower reoperation rate for surgical or adjacent segments than ACDF [8–10]. However, some studies reported that TDR has limitations such as a high rate of heterotopic ossification (HO) and spontaneous fusion [11–13].

The first-generation dynamic cervical implant (DCI) was designed by Matgé in 2002. The second-generation DCI was produced by Paradigm Spine (New York, NY, USA) in 2005, and has been used in clinical practice since 2008 [14]. Several reports have focused on the clinical and radiographic outcomes of DCI cases [15–18]; all such studies achieved satisfactory clinical and radiographic outcomes during an average follow-up period of 24 months. However, mid- to long-term follow-up results are still lacking. Therefore, we retrospectively investigated the clinical and radiographic outcomes of patients who underwent DCI arthroplasty for degenerative cervical disc disease and had a minimum follow-up of 5 years. Clinical and radiographic analyses were used to investigate the mid- to long-term efficacy of the second-generation DCI product.

Methods

This was a retrospective study. Between April 2010 to October 2010, 38 patients with single- or double-level degenerative disc disease underwent anterior cervical discectomy and DCI arthroplasty in our department. These patients were those aged over 18 years with single- or double-level cervical disc herniation for whom conservative treatment had failed. Exclusion criteria are shown in Table 1. The diagnosis and intended operative level(s) were determined from the combination of medical history, physical examination, and radiographic imaging including preoperative plain radiography (in the lateral, flexion, and extension positions), three-dimensional computed tomography (3D-CT), and magnetic resonance imaging (MRI). The general characteristics of these patients are shown in Table 2.

Table 1 Exclusion criteria for anterior cervical discectomy and DCI arthroplasty

Exclusion criteria
Segmental instability (intervertebral motion>11°or 3 mm)
Advanced degenerative changes (marked reduction or absence of intervertebral motion or height)
Facet joint arthrosis or spondylosis
Cervical kyphosis
Active infection
Osteoporosis
Inflammatory spondloarthropathies such as ankylosing spondylitis or rheumatoid arthritis
Expected cord edema and myelomalacia
Known allergy to titanium
Previous cervical spine surgery

Surgical procedure

All surgeries were performed by the same spine surgeon, who had over 20 years of experience. Surgeries were conducted using a standard anterior cervical approach and discectomy. Under general anesthesia, the patients were placed in the supine position with the neck slightly extended. Through a right cervical incision, the target segment was exposed with the assistance of intraoperative C-arm X-ray. The anterior longitudinal ligament was opened, and the discectomy procedure was then performed. Cartilaginous endplates and osteophytes on the posterior edge of the vertebral body were excised

Table 2 General information of involved patients

General information	Data
Number of patients	38
Mean age in years (range)	56.8(36~ 78)
Gender (male/female)	18/20
Mean follow-up length in months (range)	72.3(68–78)
Pathogenesis	
Simple disc herniation	18
Combined osteophyte formation	20
Diagnosis	
Radiculopathy	15
Myelopathy	11
Myeloradiculopathy	12
Implanted levels	
C3~ 4	3
C4~ 5	16
C5~ 6	18
C6~ 7	5
In total	42
Operation levels	
1 level	34
2 levels	4

with a high-speed drill while the bony endplates were protected properly. After sufficient decompression, an appropriately sized DCI was implanted into the intervertebral space under X-ray monitoring. The distance between the anterior/posterior edge of the DCI and the edge of the vertebral body was controlled within a range of 2–3 mm, and the lateral boundary did not exceed the Luschka joint. A drainage tube was left in the wound, and removed within 24 h. Patients were braced in a cervical collar for 1 week, and were then permitted to begin gradual mobilization under the guidance of doctors.

Evaluation

Clinical outcomes

As standard procedure in our department, all patients with degenerative cervical disc disease undergo a neurological examination and complete an extensive questionnaire, including the visual analogue scale (VAS), Japanese Orthopaedic Association (JOA) score, Neck Disability Index (NDI) score, and 36-Item Short Form Health Survey questionnaire (SF-36) preoperatively, at postoperative 1, 12, and 24 months, and at final follow-up.

Radiological indications

Plain radiography (in the lateral, flexion, and extension positions) and 3D-CT were conducted preoperatively, at 6, 12, and 24 months postoperatively, and at final follow-up. Pre- and postoperative cervical lordosis was measured on lateral radiographs using the cervical curvature index (Fig. 1), as described by Ishihara [19]. The intervertebral height was measured as the distance between the midpoint of the upper endplate of the upper vertebral body and the midpoint of the inferior endplate of the lower vertebral body (Fig. 1). The cervical spine range of motion (ROM), ROM of the functional spinal unit (FSU), and adjacent intervertebral space were calculated using the Cobb's method on full flexion and extension radiography [20] (Fig. 1). Migration and subsidence of the implant were measured and recorded. Subsidence was defined as a loss of height of more than 3 mm [21]. HO was also recorded.

Data were expressed as the mean ± standard deviation. Results were analyzed statistically with the paired Student's t-test using SPSS 21.0 software (SPSS Inc., Chicago, Illinois). A p value of less than 0.05 was taken to indicate a significant difference.

Results

The mean follow-up period was 72.3 months (range 68–78 months). In total, 42 levels from 38 patients were included. There were no surgical complications such as wound infection, leakage of cerebrospinal fluid, dysphagia, and/or hoarseness detected throughout the entire follow-up period. During the follow-up period, two patients (5.2%) experienced symptom recurrence at the index level due to a newly-emerging osteophyte at the posterior border of the vertebra; these symptoms were relieved after conservative treatment. A total of six adjacent operation levels had ROM > 11°, indicating that the adjacent level was unstable, but there were no symptoms.

Clinical outcomes

All patients showed significant postoperative improvement in neurological symptoms. The clinical parameters improved significantly after surgery, and the effect remained at final follow-up. The mean JOA score significantly increased from 8.5 ± 1.4 preoperatively to 15.4 ± 1.8 at final follow-up (Fig. 2). The recovery rate of the JOA score was 81.1%, which satisfied the criterion for clinical efficacy. The mean NDI score significantly decreased from 41.3 ± 4.2 preoperatively to 14.6 ± 3.4 at final follow-up (Fig. 2). The average VAS score significantly decreased from 7.5 ± 0.5 preoperatively to 1.8 ± 0.4 at final follow-up (Fig. 2). The SF-36 physical component summary (PCS) score

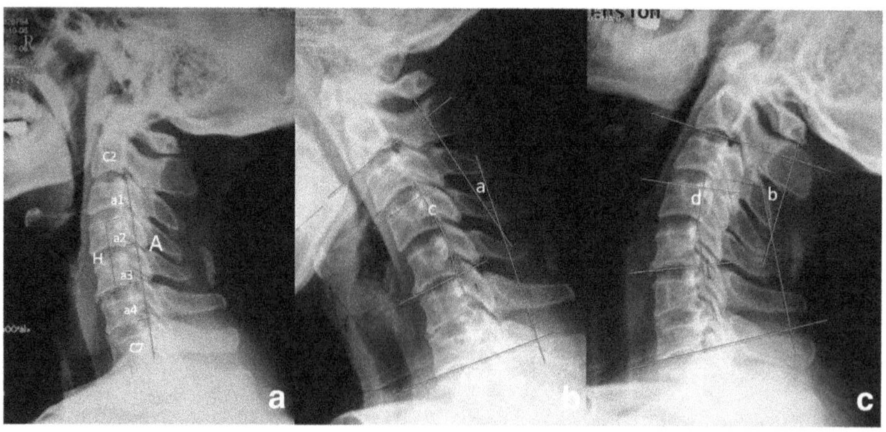

Fig. 1 Lateral radiograph showing evaluation of the cervical curvature index (CCI = (a1 + a2 + a3 + a4)/A), intervertebral height (H), the ROM of cervical spine (**a** + **b**), and the ROM of FSU (**c** + **d**)

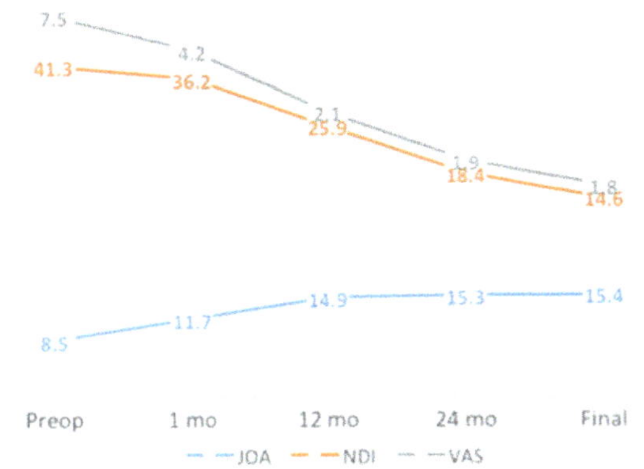

Fig. 2 JOA score, NDI score and VAS score of different time-points for involved patients

increased significantly from 30.4 ± 5.2 preoperatively to 49.3 ± 6.7 at final follow-up (Fig. 3). The SF-36 mental component summary (MCS) score increased significantly from 33.1 ± 5.1 preoperatively to 54.1 ± 7.6 at final follow-up (Fig. 3).

Radiographic analysis

Two spine surgeons evaluated all radiographs independently. When there was a difference in opinion between the two surgeons, an additional radiologist made the final decision. Ten of the 42 (23.8%) DCIs migrated forward (Fig. 4). HO was detected in 24 of the 42 (57.1%) DCI segments (Fig. 5). The mean cervical curvature index (CCI) was 0.23 ± 0.04 preoperatively, and 0.21 ± 0.04 at final follow-up (Fig. 6); however, this change was not significant.

The average intervertebral height on standard lateral radiographs increased from 35.2 ± 3.2 mm preoperatively to 39.5 ± 2.8 mm at 1 month postoperatively and 38.4 ± 3.1 mm at 24 months postoperatively, but decreased to

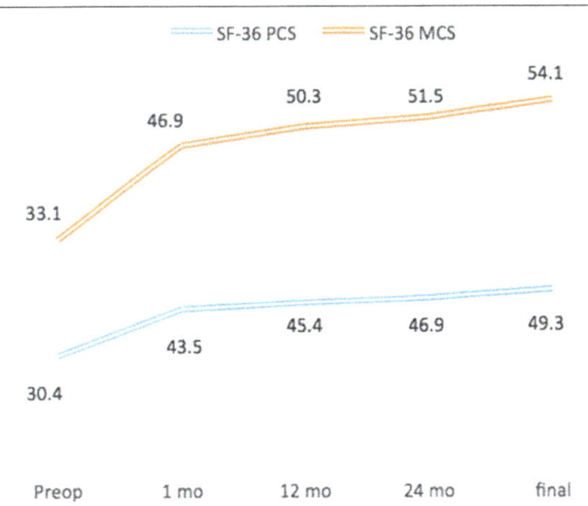

Fig. 3 SF-36 PCS and SF-36 MCS of different time-points for involved patients

36.0 ± 3.5 mm at final follow-up (Fig. 6); there was a significant difference between the value at 1 month postoperatively and that at final follow-up ($p < 0.05$). Subsidence occurred in 14 of 42 (33.3%) DCIs. An image from a representative patient is shown in Fig. 7.

The ROM of the cervical spine was 58.1° ± 5.8° preoperatively, 59.2° ± 6.7° at 24 months postoperatively, and 56.9° ± 7.1° at final follow-up (Fig. 6). There was no significant change in ROM during the follow-up period. The average ROM of the FSU was 10.7° ± 2.6° preoperatively, 9.5° ± 2.1° at 24 months postoperatively, and 4.4° ± 1.3° at final follow-up (Fig. 8). The elastic effect was well maintained at the 24-month follow-up, but had significantly decreased at the final follow-up (p < 0.05). The ROM of the upper adjacent operation level was 8.4° ± 2.4°preoperatively, and 8.6° ± 2.5°at final follow-up. The ROM of the lower adjacent operation level was 8.1° ± 1.9°preoperatively, and 8.6° ± 2.5°at final follow-up (Fig. 8). There was no significant change in the ROM of the upper and lower adjacent levels from preoperatively to final follow-up.

Discussion

DCI arthroplasty is a non-fusion technique that was first introduced by Matgé in 2002, before being improved and introduced into clinical practice by Paradigm Spine (New York, NY, USA) [14]. The two main characteristics of DCI are the U-shaped appearance with runcinate teeth at the anterior edge, and the axial elasticity. Compare with TDR, DCI arthroplasty has several reported advantages: 1) DCI arthroplasty has a wider range of indications and is a relatively simple surgical technique [18], 2) DCI functions as a shock absorber that limits axial rotation and lateral bending, thus exacerbating facet joint stress [17], 3) DCI allows for axial compression in flexion and limited extension, with motion at the index level relatively close to the intact value [22], and 4) there is no grinding of the metal when the DCI functions, and so there is no local or systemic reaction to debris [18].

Several studies have evaluated the clinical efficacy and radiographic outcomes of patients who have undergone DCI arthroplasty. Matgé et al. reported that all 47 patients who underwent DCI arthroplasty achieved satisfactory or somewhat satisfactory clinical outcomes during 2 years of follow-up; three of the 47 patients experienced implant subsidence, and 12 patients had major HO that resulted in less ROM [17]. Li et al. demonstrated that DCI arthroplasty and ACDF had the same effect in improving and maintaining clinical functions, but DCI arthroplasty resulted in a better overall cervical or segmental ROM; no subsidence of DCI was detected during the 2-year follow-up [18]. Liu et al. reported that patients who underwent TDR had a higher incidence of HO than those who underwent DCI arthroplasty during a 2-year follow-up period,

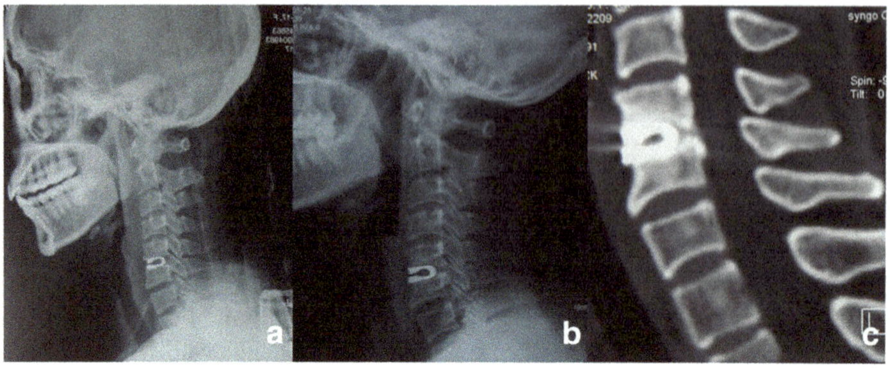

Fig. 4 A 39-year old female patient diagnosed C5/6 disc herniation underwent anterior C5/6 discectomy and DCI arthroplasty. Lateral radiographic image of 1-month postoperative (**a**) showed DCI implant was at the appropriate position. However lateral radiographic image and sagittal CT (**b, c**) at the final follow-up illustrated anterior migration of DCI implant with subsidence

but other clinical and radiographic outcomes were similar, and no DCI subsidence was detected [15]. In our previous report on the present series of patients, both clinical and radiographic outcomes were satisfactory, and were maintained for more than 2 years of follow-up [16]. The outcomes of these reports all indicate that DCI is an effective technique for treating degenerative cervical disc disease (mostly single level) in the short-term, but mid- to long-term follow-up data is still lacking.

In the present study, a minimum 5-year follow-up of 38 cases showed that satisfactory clinical outcomes were obtained irrespective of whether the patients had radiculopathy or myelopathy. Compared with preoperatively, there were significant improvements at final follow-up in VAS scores for pain in the upper body, neck, and shoulder, NDI score, JOA score, and SF-36 outcomes; the average ameliorative rate of the JOA score was 81.1%. Although DCI subsidence was detected, clinical efficacy was maintained during follow-up. The present results suggest that neurological improvement depends mainly on thorough decompression.

Motion preservation is the main purpose of the non-fusion technique. DCI arthroplasty is reportedly effective in preserving and maintaining the ROM of the cervical spine or the index level within 2 years of follow-up [15–18]. In the present study, the ROM of the index level was well maintained during the first 2 years of follow-up, but had significantly decreased at final follow-up. We consider that this may have been due to HO formation at the anterior or posterior border of the operation intervertebral space, and/or implant subsidence.

HO is reportedly very common after TDR of the cervical spine, but the mechanism is still uncertain [23]. The underlying cause of HO may be subchondral bleeding [24, 25]. HO formations are commonly seen in studies of DCI arthroplasty [15–17], but the previously reported incidences of HO are not as high as those seen in the present study (57.1%). We suggest that this may be due to the following two reasons: 1) the present study had a longer follow-up duration than these previous studies, and 2) we used a high-speed burr to remove the cartilage endplate intraoperatively, which may injure the bony endplate and

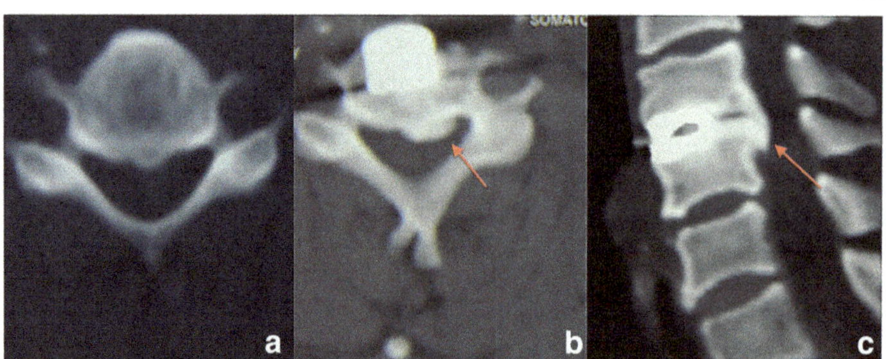

Fig. 5 A 41-year old male patient diagnosed C4/5 disc herniation underwent anterior C4/5 discectomy and DCI arthroplasty. Transaxial CT of preoperative (**a**) and final follow-up (**b**) showed HO formation at the index level during follow-up. Sagittal CT at the final follow-up (**c**) illustrated the formation of an ossified bridge, which would restrict ROM of FSU. Also, the osteophyte narrowed the nerve root canal, causing pain and numbness of left arm. Symptom relieved after conservative treatment

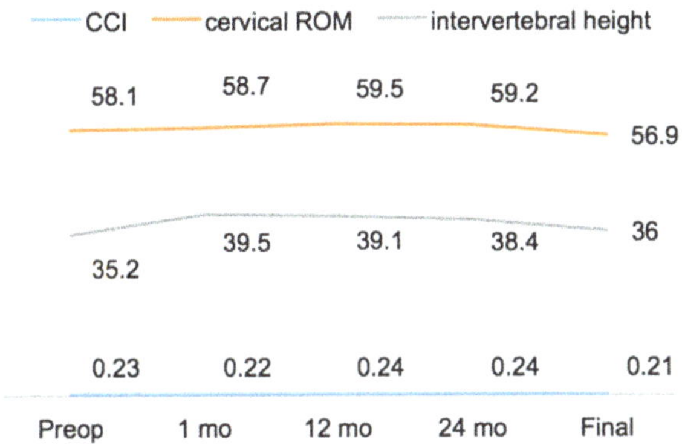

Fig. 6 CCI, cervical ROM and intervertebral height of different time-points for involved patients

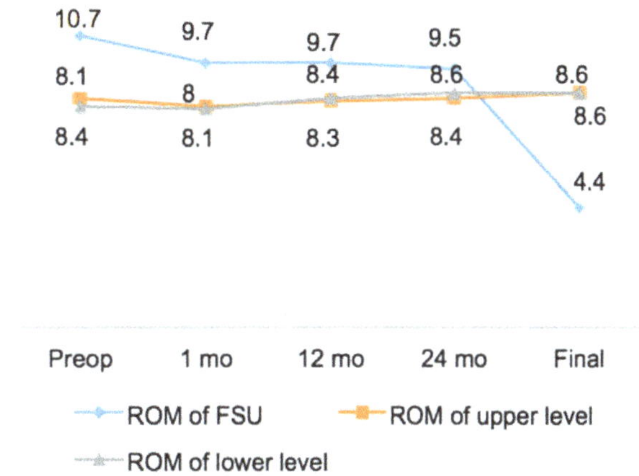

Fig. 8 ROM of FSU, upper level and lower level of different time-points for involved patients

cause subchondral bleeding. HO formations restrict segmental ROM, especially when an ossified bridge is formed at the index level. Furthermore, HO at the posterior edge of the vertebra may cause stenosis of the spinal canal or the intervertebral foramen area, leading to recurrence of symptoms. Two of the present patients (5.2%) experienced symptom recurrence at the index level due to newly-emerged osteophytes during follow-up, but these symptoms resolved after conservative treatment.

Severe implant subsidence not only causes a decrease in ROM at the index level, but also leads to a loss of vertebral height of the operated segment; the incidence of subsidence in the present study was 33.3% at final follow-up. Migration was detected in ten of the 42 DCI segments, all of which had migrated forward. Furthermore, migration was only seen at the subsided levels. The incidence of subsidence in the present study is

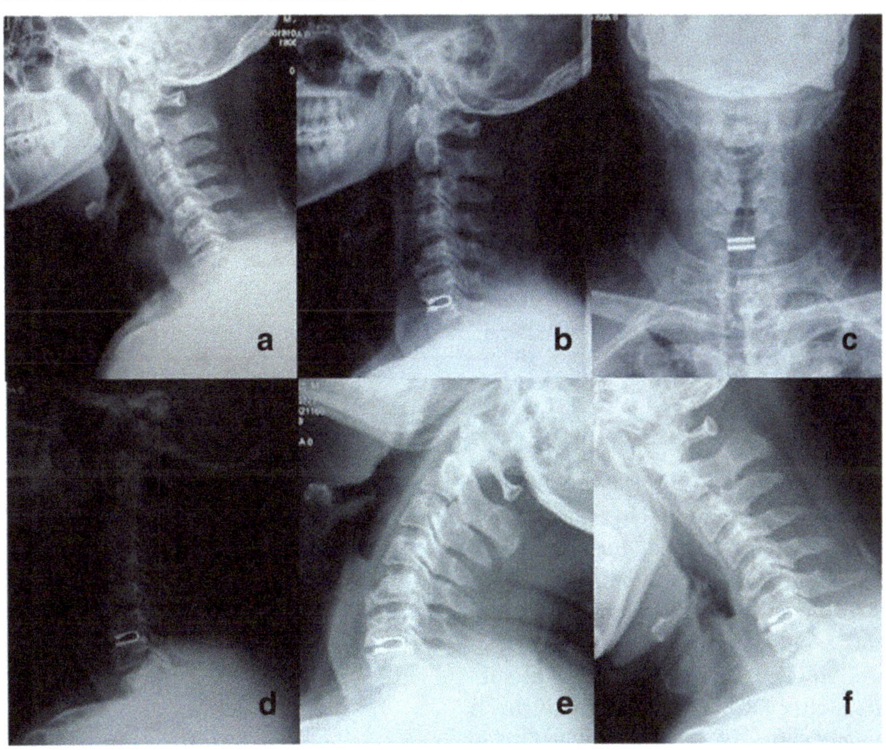

Fig. 7 A 36-year old male patient diagnosed C6/7 disc herniation underwent anterior C6/7 discectomy and DCI arthroplasty. Preoperative lateral radiographic image (**a**) showed narrowed intervertebral space. 1 month postoperative X-ray image (**b, c**) demonstrated partial restoration of intervertebral height and appropriate position of DCI implant. However, Lateral and flexion-extension radiographic image at the final follow-up (**d, e, f**) illustrated subsidence of the DCI implant with decrease of the intervertebral height and ROM of FSU

much higher than that reported in studies on TDR [23]. Unlike TDR, the anterior runcinate teeth of the DCI can help maintain stability of the operated segment, which supposedly prevents the implant from migrating or dropping off. However, the elasticity modulus of titanium alloy is much higher than that of the cortical bone of the cervical vertebrae. A relatively high degree of local stress placed on the endplate by the runcinate teeth may cause destruction of the endplate, especially in patients with osteoporosis during follow-up. Moreover, DCI allows flexion-extension motion of the operated segment, which increases the local stress at the DCI–endplate interface. We consider that subsidence occurred mainly because of persistent local stress at the segmental endplates, especially the anterior portion where the DCI–endplate interface was located. In addition, iatrogenic bony endplate injury may sometimes occur during the excision of the cartilaginous endplates. Regarding the DCI migration, the orientation of the runcinate teeth of the DCI is anteroinferior/anterosuperior, which facilitates the anterior migration during subsidence. Theoretically, a decreased intervertebral height causes reduction of the intervertebral foramen area, which is a factor affecting the formation of radiculopathy. However, no patient in the present study has so far experienced numbness, neuralgia, or paralysis of the upper extremities.

Regarding the decrease in local ROM, the index level is likely a fused part, thus leading to the likelihood of a compensatory increase in ROM at the adjacent segments. A total of six adjacent levels in the present study had a ROM > 11°, indicating instability, but these cases were asymptomatic.

The present study had several limitations. These include the lack of a control group, the relatively small sample size, and the fact that all cases were from a single center. Additionally, a longer follow-up duration is still needed to evaluate whether ASD develops over the long-term, and to evaluate the impact of implant subsidence.

Conclusion

DCI arthroplasty is a non-fusion surgical method for treating cervical spine degeneration. In the present study, clinical efficacy was maintained during mid- to long-term follow-up. HO formation is common at final follow-up, leading to a significant decrease in ROM at the index level, and a potential risk of spinal cord or nerve root compression. The incidence of implant subsidence and migration after DCI arthroplasty is relatively high, carrying a potential risk of ASD and reduction of the intervertebral foramen area. Based on the present results, we suggest that TDR or ACDF should still be the first choice for patients with degenerative cervical disc disease, rather than DCI arthroplasty.

Abbreviations

ACDF: Anterior cervical discectomy and fusion; ASD: Adjacent segment degeneration; CCI: Cervical curvature index; CT: Computed tomography; DCI: Dynamic cervical implant; FSU: Functional spinal unit; HO: Heterotopic ossification; JOA: Japanese orthopaedic association; MCS: Mental component summary; MRI: Magnetic resonance imaging; NDI: Neck disability index; PCS: Physical component summary; ROM: Range of motion; SF-36: 36-Item short form; TDR: Total disc replacement; VAS: Visual analogue scale

Acknowledgments

The authors thank the patients who generously agreed to be interviewed for this research.

Funding

This study was supported in part by the Department of Science and Technology of Sichuan Province (CN) NO.2015SZ0028.

Authors' contributions

LW and BH conceptualized and designed the study, drafted the initial manuscript. HL and XY carried out the initial analyses, reviewed and revised the manuscript. LL reviewed and revised the manuscript. YS and LW coordinated and supervised data collection, critically reviewed and revised the manuscript for important intellectual content. All authors approved the final manuscript as submitted and agree to be accountable for all aspects of the work.

Consent for publication

Not applicable.

Competing interests

The authors declare that they have no competing interests.

References

1. Eck JC, Humphreys SC, Lim TH, et al. Biomechanical study on the effect of cervical spine fusion on adjacent-level intradiscal pressure and segmental motion. Spine. 2002;27(22):2431–4.
2. Kulkarni V, Rajshekhar V, Raghuram L. Accelerated spondylotic changes adjacent to the fused segment following central cervical corpectomy: magnetic resonance imaging study evidence. J Neurosurg. 2004;100(1 Suppl Spine):2–6.
3. Goffin J, Geusens E, Vantomme N, et al. Long-term follow-up after interbody fusion of the cervical spine. J Spinal Disord Tech. 2004;17(2):79–85.
4. Bohlman HH, Emery SE, Goodfellow DB, Jones PK. Robinson anterior cervical discectomy and arthrodesis for cervical radiculopathy. Long-term follow-up of one hundred and twenty-two patients. J Bone Joint Surg Am. 1993;75(9): 1298–307.
5. Chang UK, Kim DH, Lee MC, Willenberg R, Kim SH, Lim J. Range of motion change after cervical arthroplasty with ProDisc-C and prestige artificial discs compared with anterior cervical discectomy and fusion. J Neurosurg Spine. 2007;7(1):40–6.
6. Hilibrand AS, Carlson GD, Palumbo MA, Jones PK, Bohlman HH. Radiculopathy and myelopathy at segments adjacent to the site of a previous anterior cervical arthrodesis. J Bone Joint Surg Am. 1999;81(4): 519–28.
7. Ishihara H, Kanamori M, Kawaguchi Y, Nakamura H, Kimura T. Adjacent segment disease after anterior cervical interbody fusion. Spine J. 2004;4(6): 624–8.
8. Heller JG, Sasso RC, Papadopoulos SM, et al. Comparison of BRYAN cervical disc arthroplasty with anterior cervical decompression and fusion: clinical and radiographic results of a randomized, controlled, clinical trial. Spine. 2009;34(2):101–7.
9. McAfee PC, Reah C, Gilder K, Eisermann L, Cunningham B. A meta-analysis of comparative outcomes following cervical arthroplasty or anterior cervical fusion: results from 4 prospective multicenter randomized clinical trials and up to 1226 patients. Spine. 2012;37(11):943–52.
10. Mummaneni PV, Burkus JK, Haid RW, Traynelis VC, Zdeblick TA. Clinical and radiographic analysis of cervical disc arthroplasty compared with allograft fusion: a randomized controlled clinical trial. J Neurosurg Spine. 2007;6(3): 198–209.

11. Leung C, Casey AT, Goffin A, et al. Clinical significance of heterotopic ossification in cervical disc replacement: a prospective multicenter clinical trial. Neurosurgery. 2005;57(4):759–63.
12. Mehren C, Suchomel P, Grochulla F, et al. Heterotopic ossification in total cervical artificial disc replacement. Spine. 2006;31(24):2802–6.
13. Parkinson JF, Sekhon LH. Cervical arthroplasty complicated by delayed spontaneous fusion. Case report. J Neurosurg Spine. 2005;2(3):377–80.
14. Matge' G, Eif M, Herdmann J. Dynamic cervical implant (DCITM): clinical results from an international multicenter prospective study. Paradig Spine. 2009;1:1–3.
15. Liu SC, Song YM, Liu LM, et al. Clinical and radiologic comparison of dynamic cervical implant arthroplasty and cervical total disc replacement for single-level cervical degenerative disc disease. J Clin Neurosci. 2016;27: 102–9.
16. Wang L, Song YM, Liu LM, Liu H, Li T. Clinical and radiographic outcomes of dynamic cervical implant replacement for treatment of single-level degenerative cervical disc disease: a 24-month follow-up. Eur. Spine J. 2014; 23(8):1680–7.
17. Matge' G, Berthold C, Gunness VR, Hana A, Hertel F. Stabilization with the dynamic cervical implant: a novel treatment approach following cervical discectomy and decompression. J Neurosurg Spine. 2015;22(3):237–45.
18. Li Z, Yu S, Hou S, et al. Clinical and radiologic comparison of dynamic cervical implant arthroplasty versus anterior cervical discectomy and fusion for the treatment of cervical degenerative disc disease. J Clin Neurosci. 2014;21(6):942–8.
19. Takeshita K, Murakami M, Kobayashi A, Nakamura C. Relationship between cervical curvature index (Ishihara) and cervical spine angle (C2—7). J Orthop Sci. 2001;6(3):223–6.
20. Lim MR, Girardi FP, Zhang K, et al. Measurement of total disc replacement radiographic range of motion: a comparison of two techniques. J Spinal Disord Tech. 2005;18:252–6.
21. van Jonbergen HW, Spruit M, Anderson PG, et al. Anterior cervical interbody fusion with a titanium box cage: early radiological assessment of fusion and subsidence. Spine J. 2005;5(6):645–9.
22. Mo ZJ, Bin Zhao Y, Wang LZ, et al. Biomechanical effects of cervical arthroplasty with U-shaped disc implant on segmental range of motion and loading of surrounding soft tissue. Eur Spine J. 2014;23(3):613–21.
23. Meisel HJ, Jurak L, Antinheimo J, et al. Four-year results of a prospective single-arm study on 200 semi-constrained total cervical disc prostheses: clinical and radiographic outcome. J Neurosurg Spine. 2016;25(5):556–65.
24. Yi S, Shin DA, Kim KN, et al. The predisposing factors for the heterotopic ossification after cervical artificial disc replacement. Spine J. 2013;13: 1048–54.
25. Tu TH, Wu JC, Huang WC, et al. The effects of carpentry on heterotopic ossification and mobility in cervical arthroplasty: determination by computed tomography with a minimum 2-year follow-up: clinical article. J Neurosurg Spine. 2012;16:601–9.

12

Increasing incidence of primary shoulder arthroplasty in Finland – a nationwide registry study

Jenni N. E. Harjula[1*], Juha Paloneva[2], Jaason Haapakoski[3], Juha Kukkonen[4], Ville Äärimaa[1] and the Finnish Shoulder Arthroplasty Registry Group

Abstract

Background: The incidence of shoulder arthroplasties is reportedly increasing and the types of arthroplasty are changing. The purpose of this study was to investigate the incidence of primary shoulder arthroplasty in Finland.

Methods: We analyzed nationwide data from the Finnish Arthroplasty Register (FAR) and the Finnish National Hospital Discharge Register (NHDR) during time period 2004–2015. The primary outcome variable was the incidence of shoulder arthroplasty per 100,000 person-years stratified by age, sex and year of surgery. The secondary outcome variables were surgical indication, arthroplasty type and prosthesis model.

Results: The number of primary shoulder arthroplasties was 7504 (women = 4878, men = 2625). The rate of operations increased from 6 to 15 per 100,000 person-years among men, and 11 to 26 per 100,000 person-years among women. The indication for arthroplasty was osteoarthritis in 56%, acute fracture in 21%, inflammatory arthritis in 13%, and rotator cuff arthropathy in 4% of the cases. Hemiarthroplasties accounted for 66%, total shoulder arthroplasties 8%, and reverse shoulder arthroplasties 12% of the cases, 14% of the cases was missing. During the 12-year study period the incidence of hemiarthroplasties decreased by 23% and the number of total shoulder and reverse shoulder arthroplasty increased by 500 and 4500%, respectively.

Conclusions: The incidence of primary shoulder arthroplasty has increased by 160% during the study period in Finland. The incidence of hemiarthroplasties decreased while total and reverse shoulder arthroplasties increased.

Keywords: Arthroplasty, Incidence, Shoulder joint, Finland

Background

Shoulder pain and stiffness are the third most common musculoskeletal complaints in the elderly Finnish population [1]. These symptoms may be attributable to progressive traumatic or degenerative changes in the glenohumeral joint. Eventually these symptoms can be surgically treated with shoulder arthroplasty. Generally there are two alternative surgical options for shoulder arthroplasty, an anatomic (hemi or total) or non-anatomic (reverse) arthroplasty type. The condition of the rotator cuff muscles and glenoid cartilage influence on the arthroplasty type. An anatomic arthroplasty is indicated if the rotator cuff muscles are intact.

According to registry-based studies, the incidence of shoulder arthroplasties has increased in eg. Australia, New Zealand, Denmark and United States [2–8]. Also the National Joint Registry of England, Wales, Northern Ireland and the Isle of Man has reported similar results [9]. Total anatomic and reverse shoulder arthroplasty have become increasingly common whereas the proportion of hemiarthroplasty has decreased [8]. The arthroplasty registries provide important information on country specific treatment practices and distribution of arthroplasty types. In Finland data on shoulder arthroplasties is collected in the Finnish Arthroplasty Register (FAR) founded in 1981 and also in the Finnish National Discharge Register (NHDR) founded in 1967.

* Correspondence: jnehar@utu.fi
[1]Department of Orthopedics and Traumatology, Turku University Hospital, University of Turku, Turku, Finland
Full list of author information is available at the end of the article

This study was set out to investigate the incidence of shoulder arthroplasty and arthroplasty types in Finland after 2004. We hypothesized that the incidence of primary shoulder arthroplasty in Finland would follow the previously reported increasing international trend.

Methods

We reviewed and combined nationwide data from FAR and NHDR during time period 2004–2015. FAR contains data on age, side, gender, domicile, type of hospital, arthroplasty component product coding and indication for operation. NHDR contains data on age, gender, domicile, type of hospital, and codes for diagnoses (according to ICD-10) and procedures (Nomesco Classification of Surgical Procedures, Finnish version). Data collection for both the NHDR and FAR is mandatory for all public and private hospitals. The validity of the NHDR has been found to be good regarding both the coverage and accuracy of data [10–12]. Specific data on the accuracy of the NHDR regarding shoulder arthroplasty are not available.

In order to capture all cases and assess the coverage of FAR reporting, the data in FAR and NHDR on primary shoulder arthroplasties were combined and thereafter the duplicates were removed. The indications for primary shoulder arthroplasty were categorized according to Nordic Arthroplasty Registry Association (NARA) [8] as: osteoarthritis, fracture sequelae, inflammatory arthritis, rotator cuff arthropathy, acute fracture, others and missing (Additional file 1). The FAR diagnosis was used as the primary data source. If the FAR diagnosis was not known (else or missing), we then used the combination of both FAR and NHDR diagnosis. The FAR data collecting paper is designed for hips and knees. Thus, the indications for surgery are rheumatoid arthritis, other arthritis, primary osteoarthrosis, congenital hip luxation, other illness, the change of the prothesis, the removal of the prothesis, secondary arthrosis, the removal of previous prothesis and other revision. For shoulders, the suitable indications for surgery are rheumatoid arthritis, other arthritis (else arthritis in the FAR column), primary osteoarthrosis, other illness (else in the FAR column) and secondary arthrosis. In some cases the indication for surgery was unknown and is marked as missing inthe FAR column. The data from the FAR data collecting papers were then supplemented with NHDR data. The most commonly used ICD-10 diagnosis have been marked in the NHDR column in Additional file 1. After combining FAR and NHDR databases, the NARA diagnosis was synthesized. The NARA diagnosis is based on NHDR database if the indication in FAR column is "Else" or" missing".

Arthroplasty type was categorized as hemi-, total-, reverse shoulder arthroplasty or missing, and determined by combining the data on the type of stem and glenoid component recorded in FAR, and the NHDR procedure code (NBB10 for hemi and NBB20 for total/reverse). In case of discrepancy between FAR and NDHR, the arthroplasty type was recorded based on FAR. Arthroplasty type in NBB20 procedures, without data on prosthesis model, was categorized as missing.

Statistics

We used national population data obtained from Statistics Finland [13] to calculate the incidence of primary shoulder arthroplasty. The primary outcome variable in this study was the incidence of shoulder arthroplasty per 100,000 person-years, which was analyzed with stratification by age, sex and year of surgery. The secondary outcome variables were indication, arthroplasty type and prosthesis model. Incidence rates were calculated using the annual adult population size, ranging from 4.1 (year 2004) to 4.4 million (year 2015) during the study period. Incidence of the operations per 100,000 person-years was calculated by dividing the annual number of procedures by the size of the population aged ≥18 years in the end of the year in question, multipilied by 100,000. The incidence was based on the size of the entire population of persons ≥18 years old in Finland rather than cohort – based estimates. Accordingly, confidence intervals were not calculated.

Poisson regression was used to analyze the operations per 100,000 person years. Two separate models were fitted; the first one included sex and year and the second one included age group and year. The year was considered as a continuous variable due to somewhat linear growth over years in both models. Also, the interactions of sex and year as well as age group and year were evaluated. However, the interactions were not included in the final models as they were not statistically significant. The results are quantified using relative risks with 95% confidence intervals (95% CI). *P*-values less than 0.05 were considered as statistically significant. Statistical analyses were carried out using SAS system for Windows, Version 9.4 (SAS Institute Inc., Cary, NC, USA).

Ethics

Ethics approval was granted by Finland's National Institute for Health and Wellness (Dnro THL/1743/5.05.00/2014).

Results

The number of primary shoulder arthroplasties during the 12-year study period was 4618 (women = 2976, men = 1641, missing = 1) in FAR and 7504 (women = 4878, men = 2625, missing = 1) in NHDR. The FAR coverage is shown in Table 1. 96% of the data in FAR matched the data from NHDR in terms of indication and 86% in terms of arthroplasty type (hemi or total). Of the 2886 arthroplasties not reported in FAR, 2039 (71%) had hemiarthroplasty coding and the rest 29% were missing. The diagnosis was osteoarthritis in 1332 (46%), fracture sequelae in 35 (1%), inflammatory arthritis in 201 (7%), rotator cuff arthropathy in 134 (5%), acute fracture 1054 (37%), others 80 (2%) and missing in 50 (2%) of the 2886 arthroplasties not reported on FAR.

The incidence of annual primary shoulder arthroplasty for each year during the study period is presented in Fig. 1. From 2004 to 2015 the rate of operations increased from 9 to 21 per 100,000 person-years altogether and 6 to 15 per 100,000 person-years among men, and from 11 to 26 for women. The incidence rates have increased linearly and statistically significantly over the years ($p < 0.001$). The number of operations increased 7% every year (RR 1.07, 95% CI: 1.04 to 1.11) which means that the number of operations have increased about doubled during 10 years (RR 2.01, 95% CI 1.48 to 2.74). Women had significantly more operations than men ($p < 0.001$, RR 1.76, 95% CI: 1.41 to 2.19). Over the study period, the mean patient age at the time of primary operation was 67 years (range 20–96) (men 67, women 67). The majority (64%) of patients were treated between ages 60–79 years. There was a statistically significant difference between the age-groups in the incidence of operations ($p < 0.001$). The age group 60–79 was 7.78 (95% CI 5.90 to 10.25) times as likely to have an operation than the group of 18–59 years ($p < 0.001$) and 80+ group was 6.94 (95% CI 5.25 to 9.16) as likely to have an operation than the group of 18–59 years ($p < 0.001$). There was no statistically significant difference between age groups 60–79 and 80+ ($p = 0.097$, RR 1.12, 95% CI 0.98 to 1.28). The incidence of primary shoulder arthroplasty among patients in different age groups is presented in Fig. 2.

Table 1 The Finnish Arthroplasty register coverage compared to the Finnish National Hospital Discharge Register regarding shoulder arthroplasties. The NHDR coverage compared to the FAR was 100%

YEAR	NHDR	FAR	FAR COVERAGE %
2004	357	265	74
2005	400	252	63
2006	445	303	68
2007	502	353	70
2008	570	391	69
2009	624	409	66
2010	650	409	63
2011	780	507	65
2012	790	508	64
2013	713	409	57
2014	761	401	53
2015	912	411	45
TOTAL	7504	4618	62

FAR the Finnish Arthroplasty register, *NHDR* the Finnish National Hospital Discharge Register

The most common indication for primary shoulder arthroplasty was osteoarthritis in 56% of the cases (Fig. 3). Acute fracture was the second (21%) and inflammatory arthritis the third most common (13%) indication. Rotator cuff arthropathy was recorded in 4% and fracture sequealae in 2% of cases. In 2% of cases the indication was other and in 2% of the cases the indication was missing.

Arthroplasty type could be identified in 86% of the cases. Hemiarthroplasties accounted for the majority (66%), total shoulder arthroplasties in 8%, and reverse shoulder arthroplasties in 12% of the cases. The most common arthroplasty type for osteoarthritis was hemiarthroplasty (65%). Similarly, a hemiarthroplasty was recorded in 84% of the patients with an acute fracture diagnosis. The most common arthroplasty type for inflammatory arthritis was also hemiarthroplasty in 60% of cases. The arthroplasty types and diagnosis are presented in Table 2.

The distribution of arthroplasty types is shown in Fig. 4. During the study period the total number of hemiarthroplasty decreased 23% and the number of total shoulder arthroplasty and reverse shoulder arthroplasty increased by 500 and 4500% 46, respectively.

Prosthesis model could be identified in 59% of the cases including 32 different models during the study period. The most commonly reported prosthesis models are shown in Fig. 5. Copeland was the most common hemiarthroplasty ($n = 1131$, 23%), Global AP (DePuy) the most common total shoulder ($n = 126$, 9%) and Delta Xtend the most common reverse ($n = 459$, 49%) arthroplasty model.

Discussion

The results of our study corroborate the hypothesis and show a 160% increase in primary shoulder arthroplasty during the study period between 2004 and 2015. This is in line with the previously published reports [2–9]. Accordingly, the proportion of hemiarthroplasties has decreased and total shoulder and reverse arthroplasty increased in Finland.

In our study, the incidence of shoulder arthroplasty was 21 per 100,000 at the end of the study period. This is higher than reported from the Nordic Arthroplasty Register Association (Denmark 13.3/100,000, Norway 7.1/100,000 and Sweden 9.1/100,000) [8]. The number of shoulder arthroplasties is rapidly increasing internationally. In Australia there was a 89% increase from

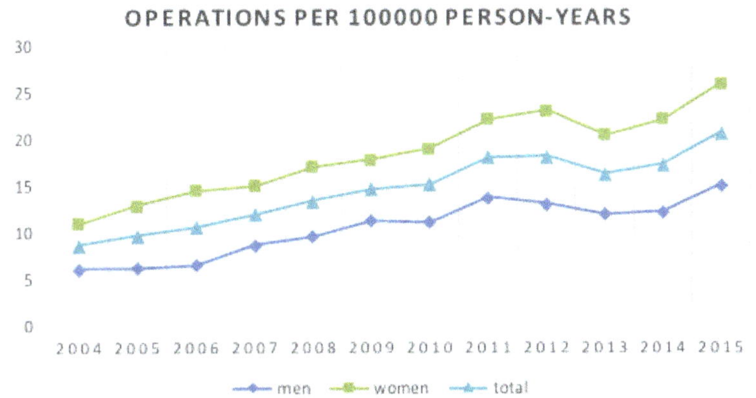

Fig. 1 The incidence per 100,000 person-years of primary shoulder arthroplasty in the Finnish adult population by year

2008 to 2015 and at the same time the proportion of total shoulder replacements increased from 58 to 82% [5]. In the National Joint Registry of England, Wales, Northern Ireland and the Isle of Man the number of primary shoulder arthroplasties has increased 118% from year 2012 to 2015 [9]. Increasing awareness of shoulder arthroplasty by both patients and physicians together with a readily available public health care may add to the detected current higher incidence of shoulder arthroplasties in Finland. Similarly, the reported incidences of other types of surgery such as total hip and knee arthroplasty, rotator cuff reconstruction and knee arthroscopy, have been relatively high in Finland compared to reports from other countries [14–18]. The mean age of the primary shoulder arthroplasty patients at the end of the study period was 67 years and it is comparable to other studies from the US as well as Nordic and British populations [3, 6, 8, 9]. Similarly to other studies, we found that the increasing majority of patients were women [6–9].

The most common and increasingly reported indication for primary shoulder arthroplasty in our cohort was osteoarthritis. The second most common was fracture that maintained a constant incidence throughout the study period. The third and fourth most common indications, inflammatory arthritis and rotator cuff arthropathy, were infrequently reported similarly to the Nordic Arthroplasty Register Association [8]. Inflammatory arthritis requiring surgical intervention is becoming a proportionally rare condition potentially due to advanced medical treatment options [19]. However, rotator cuff arthropathy is a common age-related condition [20] and the small registered number is likely due to missing diagnostic coding in FAR. In our study this indication was given only if both osteoarthritis and/or rotator cuff disease diagnosis were recorded. Therefore, it is likely that some patients with only osteoarthritis diagnosis, had in fact rotator cuff arthropathy.

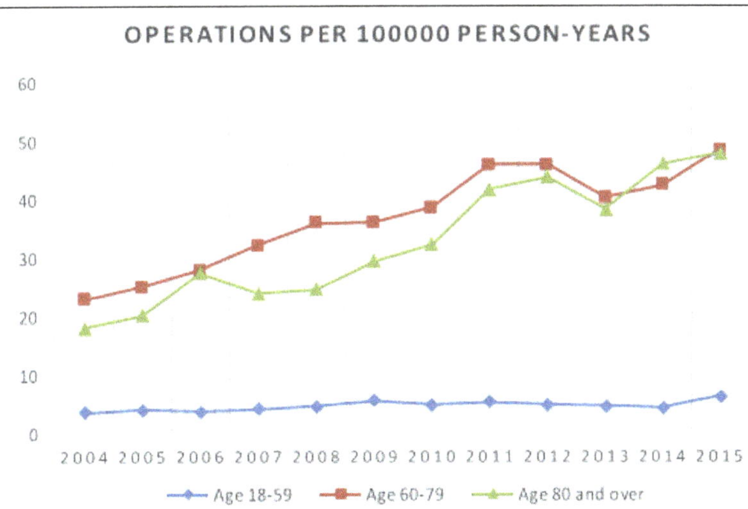

Fig. 2 The incidence of primary shoulder arthroplasty among patients in different age groups in Finland by year

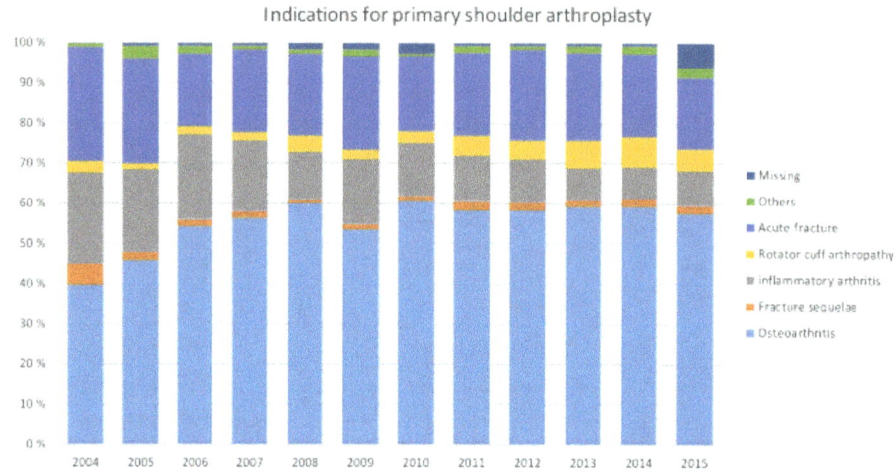

Fig. 3 Reported indications for primary shoulder arthroplasty during the study period. The number of annual indications are presented in Additional file 3

The prevalence of rotator cuff tears increases with advancing age [21]. As the oldest age group in the population grows in Finland it could be anticipated that an increasing number of patients seek treatment not only for osteoarthritis but also for rotator cuff disease. It has been shown that rotator cuff tears are increasingly often treated surgically in the elderly population [17]. These observations may be associated with the increasing incidence of reverse shoulder arthroplasty. However, the absolute and proportional number of reverse shoulder prosthesis is still low in Finland compared to other Nordic countries [8]. Nevertheless, the simultaneous decline

Table 2 The number and percentage of primary arthroplasty types, together with patient mean age and gender in categorized indications during the study period

	Osteo-arthritis	Fracture sequelae	Inflammatory arthritis	Rotator cuff arthropathy	Acute fracture	Others	Missing	Total
Hemiarthroplasty								
n	2728	79	580	85	1328	81	48	4929
(%)	55	2	11	2	27	2	1	100
Mean age	65.8	61.2	63.4	65.5	69.9	63.5	66.3	66.5
(women %)	53	56	80	41	75	62	73	62
Total arthroplasty	497	10	76	3	24	1	2	613
	81	2	12	1	4	0	0	100
	67.8	65.3	66.8	72.3	70.1	76	77.5	67.8
	60	70	80	100	79	100	100	63
Reverse arthroplasty	396	35	214	134	102	12	35	928
	43	4	23	14	11	1	4	100
	73.7	68.7	70.9	74.8	73.1	75.4	74.4	73.0
	71	89	86	69	76	83	74	76
Missing	613	21	101	103	129	27	40	1038
	59	2	10	10	12	3	4	100
	69.0	71.5	66.5	73.2	72.6	64.6	67.1	69.5
	63	76	81	76	79	59	75	68
Total	4234	145	971	325	1583	121	125	7504
	53	2	13	4	21	2	2	100
	67.2	64.8	65.6	71.8	70.3	65.0	69.0	67.8
	57	68	81	64	76	64	74	65

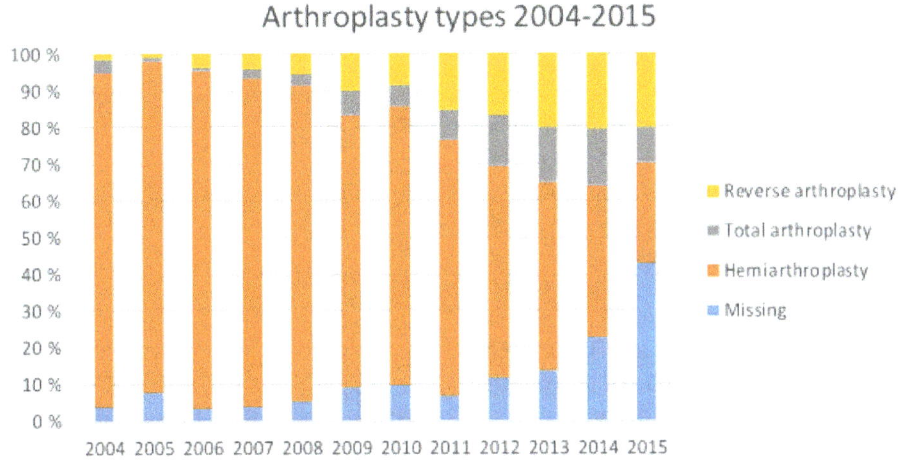

Fig. 4 The change in arthroplasty types during the study period. Y-axis indicates the annual number. The number of annual arthroplasties are presented in Additional file 4

of hemiarthroplasties and increase of total shoulder arthroplasties is noteworthy in our cohort. This is in line with the Kaiser Permanent Shoulder Arthroplasty Registry [6] and is associated with reports on superior clinical outcome of total shoulder arthroplasty compared to hemiarthroplasty [22–24].

The vast number of different prosthesis models represents non-uniform and sporadic shoulder arthroplasty practices in Finland. Copeland was the most commonly reported implant during the study period. This resurfacing implant has been associated with inferior results and high revision rates [25]. On the other hand the most common total shoulder arthroplasty Global AP and reverse shoulder arthroplasty Delta Xtend have been associated good survival on Australian Shoulder Arthroplasty registry [5]. The observed increase in total and reverse shoulder arthroplasty may be explained by the reportedly good results and survival of TSA and RSA [5].

The Finnish Arthroplasty Register (FAR) data collecting paper forms were originally designed for hip and knee arthroplasty and therefore the applicability for recording shoulder arthroplasties has been limited. The shoulder arthroplasty type coding could be reliably identified in the FAR only after 2004 after which time point we extracted the studied data. A major limitation of FAR concerning shoulder arthroplasty surgery is the increasingly poor coverage despite its national and obligatory nature. Therefore, the prosthesis model could be determined in only 59% of the cases. Also the information about the resurfacing procedure or stemmed and stemless humeral implants is limited. FAR is currently under renewal and the paper format will be replaced by shoulder specific electronic online software in the future. A second limitation is the insufficient coding for both diagnosis and operations. ICD-10 or Nomesco do not contain a universal coding for rotator cuff arthropathy, nor for reverse shoulder arthroplasty – this information was gathered by combining data from FAR and NHDR and the data may contain human error. The third limitation is the lack of patient reported

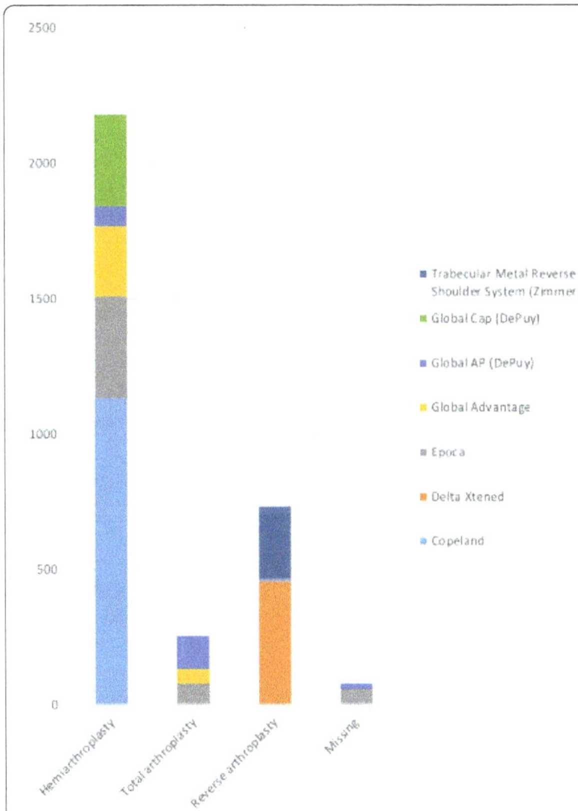

Fig. 5 The most common reported prosthesis models (= each used in over 200 cases) for primary shoulder arthroplasty in Finland during the study period

outcome measures. The future Finnish shoulder arthroplasty registry will contain a shoulder specific data set including information on eg. imaging data and PROM outcomes.

The main strength of our study is the combined information from FAR and NHDR registries. The reported information in the FAR and NHDR was 90% matching. Most of the unreported data in FAR was coded as hemiarthroplasty in NHDR and enabled reliable arthroplasty typing in 89% of the cases. The data from the NHDR have been previously shown to have good validity regarding both coverage and accuracy [26, 27]. The NHDR covers the entire country, including both public and private hospitals. The total primary shoulder arthroplasty incidence may therefore be considered representative.

Conclusion

The incidence of shoulder arthroplasty in Finland has increased almost linearly by 260% during the 12-year study period. We may therefore expect a further increase in the rate of shoulder arthroplasties, and moreover revisions, in the future. The poor coverage of FAR is alarming. New emerging treatment practices, such as reverse shoulder arthroplasty with various prosthesis designs, require meticulous tracking and communication of the outcomes and complications. Functional arthroplasty registries with obligatory input and output of comprehensive data, may provide an important mechanism for this in the future.

Additional files

Additional file 1: The protocol for combining the FAR and NHDR diagnostic data according to NARA diagnosis categories. The NHDR diagnoses for other osteoarthritis, other fracture sequelae, other inflammatory arthritis, other fracture are presented in Additional file 2.

Additional file 2: The NHDR diagnoses for other osteoarthritis, other fracture sequelae, other inflammatory arthritis, other fracture.

Additional file 3: The number of annual indications for primary shoulder arthroplasty.

Additional file 4: The number of annual arthroplasties for primary shoulder arthroplasty.

Abbreviations

FAR: The Finnish Arthroplasty Register; NHDR: The Finnish National Hospital Discharge Register; NARA: Nordic Arthroplasty Registry Association

Acknowledgements

The authors thank Anu Perälä, for decoding and maintenance of the registry material. The authors also thank the Nordic Arthroplasty Register Association for collaboration.

Finnish Shoulder Arthroplasty Registry Group: Pirjo Honkanen [5], Tapio Flinkkilä [6], Antti Joukainen [7], Konsta Pamilo [2], Mikko Salmela [8], Ville Äärimaa [1], Keijo Mäkelä [1]

[1]Department of Orthopedics and Traumatology, Turku University Hospital, University of Turku, Finland

[2]Department of Surgery, Central Finland Hospital, Jyväskylä, Finland

[3]National Institute for Health and Welfare, Helsinki, Finland

[4]Department of Surgery, Division of Orthopaedic and Trauma Surgery, Satakunta Central Hospital and University of Turku

[5]Center of Rheumatic Diseases, Tampere University Hospital, Finland and The Coxa Hospital for Joint Replacement, Tampere, Finland

[6]Department of Orthopedics and Traumatology, Oulu University Hospital, Finland

[7]Department of Orthopedics and Traumatology, Kuopio University Hospital, Finland

[8]Department of Orthopedics and Traumatology, Helsinki University Hospital, Finland

Authors' contributions

JNEH: study design, preparation of the manuscript, statistical work and analyses of the results; JP: preparation of the manuscript, statistical work and analyses of the results; JH: preparation of the manuscript, statistical work and analyses of the results; JK: study design, preparation of the manuscript, interpretation of the data; VÄ: study design, preparation of the manuscript, supervision; FSARG: preparation of the manuscript. All authors read and approved the final manuscript.

Consent for publication

Not applicable.

Competing interests

JNEH, JP, JH and JK have no competing interests; VÄ has received research grants from Turku University Hospital district, Suomen Lääketieteensäätiö and SECEC for other studies.

Author details

[1]Department of Orthopedics and Traumatology, Turku University Hospital, University of Turku, Turku, Finland. [2]Department of Surgery, Central Finland Hospital, Jyväskylä, Finland. [3]National Institute for Health and Welfare, Helsinki, Finland. [4]Department of Surgery, Division of Orthopaedic and Trauma Surgery, Satakunta Central Hospital and University of Turku, Turku, Finland.

References

1. Aromaa A, Koskinen S. Terveys ja toimintakyky Suomessa: Terveys 2000 -tutkimuksen perustulokset. Finland: Kansanterveyslaitoksen julkaisuja B: 3/2002. http://urn.fi/URN:ISBN:951-740-262-7. Accessed 19 Feb 2016.
2. New Zealand Joint Registry, The New Zealand Joint Registry: Sixteen Year Report, January 1999 to December 2014, http://www.nzoa.org.nz/system/files/Web_DH7657_NZJR2014Report_v4_12Nov15.pdf 2015; Accessed 5 May 2015.
3. Jain NB, Yamaguchi K. The contribution of reverse shoulder arthroplasty to utilization of primary shoulder arthroplasty. J Shoulder Elb Surg. 2014;23:1905–12. http://dx.doi.org.ezproxy.utu.fi:2048/10.1016/j.jse.2014.06.055.
4. Kim SH, Wise BL, Zhang Y, Szabo RM. Increasing incidence of shoulder arthroplasty in the United States. J Bone Joint Surg Am. 2011;93:2249–54. https://doi.org/10.2106/JBJS.J.01994.
5. Australian Orthopaedic Association National Joint Replacement Registry, Annual report from the Australian Joint Replacement Registry. Demographics and outcome of shoulder arthroplasty, Supplementary report https://aoanjrr.sahmri.com/documents/10180/217645/Shoulder%20Arthroplasty 2013.
6. Dillon MT, Ake CF, Burke MF, Singh A, Yian EH, Paxton EW, Navarro RA. The Kaiser Permanente shoulder arthroplasty registry: results from 6,336 primary shoulder arthroplasties. Acta Orthop. 2015;86(3):286–92. https://doi.org/10.3109/17453674.2015.1024565. Epub 2015 Mar 2
7. Rasmussen JV, Jakobsen J, Brorson S, Olsen BS. The Danish shoulder arthroplasty registry: clinical outcome and short-term survival of 2,137 primary shoulder replacements. Acta Orthop. 2012;83(2):171–3. https://doi.org/10.3109/17453674.2012.665327. Epub 2012 Feb 13
8. Rasmussen JV, Brorson S, Hallan G, Dale H, Äärimaa V, Mokka J, Jensen SL, Fenstad AM, Salomonsson B. Is it feasible to merge data from national shoulder registries? A new collaboration within the Nordic Arthroplasty Register Association. J Shoulder Elb Surg. 2016;25(12):e369–77. https://doi.org/10.1016/j.jse.2016.02.034. Epub 2016 Apr 20
9. The National Joint Registry for England, Wales, Northern Ireland and the Isle of Man: 14th Annual Report: https://doi.org/10.1016/j.jse.2014.06.055

10. Mattila VM, Sillanpaa P, Iivonen T, Parkkari J, Kannus P, Pihlajamaki H. Coverage and accuracy of diagnosis of cruciate ligament injury in the finnish national hospital discharge register. Injury. 2008;39(12):1373–6.
11. Sund R. Quality of the Finnish hospital discharge register: a systematic review. Scand J Public Health. 2012;40(6):505–15.
12. Huttunen TT, Kannus P, Pihlajamäki H, Mattila VM. Pertrochanteric fracture of the femur in the Finnish National Hospital Discharge Register: validity of procedural coding, external cause for injury and diagnosis. BMC Musculoskelet Disord. 2014;15(1):98.
13. Statistics Finland. Population Structure [http://www.stat.fi/til/vaerak/index_en.html].
14. Niemeläinen M, Mäkelä K, Robertsson O, W-Dahl A, Fenstad AM, Pedersen AB, Schrøder H, Huhtala H, Eskelinen A. Differences between incidences of knee arthroplasties in the Nordic countries a population-based study of data from the Nordic arthroplasty register association. Acta Orthop. 2017:1–6. [Epub ahead of print]
15. Ackerman IN, Bohensky MA, de Steiger R, Brand CA, Eskelinen A, Fenstad AM, Furnes O, Graves SE, Haapakoski J, Mäkelä K, Mehnert F, Nemes S, Overgaard S, Pedersen AB, Garellick G. Lifetime risk of primary total hip replacement surgery for osteoarthritis from 2003-2013: a multi-national analysis using national registry data. Arthritis Care Res. 2017; [Epub ahead of print]
16. Paloneva J, Lepola V, Karppinen J, Ylinen J, Äärimaa V, Mattila VM. Declining incidence of acromioplasty in Finland. Acta Orthop. 2015a;86(2):220–4.
17. Paloneva J, Lepola V, Äärimaa V, Joukainen A, Ylinen J, Mattila VM. Increasing incidence of rotator cuff repairs–a nationwide registry study in Finland. BMC Musculoskelet Disord. 2015b;12(16):189. https://doi.org/10.1186/s12891-015-0639-6.
18. Mattila VM, Sihvonen R, Paloneva J, Felländer-Tsai L. Changes in rates of arthroscopy due to degenerative knee disease and traumatic meniscal tears in Finland and Sweden. Acta Orthop. 2016;87(1):5–11.
19. Young BL, Watson SL, Perez JL, McGwin G, Singh JA, Ponce BA. Trends in joint replacement surgery in patients with rheumatoid arthritis. J Rheumatol. 2018;45(2):158–64. https://doi.org/10.3899/jrheum.170001. Epub 2017 Dec 1
20. Hashimoto T, Nobuhara K, Hamada T. Pathologic evidence of degeneration as a primary cause of rotator cuff tear. Clin Orthop Relat Res. 2003;415:111–20.
21. Tashjian RZ. Epidemiology, natural history, and indications for treatment of rotator cuff tears. Clin Sports Med. 2012;31:589–604. PMID: 23040548*
22. Bryant D, Litchfield R, Sandow M, Gartsman GM, Guyatt G, Kirkley A. A comparison of pain, strength, range of motion, and functional outcomes after hemiarthroplasty and total shoulder arthroplasty in patients with osteoarthritis of the shoulder. A systematic review and meta-analysis. J Bone Joint Surg Am. 2005;87(9):1947–56.
23. Edwards TB, Kadakia NR, Boulahia A, Kempf JF, Boileau P, Némoz C, Walch G. A comparison of hemiarthroplasty and total shoulder arthroplasty in the treatment of primary glenohumeral osteoarthritis: results of a multicenter study. J Shoulder Elb Surg. 2003;12(3):207–13.
24. Gartsman GM, Roddey TS, Hammerman SM. Shoulder arthroplasty with or without resurfacing of the glenoid in patients who have osteoarthritis. J Bone Joint Surg Am. 2000;82(1):26–34.
25. Rasmussen JV, Polk A, Brorson S, Sørensen AK, Olsen BS. Patient-reported outcome and risk of revision after shoulder replacement for osteoarthritis. 1,209 cases from the Danish shoulder arthroplasty registry, 2006-2010. Acta Orthop. 2014;85(2):117–22. https://doi.org/10.3109/17453674.2014.893497.
26. Huttunen TT, Kannus P, Pihlajamaki H, Mattila VM. Pertrochanteric fracture of the femur in the Finnish National Hospital Discharge Register: validity of procedural coding, external cause for injury and diagnosis. BMC Musculoskelet Disord. 2014;15(98) https://doi.org/10.1186/1471-2474-15-98. [PMC free article]
27. Sund R. Quality of the Finnish hospital discharge register: a systematic review. Scand J Public Health. 2012;40:505–15. https://doi.org/10.1177/1403494812456637.

13

Optimising perioperative care for hip and knee arthroplasty in South Africa: a Delphi consensus study

U. Plenge[1*], M. B. Nortje[2], L. C. Marais[3], J. D. Jordaan[4], R. Parker[1], N. van der Westhuizen[5], J. F. van der Merwe[6], J. Marais[7], W. V. September[7], G. L. Davies[8], T. Pretorius[8], C. Solomon[9], P. Ryan[10], A. M. Torborg[11], Z. Farina[12], R. Smit[13], C. Cairns[14], H. Shanahan[15], S. Sombili[16], A. Mazibuko[17], H. R. Hobbs[2], O. S. Porrill[1], N. E. Timothy[18], R. E. Siebritz[18], C. van der Westhuizen[19], A. J. Troskie[20], C. A. Blake[20], L. A. Gray[21], T. W. Munting[22], H. K. S. Steinhaus[23], P. Rowe[24], J. G. van der Walt[25], R. Isaacs Noordien[26], A. Theron[27] and B. M. Biccard[1]

Abstract

Background: A structured approach to perioperative patient management based on an enhanced recovery pathway protocol facilitates early recovery and reduces morbidity in high income countries. However, in low- and middle-income countries (LMICs), the feasibility of implementing enhanced recovery pathways and its influence on patient outcomes is scarcely investigated. To inform similar practice in LMICs for total hip and knee arthroplasty, it is necessary to identify potential factors for inclusion in such a programme, appropriate for LMICs.

Methods: Applying a Delphi method, 33 stakeholders (13 arthroplasty surgeons, 12 anaesthetists and 8 physiotherapists) from 10 state hospitals representing 4 South African provinces identified and prioritised i) risk factors associated with poor outcomes, ii) perioperative interventions to improve outcomes and iii) patient and clinical outcomes necessary to benchmark practice for patients scheduled for primary elective unilateral total hip and knee arthroplasty.

Results: Thirty of the thirty-three stakeholders completed the 3 months Delphi study. The first round yielded i) 36 suggestions to preoperative risk factors, ii) 14 (preoperative), 18 (intraoperative) and 23 (postoperative) suggestions to best practices for perioperative interventions to improve outcomes and iii) 25 suggestions to important postsurgical outcomes. These items were prioritised by the group in the consecutive rounds and consensus was reached for the top ten priorities for each category.

Conclusion: The consensus derived risk factors, perioperative interventions and important outcomes will inform the development of a structured, perioperative multidisciplinary enhanced patient care protocol for total hip and knee arthroplasty. It is anticipated that this study will provide the construct necessary for developing pragmatic enhanced care pathways aimed at improving patient outcomes after arthroplasty in LMICs.

Keywords: Delphi study, Enhanced recovery pathways, Low middle income countries, Total hip and knee arthroplasty, Total hip and knee replacement, Patient outcomes

* Correspondence: ullaplenge@gmail.com
[1]Department of Anaesthesia and Perioperative Medicine, Groote Schuur Hospital and Faculty of Health Sciences, University of Cape Town, Cape Town, South Africa
Full list of author information is available at the end of the article

Background

In the past 20 years, enhanced recovery pathways (ERPs) have become increasingly integrated into most surgical fields as standard care in high income countries, as is exemplified by national priority programs [1–3], and the widespread acceptance of the Enhanced Recovery After Surgery (ERAS) society network [4]. ERPs represent a fundamental shift towards a patient-centred, multidisciplinary-driven continuity of care that aim to attenuate surgical stress and expedite recovery [5]. Studies on total joint arthroplasty (TJA) for both hips and knees have shown that implementation of an evidence-based, structured approach to patient care decreases postoperative morbidity and consequently length of stay without increasing readmission rate [6–8].

However, in low- and middle-income countries (LMICs) , the value of implementing ERPs is yet to be explored. This may be because: i) the perception that current hospital resources may make it difficult to develop and implement structured and sustainable protocols to enhance postoperative recovery, and ii) short and long-term data collection on the quality of the work provided is scarce, inhibiting the ability to benchmark clinical results and improve the service provided to patients. Despite these challenges, a healthcare system in a middle-income country such as South Africa may benefit from the implementation of ERPs through reduced postoperative morbidity and the associated cost reductions, as has been demonstrated in high-income countries (HICs) [9].

While the goals of implementing ERPs can be expected to be independent of a country's economic status, we believe the differences in patient demographics, healthcare infrastructure and healthcare resources between HICs and LMICs warrants a LMIC derived programme of enhanced care to facilitate practice change and improve patient outcomes in these settings. The aim of our study was therefore to establish multidisciplinary consensus on; i) preoperative risk factors associated with poor outcomes, ii) perioperative interventions considered necessary to improve outcomes, and iii) important postsurgical patient and clinical outcomes. This study was conducted in South Africa, which represents an upper-middle-income country, as defined by the World Bank [10]. However, as this work was conducted in the public healthcare sector, and South Africa has one of the world's highest levels of inequality [11], it is likely that this work reflects the state funded healthcare system of a LMIC, as opposed to high-middle-income countries. This assumption is supported by the South African public healthcare service data from the African Surgical Outcomes Study, where the median number of specialists per 100,000 population was 0.9 (IQR 0.2-1.9) (unpublished data) [12], which is well below the recommended 20–40 specialists per 100,000 population [13].

Methods

We conducted a Delphi survey with experts from different fields involved in the care of arthroplasty surgical patients in South Africa. The Delphi study is an accepted method for achieving convergence of opinions concerning knowledge solicited from experts within specific fields, and has been adopted for priority-setting in medicine [14]. The technique is an iterative process which allows the participant to refine his or her prioritization of items, in an anonymous manner, based on the group's work from round to round and with controlled feedback of opinions [15].

Participant recruitment

Participants were recruited from all the hospitals which we knew had a history of performing elective TJAs. This approach was necessary, as currently there is no national arthroplasty database of public hospitals performing TJAs in South Africa. We invited orthopaedic arthroplasty surgeons, anaesthetists and physiotherapists from 18 regional and central hospitals in the public sector covering seven of the nine provinces in South Africa. They were contacted by email and asked to participate in four sequential studies aimed at improving perioperative care for patients scheduled for primary elective unilateral hip and knee TJA in South Africa. The Delphi study is the first of these four studies. For a hospital to participate we required participation of both the Anaesthesia and the Orthopaedic Departments in the project. With the use of telephone calls, face-to-face meetings and further email correspondence, 33 experts in the perioperative management of arthroplasty patients from 10 hospitals representing four provinces accepted the invitation to participate in these four studies. Reasons for exclusion from the study where i) not confirming their participation (5) or ii) declining to participate due to lack of interest or lack of resources to participate in this and future studies (3). Prior to commencement of the Delphi study, the participants were given detailed information of the Delphi process and how consensus would be defined.

The Delphi process

This Delphi survey was conducted over 3 months from December 2016 to March 2017. In the first round participants submitted suggestions for; i) risk factors associated with poor outcome, ii) best practices for preoperative, intraoperative and postoperative interventions to improve postoperative outcomes and iii) important patient and clinical outcomes to benchmark care, deemed relevant in the South African context for patients scheduled for primary elective unilateral hip and knee TJA. Participants were encouraged to elaborate on how to quantify these components and provide supporting references. UP and BMB grouped the responses in each category into statements. The category statements and supporting references were shared with all participants. In the second Delphi round, the participants were asked to rank the top-ten statements in each category, and where possible, add further comments or relevant references. Based on participants' responses, statements that overlapped were grouped together prior to the third Delphi round. In the third round the participants were presented with their individual as well as the overall group ranking of the prioritised statements within each category. They were asked to re-evaluate their previous round's ranking, considering the group ranking and where possible when their rankings differed greatly from that of the group, to add further comments or references supporting their decision. In the fourth and final round, participants were given an opportunity to present any strong disagreement with the priority rankings from the third Delphi round with a Skype teleconference. Non-participation in the fourth round indicated agreement with the proposed Delphi priorities from the third round. Following the teleconference, the consensus of the group was taken as final. UP and BMB were neutral in the prioritization of statements throughout the study.

Statistical analysis

The rank order of the research priorities for each round was established using a reverse scoring system i.e. a respondent's rank of 1 received 10 points, down to a rank of 10, which received 1 point. The scores of the respondents were combined for each round to develop the research priority rank order.

Results

Participants and response rate

The recruited participants included 13 arthroplasty surgeons, 12 anaesthetists and 8 physiotherapists involved in hip and knee arthroplasty. Response rate in the first round was 97% (32/33), 91% (30/33) in the second round and 91% (30/33) in the third round. In the fourth round, all 33 participants accepted the ranking of the prior third Delphi round. However, three participants contributed in the fourth round to a refinement of two of the Delphi statements. The first was an amalgamation of "peripheral nerve blocks" with "multimodal opioid-sparing analgesia regimen" in the postoperative intervention category, which changed the overall ranking in this category. This change clarified that non-opioid analgesic regimens can include regional anaesthesia. The second change was to define "long term survival" in the outcome category as "1-year mortality", to ensure an objective outcome variable.

Preoperative risk factors

Two hundred forty-seven suggestions were submitted for round 1 for preoperative risk factors believed to be associated with poor outcomes in patients scheduled for primary elective unilateral hip and knee TJA. The suggestions were categorised into 36 broad statements for round 2 which were refined to 28 statements for round 3. The ten prioritised risk factors identified after the second round did not change in the subsequent rounds (Table 1).

Preoperative interventions

Round 1 yielded 166 suggestions of preoperative interventions judged to be important to improve outcomes following primary elective unilateral hip and knee TJA. These were amalgamated into 14 statements in round 2 and further refined to 11 different statements for round 3. The ten priorities identified after the second round did not change in subsequent rounds (Table 2).

Intraoperative interventions

One hundred forty-four suggestions for intraoperative interventions believed to improve postoperative outcomes following primary elective unilateral hip and knee TJA were submitted in round 1. These were amalgamated into 18 statements for the second round and further refined to 11 statements for round 3. The ten priorities identified by the second round, did not change in the fourth round (Table 3).

Postoperative interventions

The first Delphi round yielded 181 suggestions of important postoperative interventions to possibly improve outcomes following primary elective unilateral hip and knee TJA. These were amalgamated into 23 statements for the second Delphi round and further refined to 17

Table 1 The ten prioritised preoperative risk factors considered most important determinants of poor outcomes in patients scheduled for primary elective unilateral hip and knee total joint arthroplasty in South Africa

1. Poor general health (ASA 3 and above)
2. Impaired cardiovascular functional status
3. Advanced age
4. Preoperative mobility
5. Obesity or chronic malnutrition
6. Recent or current sources of infection (e.g. bladder, respiratory, dental etc.)
7. Preoperative chronic pain
7. Matching surgical complexity with surgical experience or skill
9. Psychiatric disorders and/or cognitive impairment
10. Preoperative anaemia

ASA American Society of Anesthesiologists

Table 2 The ten prioritised preoperative interventions considered most important determinants to improve outcomes following primary elective unilateral hip and knee total joint arthroplasty in South Africa

1. A patient optimisation clinic
2. Multidisciplinary planning
3. Patient education
4. Infection prevention
5. Establishing high-volume units
6. Smoking cessation
7. Optimisation of preoperative analgesia regimen
8. Minimise preoperative fasting
9. Establish a patient blood management programme
10. Alcohol cessation

Table 4 The ten prioritised postoperative interventions considered most important determinants to improve outcomes following primary elective unilateral hip and knee total joint arthroplasty in South Africa

1. Early mobilisation after surgery
2. Standardised orthopaedic nursing care
3. Multimodal opioid-sparing analgesia regimen
4. Active management of medical co-morbidities
5. DVT prophylaxis
6. A pain management team
7. Patient empowerment in his or her recovery
8. Patient controlled analgesia
9. Multidisciplinary ward rounds
10. Postoperative rehabilitation

statements for the third Delphi round. The final ten priorities were agreed upon in the fourth round of the Delphi process, following amalgamation of "peripheral nerve blocks" into "multimodal opioid-sparing analgesia regimen" (Table 4).

Important patient and clinical outcomes

One hundred sixty-four suggestions were made in the first Delphi round for important patient and clinical outcomes following primary elective unilateral hip and knee TJA. These were categorised into statements for the second Delphi round and further refined to 23 statements for the third Delphi round. The ten prioritised outcomes did not change after the second round (Table 5).

Discussion

This study reports a national consensus of the predictors of morbidity, perioperative interventions to improve surgical outcomes, and the clinical outcomes necessary to document perioperative success for patients scheduled for primary elective unilateral hip and knee TJA in South Africa. These findings provide the information necessary to develop a feasible enhanced care programme for South African arthroplasty patients.

The multidisciplinary involvement of regional and central hospitals performing TJAs across South Africa provides a realistic consensus of the factors needed for an enhanced care arthroplasty programme in the public service in South Africa. We believe that the "buy-in" by the participants was high, and this is important for successful organisational change [16]. Furthermore, consensus on the priorities was established early (within Delphi round 2) in four of the five categories, supporting the validity of the final consensus document [17].

However, this study also has limitations. Firstly, while expert consensus is the lowest level of evidence, it is an established method to facilitate clinical guidelines when the evidence is limited [18], particularly when study interventions and study results might not be transferable to settings with a different socio-economic and demographic structure. Furthermore, group consensus studies

Table 3 The ten prioritised intraoperative interventions considered most important determinants to improve outcomes following primary elective unilateral hip and knee total joint arthroplasty in South Africa

1. Meticulous surgical technique
2. Infection prevention
3. Optimisation of prosthesis choice and placement
4. Multimodal opioid-sparing analgesia regimen
5. Monitoring and optimisation of haemodynamics
6. Central neuraxial anaesthesia
7. Establish a patient blood management programme
8. Temperature regulation
9. Glycaemic control
10. Deep vein thrombosis prophylaxis

Table 5 The ten prioritised patient and clinical outcomes considered most important following primary elective unilateral hip and knee total joint arthroplasty in South Africa

1. Patient reported outcome measures
2. Postoperative pain at rest and during movement
3. 1-year mortality
4. Early mobilisation
5. Prosthetic joint infection rate
6. Joint range of motion
7. Major adverse cardiac events
8. Hospital length of stay
9. Implant longevity
10. Cost of care

can expedite the transformation of evidence-based knowledge gained in HICs into practical implementation in LMICs [19], which is why we believe this process is entirely appropriate for the public health service in South Africa, and may be applicable to other LMICs. In our study we have: i) identified feasible interventions which may improve patient outcomes in a resource limited environment, and ii) prioritized which interventions are preferable for implementation if resources do not allow for adoption of all suggested interventions in clinical practice. We believe this approach will allow all sites to focus their resources on developing a pragmatic multidisciplinary programme of enhanced care.

A second limitation is the possibility that we did not invite all sites which performs TJAs in South Africa to participate in the study, as the public health care sector currently does not have a national arthroplasty database. Nevertheless, we succeeded in enrolling both regional and central hospitals from different provinces, which ensured a broad representation of specialists involved in TJAs in South Africa. Finally, we did not include the full spectrum of stakeholders involved in the perioperative management of joint arthroplasty patients or patients themselves. However, we believe our consensus document does represent stakeholders who were not participants in this study, as patient relevant outcomes and parameters important to nursing care, physicians, nutritionists and geriatricians are included (Tables 1, 2, 3, 4 and 5).

Identification of modifiable and non-modifiable risk factors is essential to guide surgical decision making and prepare the patient optimally ensuring safe perioperative care [20]. This is important in a country such as South Africa, which has a medium Human Development Index (HDI)[1] suggesting a higher risk for perioperative mortality compared to countries with high HDI [21]. Hence, addressing the prioritised preoperative risk factors (Table 1) may improve patient outcomes [22]. Additionally, introducing a best practice protocol in the perioperative period (Tables 2, 3 and 4) aims to provide continuity of care with emphasis on less variability and better quality of service provided [23]. Finally, identifying and standardising procedure specific outcomes facilitates benchmarking, which is crucial to improve the quality of patient care [24]. Only recently have such multinational collaborative efforts been instituted for TJAs to guide future trials towards comparable outcomes [25]. Importantly, this international group of patient partners, orthopaedic surgeons, physical therapists, rheumatologists and methodologists successfully achieved consensus for six core outcome domains; i) pain, ii) function, iii) patient satisfaction, iv) revision, v) adverse events and vi) death, which are all represented in our consensus document (Table 5). While this similarity provides external validity to the work of our Delphi group, it also suggests that aspirations for best patient practice is independent of a country's income status. However, the novelty of our Delphi study remains with the prioritised preoperative risk factors and perioperative interventions, which we hope will facilitate a pragmatic approach to achieving these postoperative goals in our resource limited settings.

Conclusion

This national multidisciplinary consensus Delphi study has produced priorities for preoperative risk stratification, perioperative interventions, and outcome assessments necessary for benchmarking, from which a pragmatic enhanced care programme for primary elective unilateral hip and knee TJA in South Africa can be developed. It is anticipated that these priorities may either be applicable or encourage other LMICs to initiate a similar Delphi process. The next phase will involve an audit of current perioperative care addressing the prioritised statements, followed by implementation of the Delphi group's proposed interventions.

Endnotes

[1*] Human Development Index (HDI) is an index based on i) life expectancy, ii) education and iii) per capita income indicators, which is used to determine whether a nation is a developed or a developing country.

Abbreviations

ASA: American Society of Anesthesiologists; DVT: Deep vein thrombosis; ERAS: Enhanced recovery after surgery; ERPs: Enhanced recovery pathways; HDI: Human Development Index; HICs: High-income countries; LMICs: Low- and middle-income countries; PBM: Patient blood management; TJA: Total joint arthroplasty

Authors' contributions

UP and BMB were responsible for overall conception and design of the Delphi study; acquisition, analysis and interpretation of data; drafting the manuscript and critical revising of the work. MBN, LCM, JDJ, RP, NvdW, JFvdM, JM, WVS, GLD, TP, CS, PR, AMT, ZF, RS, CC, HS, SS, AM, HRH, OSP, NET, RES, CvdW, AJT, CAB, LAG, TWM, HKSS, PR, JGvdW, RIN and AT made substantial contributions to acquisition, analysis and interpretation of data and critical revising of the work. All authors approved the final version and agreed to be accountable for all aspects, accuracy and integrity of the work.

Competing interests

The authors declare that they have no competing interests.

Author details

[1]Department of Anaesthesia and Perioperative Medicine, Groote Schuur Hospital and Faculty of Health Sciences, University of Cape Town, Cape Town, South Africa. [2]Department of Orthopaedic Surgery, Groote Schuur Hospital and Faculty of Health Sciences, University of Cape Town, Cape Town, South Africa. [3]Department of Orthopaedic surgery, School of Clinical Medicine, University of KwaZulu-Natal, Pietermaritzburg, South Africa. [4]Department of Orthopaedic Surgery, Tygerberg Medical School, University of Stellenbosch, Cape Town, South Africa. [5]Department Anaesthesia,

University of the Free State, Bloemfontein, South Africa. [6]Department of Orthopaedic surgery, University of the Free State, Bloemfontein, South Africa. [7]Department of Physiotherapy, Paarl Provincial Hospital, Paarl, South Africa. [8]Department of Anaesthesia, Paarl Provincial Hospital, Paarl, South Africa. [9]Department of Orthopaedics, Paarl Provincial Hospital, Paarl, South Africa. [10]Arthroplasty and Sports Medicine unit, Department of Orthopaedics, Inkosi Albert Luthuli Central Hospital, University of KwaZulu-Natal, Durban, South Africa. [11]Department of Anaesthesia, Inkosi Albert Luthuli Central Hospital, University of KwaZulu-Natal, Durban, South Africa. [12]Department of Anaesthesia, Critical Care and Pain Management, Grey's Hospital, Pietermaritzburg, South Africa. [13]Department of Orthopaedic surgery, Grey's Hospital, Pietermaritzburg, South Africa. [14]Greys Pain clinic, Department of Anaesthesia, Grey's Hospital, Pietermaritzburg, South Africa. [15]Department of Physiotherapy, Grey's Hospital, Pietermaritzburg, South Africa. [16]Department of Orthopaedic surgery, Steve Biko Academic Hospital, University of Pretoria, Pretoria, South Africa. [17]Department of Anaesthesia, Steve Biko Academic Hospital, University of Pretoria, Pretoria, South Africa. [18]Department of Physiotherapy, Groote Schuur Hospital and Faculty of Health Sciences, University of Cape Town, Cape Town, South Africa. [19]Department of Anaesthesia, Worcester Hospital, Worcester, South Africa. [20]Department of Orthopaedic Surgery, Worcester Hospital, Worcester, South Africa. [21]Department of Physiotherapy, New Somerset Hospital, Cape Town, South Africa. [22]Department of Orthopaedics, New Somerset Hospital and Christiaan Barnard Memorial Hospital, Cape Town, South Africa. [23]Department of Anaesthesia, New Somerset Hospital, Cape Town, South Africa. [24]Department of Orthopaedic surgery, Victoria Hospital, Cape Town, South Africa. [25]Department of Anaesthesia, Victoria Hospital, Cape Town, South Africa. [26]Department of Physiotherapy, Victoria Hospital, Cape Town, South Africa. [27]Department of Anaesthesiology and Critical Care, Tygerberg Academic Hospital, University of Stellenbosch, Cape Town, South Africa.

References

1. Alfonsi P, Slim K, Chauvin M, Mariani P, Faucheron JL, Fletcher D. French guidelines for enhanced recovery after elective colorectal surgery. J Visc Surg. 2014;151(1):65–79.
2. Simpson JC, Moonesinghe SR, Grocott MP, Kuper M, McMeeking A, Oliver CM, Galsworthy MJ, Mythen MG, National Enhanced Recovery Partnership Advisory B. Enhanced recovery from surgery in the UK: an audit of the enhanced recovery partnership programme 2009-2012. Br J Anaesth. 2015; 115(4):560–8.
3. Scott MJ, McEvoy MD, Gordon DB, Grant SA, Thacker JKM, Wu CL, Gan TJ, Mythen MG, Shaw AD, Miller TE. American Society for Enhanced Recovery (ASER) and Perioperative Quality Initiative (POQI) joint consensus statement on optimal analgesia within an enhanced recovery pathway for colorectal surgery: part 2-from PACU to the transition home. Perioper Med (Lond). 2017;6:7.
4. The ERAS Society. http://www.erassociety.org. Assessed on 20th March 2018.
5. Kehlet H. Multimodal approach to control postoperative pathophysiology and rehabilitation. Br J Anaesth. 1997;78(5):606–17.
6. Scott NB, McDonald D, Campbell J, Smith RD, Carey AK, Johnston IG, James KR, Breusch SJ. The use of enhanced recovery after surgery (ERAS) principles in Scottish orthopaedic units–an implementation and follow-up at 1 year, 2010-2011: a report from the musculoskeletal audit, Scotland. Arch Orthop Trauma Surg. 2013;133(1):117–24.
7. Kehlet H. Fast-track hip and knee arthroplasty. Lancet (London, England). 2013;381(9878):1600–2.
8. Zhu S, Qian W, Jiang C, Ye C, Chen X. Enhanced recovery after surgery for hip and knee arthroplasty: a systematic review and meta-analysis. Postgrad Med J. 2017;93:736.
9. Kash BA, Zhang Y, Cline KM, Menser T, Miller TR. The perioperative surgical home (PSH): a comprehensive review of US and non-US studies shows predominantly positive quality and cost outcomes. Milbank Q. 2014;92(4): 796–821.
10. The World Bank data on upper-middle-income countries. https://data.worldbank.org/income-level/upper-middle-income. Assessed on 20th March 2018.
11. United Nations Human Development Report. http://hdr.undp.org/en/composite/IHDI. Assessed on 20th March 2018.
12. Biccard BM, Madiba TE, Kluyts HL, Munlemvo DM, Madzimbamuto FD, Basenero A, Gordon CS, Youssouf C, Rakotoarison SR, Gobin V, et al. Perioperative patient outcomes in the African surgical outcomes study: a 7-day prospective observational cohort study. Lancet (London, England). 2018; 391:1589.
13. Meara JG, Leather AJ, Hagander L, Alkire BC, Alonso N, Ameh EA, Bickler SW, Conteh L, Dare AJ, Davies J, et al. Global surgery 2030: evidence and solutions for achieving health, welfare, and economic development. Lancet (London, England). 2015;386(9993):569–624.
14. The James Lind Alliance. http://www.jla.nihr.ac.uk. Assessed on 20th March 2018.
15. Hsu C-C, Sandford BA. The Delphi technique: making sense of consensus. Pract Assess Res Eval. 2007;12(10):1–8.
16. Campbell RJ. Change management in health care. Health Care Manag (Frederick). 2008;27(1):23–39.
17. Boulkedid R, Abdoul H, Loustau M, Sibony O, Alberti C. Using and reporting the Delphi method for selecting healthcare quality indicators: a systematic review. PLoS One. 2011;6(6):e20476.
18. Murphy MK, Black NA, Lamping DL, McKee CM, Sanderson CF, Askham J, Marteau T: Consensus development methods, and their use in clinical guideline development. Health Technol Assess 1998, 2(3):i-iv, 1-88.
19. Minas H, Jorm AF. Where there is no evidence: use of expert consensus methods to fill the evidence gap in low-income countries and cultural minorities. Int J Ment Health Syst. 2010;4:33.
20. Pearse RM, Holt PJ, Grocott MP. Managing perioperative risk in patients undergoing elective non-cardiac surgery. BMJ. 2011;343:d5759.
21. Bainbridge D, Martin J, Arango M, Cheng D, Evidence-based Peri-operative Clinical Outcomes Research G. Perioperative and anaesthetic-related mortality in developed and developing countries: a systematic review and meta-analysis. Lancet. 2012;380(9847):1075–81.
22. Levett DZH, Edwards M, Grocott M, Mythen M. Preparing the patient for surgery to improve outcomes. Best Pract Res Clin Anaesthesiol. 2016;30(2):145–57.
23. Garson L, Schwarzkopf R, Vakharia S, Alexander B, Stead S, Cannesson M, Kain Z. Implementation of a total joint replacement-focused perioperative surgical home: a management case report. Anesth Analg. 2014;118(5):1081–9.
24. Myles PS, Grocott MP, Boney O, Moonesinghe SR, Group CO-S. Standardizing end points in perioperative trials: towards a core and extended outcome set. Br J Anaesth. 2016;116(5):586–9.
25. Singh JA, Dowsey MM, Dohm M, Goodman SM, Leong AL, Scholte Voshaar MM, Choong PF. Achieving consensus on total joint replacement trial outcome reporting using the OMERACT filter: endorsement of the final core domain set for total hip and total knee replacement trials for endstage arthritis. J Rheumatol. 2017;44:1723.

14

A systematic review of psychological interventions in total hip and knee arthroplasty

Samantha Bay[1*], Lukas Kuster[2], Neil McLean[1], Michelle Byrnes[3] and Markus Stefan Kuster[2,4]

Abstract

Background: The current practice in elective orthopaedics does not routinely include psychological interventions despite evidence that psychological factors such as personality, anxiety, depression and negative thinking styles can influence outcomes and recovery from surgery. The objective of this paper was to review the effectiveness of psychological interventions used in conjunction with total hip (THA) and knee arthroplasty (TKA), in improving patient reported joint outcomes.

Methods: An extensive literature search was conducted according to Preferred Reporting Items for Systematic reviews and Meta-Analyses guidelines. Search terms included psychology, interventions, and orthopaedics. Articles were included if they were randomised controlled trials (RCTs) of psychological interventions involving active patient participation measured with patient reported joint outcomes in patients undergoing hip or knee arthroplasty.

Results: A total of 19,489 titles were screened. Seven studies met the inclusion criteria and were included. Five of seven studies did not show improvements in patient reported outcomes after surgery. Specifically, psycho-education alone was not effective at improving patient reported joint outcomes in two out of two studies.

Conclusion: The current literature does not support routine psychological interventions for TKA and THA. However, it should be noted that the literature for psychological interventions in conjunction with TKA and THA is still in its infancy. This gap in the literature is surprising, considering the importance of the role of psychological factors in recovery. Further RCTs with long term follow ups, multidisciplinary involvement, and more comprehensive and focused interventions that go beyond educating patients are needed. Future studies should account for the demand effect, include measures of psychological variables to determine whether psychological interventions are more beneficial for some patients compared to others, and compare the different modes of delivery and timing of interventions to determine the optimal nature and duration of psychological interventions for TKA and THA.

Keywords: Arthroplasty, Knee, Hip, Psychology, Intervention

Background

The current practice in elective orthopaedics does not involve routine psychological interventions, despite evidence that psychological factors influence outcome and recovery from surgery [1–3]. One in eight patients experience moderate to severe levels of pain one year after total knee arthroplasty (TKA) despite having normal clinical and radiographic findings [4]. Many studies have suggested that psychological factors such as personality, anxiety, depression and negative thinking styles influence outcomes and recovery from surgery [1–3, 5, 6]. Giesinger et al. documented that psychological and demographic factors accounted for more variance in patient reported outcomes after hip and knee arthroplasty, than surgical factors [1]. Therefore, it would seem logical that inclusion of psychological interventions to facilitate recovery from arthroplasty may enhance patient satisfaction and outcomes, as psychological factors can influence

* Correspondence: samantha.bay@research.uwa.edu.au
[1]M304, School of Psychological Science, The University of Western Australia, 35 Stirling Highway, Perth, Western Australia 6009, Australia
Full list of author information is available at the end of the article

perception of pain, participation in rehabilitation and other outcomes after surgery [7].

Previous meta-analyses and systematic reviews [8–10] of psychological interventions found some to be effective in improving physical and psychological outcomes after surgeries. For example, in the most recent review, Nelson et al. investigated 20 studies with patients undergoing abdominal, cardiac, and orthopaedic surgery, and documented that there was some evidence for relaxation therapy in improving psychological well-being, such as reducing tension, anger, anxiety and pain, and evidence that guided imagery reduced post-surgical pain levels, and reducing analgesic intake [9].

Most reviews include a wide range of surgical procedures, which makes it difficult to draw conclusions and frame recommendations specific to TKA and total hip arthroplasty (THA). Arthroplasty is an elective surgery and is often undergone by healthy individuals with relatively low rates of comorbidities [11], and is thus very different from other surgeries, for example, coronary artery bypass grafting where patients require surgery in order to prolong life.

This systematic review aimed to bring more clarity with respect to the effectiveness of psychological interventions in improving joint outcomes following hip and knee arthroplasty. The following questions were addressed: Are psychological interventions beneficial in improving recovery and joint outcomes after TKA and THA? If so, are all types of psychological interventions equally effective?

Descriptions of psychological interventions in reviewed articles:

Cognitive behaviour therapy, psycho-education, motivational interviewing, relaxation therapy and guided imagery are some examples of well-established evidence-based psychological therapies in the literature.

Cognitive behaviour therapy

Cognitive behaviour therapy seeks to reduce symptoms by modifying maladaptive thought patterns and behaviours [12, 13]. It is based on the works of Beck [14] and Ellis [15]. Ellis proposed the ABC model of irrational beliefs, which cognitive behaviour therapy is based upon [16]. In the ABC model, an activating event (A), such as pain after surgery, in combination with a negative/irrational Belief (B), thinking that surgery is only successful if there is no pain at all, leads to a maladaptive behavioural or cognitive consequence (C), thinking that the pain will last forever and that the procedure had failed [16]. Cognitive behaviour therapy aims to help the patient understand and alter beliefs and thought processes, in order to positively influence consequences [15, 17, 18]. The therapist guides the patient to actively recognise maladaptive beliefs and thoughts, and to effect changes in emotional and behavioural consequences [18].

Psycho-education

Psycho-education is the systematic education of patients about their condition, along with discussion of coping strategies that might be used to manage and cope with current and future problems [19–21]. Psycho-education is often part of cognitive behaviour therapy [22, 23], but unlike cognitive behaviour therapy, Psycho-education does not aim to change emotional and behavioural consequences by exploring and changing a patient's belief, but rather gives the patient information about their condition and offers suggestions of behaviour changes that they can implement when faced with problems.

Motivational interviewing

Motivational interviewing is a counselling style that is targeted at eliciting behaviour changes [24]. Unlike persuasion, which generally increases resistance from the patient, motivational interviewing aims to explore and resolve the patient's ambiguity to change [24]. The counsellor uses empathy and acknowledges resistance, to guide the patient to create a discrepancy between reasons for and against change [25]. It is paramount that the patient reaches the conclusion on their own accord, with guidance from the counsellor [25].

Relaxation therapy

Relaxation therapy encompasses a range of techniques designed to reduce muscle tension and autonomic arousal [26]. This is achieved by using skills that focus on the internal state of the individual such as controlled breathing, focused muscle relaxation and postural awareness and management. [26]. Techniques typically focus on the redirection of attention of the patient from their thoughts and emotions [27].

Guided imagery

Guided imagery is a type of relaxation therapy in which patients deliberately form mental representations of positive images to promote relaxation and body awareness [28, 29]. While many relaxation therapies focus on physical components such as breathing and muscle tension, guided imagery most commonly focuses on sensory information such as sound, smell, touch, vision and taste [29, 30].

Methods

Preferred Reporting Items for Systematic reviews and Meta-Analyses (PRISMA) guidelines were applied. There was no published protocol for this review.

Search strategy

The search included empirical articles published in peer-reviewed journals, conference abstracts, and unpublished articles between January 1980 and mid-May 2017. An extensive literature search was conducted by searching electronic databases (Keyword and MeSH explode) for published articles and conference abstracts (MEDLINE, PsycInfo, EBSCO, PubMed, CINAHL, Web of Science, Scopus), grey literature (PsycExtra, Cochrane Library), and dissertations and theses (ProQuest Dissertations and Theses). Hand-searching was also conducted by reviewing the references cited in previous systematic reviews, and articles included in this study.

Unpublished dissertations, theses and grey literature were included in the search in order to avoid publication bias. Authors of conference abstracts, who reported collecting data on patient reported outcomes in elective orthopaedic surgery after psychological interventions were contacted by email for further information about their studies. The date of the last search was 17 May 2017. The search methodology is detailed in Fig. 1.

The following search terms were used: (psychological OR cognitive OR behavioural) AND (intervention OR therapy OR treatment OR program OR education OR information OR teaching OR skill OR learning) AND (orthopaedic OR orthopedic OR knee surgery OR hip surgery OR shoulder surgery OR spine surgery). Boolean truncations were used to allow for a more expansive search (see in Appendix for an example).

The terms chosen covered were broad in focus to allow inclusion of all studies that investigated the role of

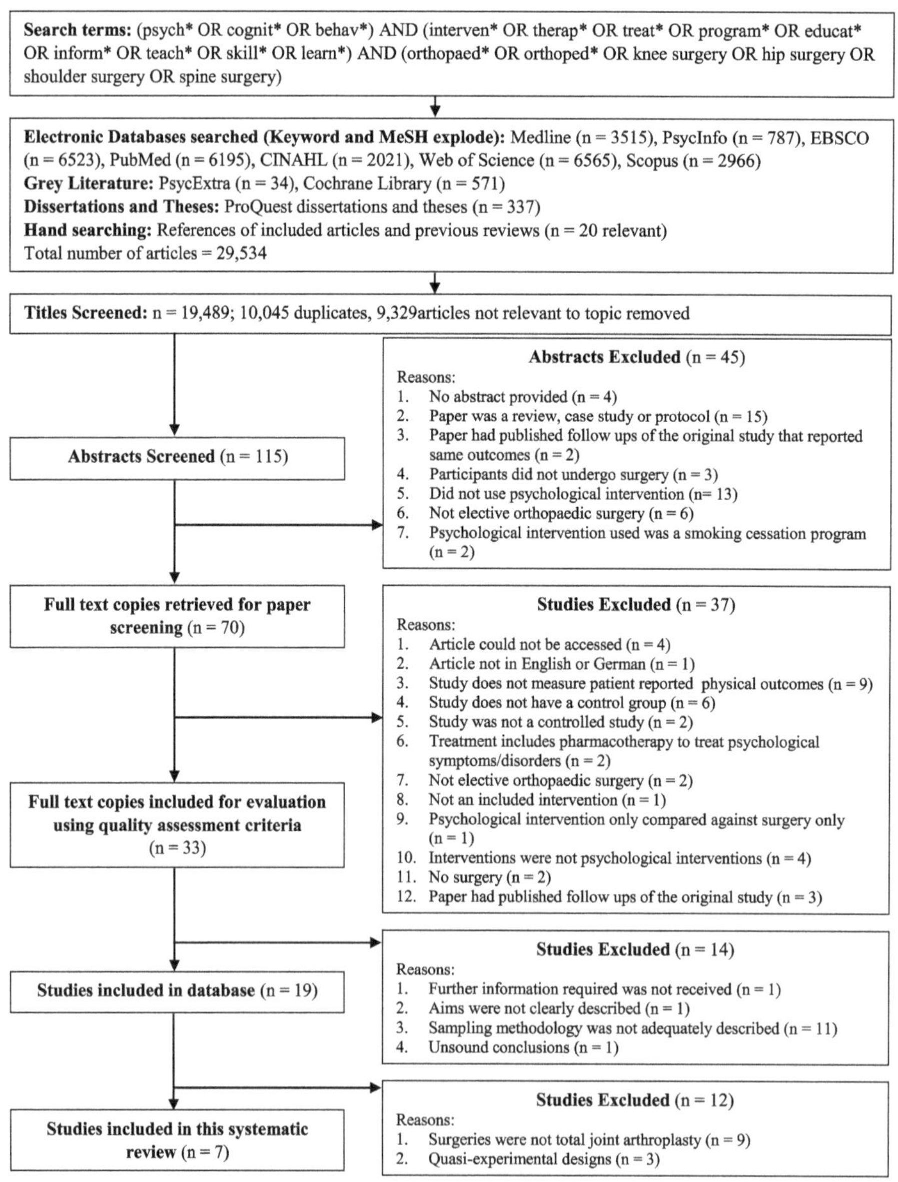

Fig. 1 Flow chart of search, retrieval and inclusion process

psychological intervention in elective orthopaedic surgery. However, in order to understand the more specific effects of psychological interventions on patients undergoing hip and knee arthroplasty, articles included in this review were further restricted.

Selection criteria

Studies included in this review satisfied the PICOS criteria:

Participants: elective orthopaedic patients undergoing knee or hip arthroplasty;

Interventions: psychological interventions involving active patient participation;

Comparisons: control groups including placebos, sham treatments, treatment as usual, education only or physical exercise only;

Outcome: Patient reported joint outcomes including pain, and/or functionality, and/or disability;

Study designs: Randomised controlled trials (RCTs).

Studies were excluded if participants did not undergo surgery, and/or if psychological intervention was compared to surgery. Studies were also excluded if they did not include a control group, and if a patient reported joint outcome was not measured. Articles that were in languages other than English and German were excluded. Only randomised control trials were reviewed.

Quality assessment

Only articles that fulfilled the requirements of the quality assessment were included in the review. In order to be considered good quality, an article must: 1) clearly describe the aims of the study; 2) adequately describe the methods undertaken in the study such that it may be replicated, which required clear descriptions of the recruitment of participants, timeline of interventions and data collection; and 3) have logical and sound conclusions drawn from results of the study.

Two authors (SB and LK) conducted the systematic searches and reviewed articles independently, according to the selection criteria. When there were disagreements regarding whether an article should be included, the issue was discussed with a third author (MSK), and a decision was made when all authors came to an agreement.

Data extraction

Data on participants, type of surgery, type of intervention, intervention timeline, sample size, follow ups, drop outs, outcome measures, professional backgrounds of therapists, power calculations, and major findings regarding patient reported joint outcomes were documented on pre-designed spreadsheets. Interventions were classified as effective if at least one outcome related to the arthroplasty was significantly improved for the treatment group compared to control group, after surgery. Data was extracted by the first author and checked by the second author.

Risk of Bias assessment

All included papers were reviewed for risk of bias, by assessing seven criteria adapted from the Cochrane Risk of Bias Tool [31]: 1) adequate randomization (selection bias); 2) dropout rate was not a threat to power (attrition bias); 3) demand effect - assessor of outcomes should not be the therapist/clinician (detection bias); 4) complete reporting of outcome data in results section; 5) significant and non-significant findings reported appropriately in the discussion section (reporting bias); 6) monitored intervention integrity; and 7) appropriate use of statistical analyses. Advice from a statistician about the appropriateness of statistical analyses was obtained.

There were two stages in defining risk of bias. Firstly, the articles were assessed according to the seven criteria, and rated with a risk score of "high" or "low" for each criterion. If there was inadequate information in articles to determine whether a criterion was satisfied, then a risk score of "high" was given. Secondly, a pre-defined classification of overall risk of bias assessment was agreed upon by the authors. Each article was rated to have either low, moderate or high overall levels of risk of bias, according to the following classification: low risk (A) where the article satisfies all 7 criteria in stage one; moderate risk (B) where 1–3 criterion were not satisfied in stage one; and high risk (C) where more than 3 criterion were not satisfied in stage one.

Results

Study selection

A total of 19,489 titles of studies were screened. Seven studies met criteria, and were included in this review (Fig. 1).

Study characteristics

Characteristics of the included studies are presented in Table 1.

Participants

The 7 reviewed studies consisted of 7 randomized controlled trials [32–38]. A total of 573 participants were involved, where 280 participants underwent a total knee arthroplasty (TKA), while 293 underwent a total hip arthroplasty (THA).

Analysis of studies

The data extracted from studies were categorised according to effectiveness in improving patient reported outcomes, and are presented in Table 2. Table 2 also

Table 1 Summary of reviewed studies

Author (Year)	Participants	Type of surgery	Control group	Psychological intervention (Type)	Frequency of sessions + (Mode of delivery)	Pre or Post surgery	Data collection points	Outcome measures (Note: Patient reported joint outcomes in bold)	Main findings about patient reported joint outcomes
Berge, Dolin, Williams & Harman (2004) [32]	Total *N* = 44 Mean age = 71.6 (PMP), 71.0 (controls) Age range = NS	THA	*N* = 21 TAU	Pain Management Training: education, cognitive behaviour therapy, relaxation **(CBT + RT)**	Total = 21.5 h; Occurred over 6 weeks; 1 to 2 mornings a week **(In-person)**	Pre; at least 6 months before surgery	Total = 3; Pre intervention, 3 and 12 months after PMP	**Pain (numerical rating scales)**, Analgesic drug use, **function (Arthritis Impact Measurement Scale),** metres walked in 4 min	Treatment group had sig. Better function than controls at 12 month follow up. No sig. Difference in pain was found between groups at 12 month follow up.
Doering et al. (2000) [33]	Total *N* = 100 Mean age = 58.7 (treatment), 60.4 (control) Age range = NS	THA	*N* = 54 TAU	Educational video + discussion **(PE)**	Total = 1 × 12 min video watched with psychologist/psychiatrist **(Video recording)**	Pre: afternoon of the pre-operative day	Total = 8; 5 consecutive days starting on pre-operation day, 3 months post-surgery	Anxiety (STAI), Depression (Von Zerssen Depression Scale), **Pain (VAS),** Blood pressure, Heart rate, Stress hormones (Urine samples), intake of analgesics and sedatives	No sig. Difference in pain was found between groups at all time points.
Forward et al. (2015) [38]	Total N = 224 TKA = 154 THA = 70 Mean age = NS Age range = NS	THA + TKA	*N* = 75 TAU TKA = NS THA = NS	Guided Imagery: Guided Meditation for Procedures or Surgery **(GI)**	Total = 4 × 18-20 min sessions: pre-surgery day, post-surgery day 0, 1 and 2 **(Audio recording)**	Pre and Post: began after admission	Total = 8; pre and post intervention on pre-surgery day, post-surgery day 0, 1 and 2	**Pain (Numeric Rating Scale)**, Anxiety (Numeric Visual Anxiety Scale, Hamilton Anxiety Scale)	No sig. Differences in pain between GI and controls during overall hospital stay.
Frost (2003) [34]	Total *N* = 24 Mean age = 66.2 (treatment), 65.9 (control) Age range = 57–75	THA	*N* = 11 Telephone contact only	Motivational Interviewing **(MI)**	Total = 3 sessions; 1 × 1 h in person, 2 x bi-monthly 15-30 min telephone session **(In-person and over the telephone)**	Post: began 3 months post-surgery	Total = 2; Pre intervention, 5 months post-surgery	Exercise (diary), Physical activity (Modifiable Activity Questionnaire), Mobility (Gait Speed), Muscle force/balance (Timed Chair Rise), **Pain/ Stiffness/physical function (WOMAC), physical health and mental health (SF-36),** Self-efficacy (Self Efficacy for Exercise Questionnaire), Depression (CESD-10)	No sig. Differences found between groups for all measures at 5 months post-surgery.
Grossman (2016) [37]	Total *N* = 60 TKA = 44 THA = 16 Mean age = 66.1 Age range = NS	THA + TKA	*N* = 15 Education only TKA = 10 THA = 5	Guided Imagery **(GI)**	Total = not standardised: 6 min recording pre-surgery twice a day for 1–2 weeks (At least once on day of surgery), encouraged to listen to recording post-surgery but no specific instruction. **(Audio recording)**	Pre: before admission and before surgery	Total = 3; pre intervention, post intervention (during hospital admission), post-surgery (before discharge)	Anxiety (STAI-S), Stress (Perceived Stress Scale), Coping Strategies (CSQ), **Pain (VAS)**, compliance (Training survey), medication use, length of hospital admission	No sig. Differences between groups for pain overall.

Table 1 Summary of reviewed studies *(Continued)*

Author (Year)	Participants	Type of surgery	Control group	Psychological intervention (Type)	Frequency of sessions + (Mode of delivery)	Pre or Post surgery	Data collection points	Outcome measures (Note: Patient reported joint outcomes in bold)	Main findings about patient reported joint outcomes
Jacobson et al. (2016) [36]	Total *N* = 82 Mean age = 65.0 Age range = 41–81	TKA	*N* = 40 Placebo audio recordings	Guided Imagery **(GI)**	Total = 35 self-directed sessions; Every day for 2 weeks before, and 3 weeks after surgery; 19-21 min each session for treatment, 17-21 min each session for control **(Audio recording)**	Pre and post: began 2 weeks pre- surgery	Total = 4; 2-3 weeks before surgery (pre-intervention), day of surgery, 3 weeks after surgery (post-intervention), 6 months after surgery	Gait velocity (Timed 10-Meter Walk), **functional status (SF-36), Pain/ stiffness/function (WOMAC),** imaging ability (Imaging Ability Questionnaire), optimism/pessimism (TKR Outcome Expectancy), **daily pain (VAS)**, self-efficacy (Self-Efficacy for Rehabilitation Scale), pain catastrophizing (PCS), fear of movement (Tampa Kinesophobia Scale), CD use questionnaire, Physiological variables (Lymphocytes, macrophages and cytokines)	Treatment group had sig. Reduced pain levels compared to baseline 3 weeks after surgery than control group. No sig. Differences between groups in improvements of knee function at 6 months post-surgery.
McGregor et al. (2004) [35]	Total *N* = 39 Mean age = 71.9 Age range = 51–92	THA	*N* = 20 TAU	Education + discussion **(PE)**	Total = 1 x advise class **(In-person)**	Pre surgery: 2-4 weeks before surgery	Total = 4; Pre-intervention, at admission, at discharge, 3 months post-surgery	**Function (WOMAC, Harris Hip Score, Berthel Activities of Daily Living Index), Pain (VAS),** Mood states (Positive Affect Negative Affect Scale), helplessness (subscale of Rheumatology Attitudes Index), **Fatigue (VAS),** expectations of pain/ function/satisfaction (VAS), Life satisfaction (Cantril Life Satisfaction Ladder)	No sig. Difference was found between groups for pain and function 3 months post-surgery. No results were reported for differences between groups in fatigue.

Note. "NS" indicates information not specified by papers. The word "significant" was abbreviated with "sig.". CBT = Cognitive Behaviour Therapy, MI = Motivational Interviewing, GI = Guided Imagery, PE = Psycho-education, RT = Relaxation Therapy, TAU = Treatment as usual, PMP = Pain management program, STAI = State-Trait Anxiety Inventory, VAS = visual analogue scale, WOMAC = Western Ontario and McMaster Universities Osteoarthritis Index, PCS = Pain Catastrophizing Scale, CESD-10 = The Centre for Epidemiologic Studies Depression scale 10

Table 2 Effectiveness of interventions in improving patient reported outcomes after surgery

Not effective					Effective					
Study	*Psychological intervention (Surgery)*	*Mode of delivery*	*Timing of Intervention*	*Joint outcomes measured*	Study	Psychological intervention (Surgery)	Mode of delivery	Timing of intervention	Joint outcome improved	Joint outcomes measured but not sig.
Doering et al. (2000) [33]	*Psycho-education (THA)*	*Video*	*Pre-surgery*	*Pain*	Berge et al. (2004) [32]	CBT + Relaxation (THA)	In-person	Pre-surgery	Function	*Pain*
Grossman (2016) [37]	*Guided Imagery (THA + TKA)*	*Audio*	*Pre-surgery*	*Pain*	Jacobson et al. (2016) [36]	Guided Imagery (TKA)	Audio	Pre- and Post-surgery	Pain	*Function, Stiffness*
Frost (2003) [34]	*Motivational Interviewing (THA)*	*In-Person + Telephone*	*Post-surgery*	*Pain, Stiffness, Function, Physical Health*						
Forward et al. (2015) [38]	*Guided Imagery (THA + TKA)*	*Audio*	*Pre- and post-surgery*	*Pain*						
McGregor et al. (2004) [35]	*Psycho-education (THA)*	*In-person*	*Pre-surgery*	*Function, Pain*						

Note. The word "significant" was abbreviated with "sig."

summarises the joint outcomes that were found to be improved by interventions, and joint outcomes that were not found to be improved by interventions.

Types of psychological interventions

Two studies used psycho-education [33, 35], one used motivational interviewing [34], and three used guided imagery [36–38]. One study used a combination of cognitive behaviour therapy and relaxation therapy [32].

Effectiveness of interventions

Patient reported outcomes included pain, physical health status, physical function, stiffness and fatigue. The most common parameter was pain, either measured on a numerical rating scale, visual analogue rating scale (VAS), or as part of the Western Ontario and McMaster Universities Arthritis Index (WOMAC).

Overall, two out of seven studies (total $n = 126$, 65 treated) found psychological interventions to be effective in improving at least one patient reported joint outcome [32, 36]. Of these two studies, one study (total $n = 44$, 23 treated) used a combination of cognitive behaviour therapy and relaxation therapy and was found to significantly improve hip function at the 12 month follow-up [32], and one study (total $n = 82$, 42 treated) used guided imagery and was found to significantly decrease knee pain 3 weeks after surgery [36]. Psycho-education, guided imagery, and motivational interviewing were amongst the types of interventions that were found to be ineffective in improving patient outcomes after TKA and THA.

The number of sessions of interventions varied widely, ranging from 1 to 35 sessions. Interventions that were effective in improving patient reported joint outcomes ranged from 6 to 35 sessions [32, 36]. All interventions with less than six sessions were not effective in improving patient reported outcomes [33–35, 38], and one intervention with more than 14 sessions was found to be ineffective [37]. However one intervention with 6 to 12 sessions [32] and another intervention with 35 self-directed sessions [36] were found to improve patient reported outcomes.

Mode of delivery

Mode of delivery varied across the studies with interventions delivered face to face, by video, by audio and by a mix of telephone and face to face contact. Effective interventions were delivered face to face [32], and by audio recording [36]. However, not all interventions delivered face to face and by audio recording were effective. Of two studies that delivered psychological interventions in-person (i.e. face to face) [32, 35], one [32] was effective (total $n = 44$, 23 treated). One study delivered interventions partially over the telephone and partially in-person [34], and was found to be ineffective. One study used video recordings [33], and was found to be ineffective. Three studies used audio recordings to deliver psychological interventions [36–38], and one [36] was effective (total $n = 82$, 42 treated).

Timing of interventions

Interventions were delivered either pre-surgery, post-surgery, or both pre and post-surgery, and varied considerably in terms of the number of sessions conducted. Four studies delivered psychological intervention sessions pre-surgery [32, 33, 35, 37], while one study delivered sessions post-surgery [34]. The number of sessions in pre-surgery interventions ranged from 1 to 28 sessions [32, 33, 35, 37], while the post-surgery intervention had 3 sessions [34]. Two studies [36, 38] delivered psychological intervention sessions both pre-surgery and post-surgery. The number of pre-surgery sessions ranged from 1 to 14 sessions, and post-surgery sessions ranged from 3 to 21 sessions [36, 38].

There was no clear trend as to the effectiveness of interventions according to the timing in which interventions were delivered. One intervention that was effective in improving at least one patient-reported outcome after surgery [36] was delivered both pre- and post-surgery (total $n = 82$, 42 treated), while the other intervention that was effective (total $n = 44$, 23 treated) was delivered pre-surgery [32]. The intervention delivered post-surgery only was not found to be effective [34], the other intervention delivered both pre and post-surgery was found to be ineffective [38], and the other three interventions delivered pre-surgery only were found to be ineffective [33, 35, 37].

Length of follow up

The timing of follow up measurements was variable and ranged between 1 day and 12 months post-surgery. One study conducted a follow up 12 months post-surgery [32], one study at 6 months post-surgery [36], one study at 5 months post-surgery [34], two studies at 3 months post-surgery [33, 35], and two studies conducted follow ups less than 1 week post-surgery [37, 38].

Risk of bias across studies

Of 7 studies, 5 had moderate risk of bias [32–34, 36, 38] and 2 had high risk of bias [35, 37].

The most adhered to criteria were adequate randomization and complete reporting of findings in the discussion section. The least adhered to criterion was having an independent researcher (i.e. not therapist or clinician) to collect outcome measures, which increased detection bias. As expected, none of the studies blinded participants or clinicians providing the interventions, as it is not possible due to the nature of psychological interventions. A summary of the risk of bias assessment is displayed in Table 3.

Discussion

Five out of seven RCTs did not show a benefit for psychological interventions in TKA and THA, questioning whether psychological interventions should be part of routine arthroplasty surgery. However, it should be noted that the literature for psychological interventions in conjunction with TKA and THA is still in its infancy, considering that 10 data-bases were searched, and only 7 RCTs met criteria to be reviewed. Many studies had small sample sizes and moderate levels of risk of bias despite being RCTs. The sub-optimal quality of articles exploring the effects of psychological interventions on patient reported joint outcomes is concerning, and the gap in the literature is surprising, considering the importance of the role of psychological factors in recovery.

Across the 7 studies, many different types of interventions were applied, and the timing and mode of delivery was variable, making comparisons difficult. Despite this, some interesting conclusions and directions for future research can be drawn.

Firstly, psycho-education was found to be ineffective in improving patient reported joint outcomes. Both RCTs applying psycho-education only found no significant differences between treatment and control groups [33, 35]. Imparting information alone to patients, while necessary, seems insufficient to change behaviour and therefore does not improve outcomes. This is in keeping with previous findings [39, 40]. Many studies have shown that psychological factors such as personality, anxiety, depression, and negative thinking styles influence the outcomes after surgeries [1–3, 5, 6]. Given that psycho-education alone is not effective in improving patient-reported joint related outcomes after surgery, these psychological factors need to be addressed using more comprehensive

Table 3 *Risk of bias assessment*

Authors	Risk of bias	Selection bias	Attrition bias	Detection bias	Complete outcome data (results)	Reporting bias	Compromised Intervention integrity?	Appropriate use of statistics?
Berge et al. (2004) [32]	B	Low risk	**High risk**	**High risk**	Yes	Low risk	**High risk**	Yes
Doering et al. (2000) [33]	B	Low risk	Low risk	**High risk**	**No**	Low risk	Low risk	Yes
Forward et al. (2015) [38]	B	Low risk	Low risk	**High risk**	**No**	**High risk**	Low risk	Yes
Frost (2003) [34]	B	Low risk	**High risk**	Low risk	Yes	Low risk	Low risk	Yes
Grossman (2016) [37]	C	Low risk	**High risk**	**High risk**	Yes	Low risk	**High risk**	**No**
Jacobson et al. (2016) [36]	B	Low risk	**High risk**	Low risk	Yes	Low risk	Low risk	**No**
McGregor et al. (2004) [35]	C	**High risk**	Low risk	**High risk**	**No**	Low risk	**High risk**	Yes

Note. Overall risk of bias: low risk (A), moderate risk (B) and high risk (C). Highlighted cells indicate unsatisfied criterion. No = high risk

interventions that go beyond educating patients. In other words, changing patients' thinking styles and providing strategies for managing physiological states are important in achieving improved patient reported outcomes after TKA and THA.

Secondly, interventions with less than six sessions were found to be ineffective, but beyond this, there was no clear relationship between the number of sessions and effectiveness of interventions. There was also no clear indication for the effectiveness of the different modes of delivery, or timing of interventions (i.e. pre/post-surgery). Further research is needed to define the optimal nature and duration of psychological intervention for TKA and THA.

There was promising evidence from two RCTs which integrated some form of relaxation therapy in their interventions, that psychological interventions improved outcomes post-surgery [32, 36]. Both studies showed a lasting effect beyond the allocated therapy period. One study that delivered cognitive behaviour therapy and relaxation therapy with a clinical psychologist found improvements in patient-reported functionality 12 months after surgery [32], and the other study found that guided imagery improved patient-reported pain 3 weeks after surgery [36].

Limitations

This systematic review identified a growing body of literature that explored the use of psychological interventions in TKA and THA. The quality of studies was sub-optimal with various sources of bias identified. Most studies did not account for a demand effect, where therapists or clinicians that administered interventions also collected outcome data. The demand effect is related to response-biases, where patients respond to questions in order to maintain socially desirable appearances [41]. It is possible that patients report improvements in order not to disappoint their therapist, or to maintain an image of being a "good patient". Future studies can account for the demand effect by having an independent researcher administer the questionnaires to patients and by including objective measures of outcomes, for example, measuring the range of motion to assess functionality of the knee or hip.

One of the main limitations of the current literature is the lack of long-term follow ups. Many studies focused on early postoperative outcomes, often only exploring outcomes during hospitalisation. It has been found that majority of patients experience low to mild levels of pain immediately after TKA [42], which mostly declines to half the intensity after 3 months [4]. Subjective perception of pain and functionality of the knee improves over a period of two years, and reaches a plateau after this period [43]. Thus, it would be important for studies to monitor patient outcomes over a longer period, as the rate of recovery varies over months [4, 42, 43].

Only one study in this review conducted a follow up at 12 months post-surgery [32] and one study conducted a follow up at 6 months post-surgery [36]. Thus, a conclusion as to whether psychological interventions have a lasting influence on patient outcomes cannot be drawn.

Most studies in the literature did not have specific intervention programs targeting different groups of patients in recovery from TKA and THA, rather, they were implemented as general concepts to every patient. Many patients will do well after TKA and THA, and psychological interventions may be more beneficial for patients with higher levels of catastrophic thinking styles, depression or anxiety as patients with these traits tend to have worse outcomes after surgery [1–3, 5, 6]. Future studies may wish to include measures of these psychological variables, to gauge whether psychological interventions are more beneficial for some patients compared to others. Additionally, most studies lacked a multi-disciplinary approach, where there was a lack of input from both mental health practitioners (e.g. psychologist or psychiatrist) and a surgical team member (e.g. surgeon). Future studies may wish to explore whether psychological interventions targeting recovery from TKA and THA specifically, with involvement of a multi-disciplinary team are effective.

Conclusions

The current literature does not support the effectiveness of psychological interventions in improving patient reported joint outcomes after TKA and THA as most interventions explored by studies were found to be ineffective. Specifically, psycho-education alone was shown to be ineffective. It should be noted that the literature for psychological interventions in conjunction with TKA and THA is still in its infancy. This gap in the literature is surprising, considering the importance of the role of psychological factors in recovery. Further RCTs with long term follow ups (e.g. at least 1 year), with more comprehensive and focused interventions that go beyond educating patients are needed. Future studies should account for the demand effect by involving an independent researcher and including objective measures of joint outcomes, include measures of psychological variables to determine whether psychological interventions are more beneficial for some patients compared to others, involve a multidisciplinary team, and compare the different modes of delivery and timing of interventions to determine the optimal nature and duration of psychological interventions for TKA and THA.

Appendix

Table 4 Example of search terms

Search terms in MEDLINE	
All fields Limit to yr. = "1980–2017"	(Psychiatry/ or psych*.mp. OR exp. Cognition/ or exp. Cognitive Processes/ or cognit*.mp. OR behav*.mp. or exp. Behavior/) AND
	(interven*.mp. OR exp. Psychotherapy/ OR therap*.mp. OR exp. Treatment/ or treat*.mp. OR program*.mp. OR educat*.mp. OR exp. Information/ or inform*.mp. OR exp. Teaching/ or teach*.mp. OR exp. Skill learning/ or skill*.mp. OR exp. Learning/ or learn*.mp.) AND
	(Orthopedics/ or Orthopedic Procedures/ OR exp. Knee/ or knee arthroplasty.mp. OR exp. Hips/ or hip arthroplasty.mp. OR shoulder surgery.mp. OR Spinal Fusion/ or spine surgery.mp. or Spine/)

Abbreviations

CBT: Cognitive Behaviour Therapy;; CESD-10: the Centre for Epidemiologic Studies Depression scale-10.; GI: Guided Imagery;; MI: Motivational Interviewing;; PCS: Pain Catastrophizing Scale;; PE: Psycho-education;; PMP: Pain management program;; PRISMA: Preferred Reporting Items for Systematic reviews and Meta-Analyses; RCTs: Randomised Control Trials; RT: Relaxation Therapy;; Sig. : Significant;; STAI: State-Trait Anxiety Inventory;; TAU: Treatment as usual;; THA: Total Hip Arthroplasty;; TKA: Total Knee Arthroplasty;; VAS: Visual analogue scale;; WOMAC: Western Ontario and McMaster Universities Osteoarthritis Index;

Acknowledgements

Authors would like to acknowledge the University of Western Australia for providing access to articles and computers to facilitate the completion of this paper. Authors would also like to acknowledge the Centre for Applied Statistics at the University of Western Australia for consulting with SB about the appropriateness of statistics in reviewed papers to assist with risk of bias assessments.

Funding

This project does not have any external funding. Access to articles and any materials used were provided by the School of Psychological Science at the University of Western Australia.

Authors' contributions

SB was the primary author, who conducted the comprehensive search of terms, data collection, analysis and writing of each section. LK was the secondary author who did an independent search of the literature to match SB's search terms, checked SB's data and contributed to the writing of each section. NM, MB, and MK are SB's PhD supervisors, whom SB consulted with while writing the review. NM and MB also contributed ideas in the development of this systematic review, and edited manuscript drafts. The idea of this systematic review originated from MK, who was consulted by SB and LK while writing the review, resolved SB and LK's disagreements about data, contributed major ideas to the discussion section and edited manuscript drafts. All authors read and approved the final manuscript.

Competing interests

MK declares that he has received royalties and research support from Zimmer Trauma, and Springer. All other authors declare no conflicts of interests.

Author details

[1]M304, School of Psychological Science, The University of Western Australia, 35 Stirling Highway, Perth, Western Australia 6009, Australia. [2]Sir Charles Gairdner Hospital, Hospital Ave, Perth, Western Australia 6009, Australia. [3]Perron Institute for Neurological and Translational Science, The University of Western Australia, RR Block, QEII Medical Centre, 8 Verdun Street, Perth, Western Australia 6009, Australia. [4]Medical School, The University of Western Australia, 35 Stirling Hwy, Perth, Western Australia 6009, Australia.

References

1. Giesinger JM, Kuster MS, Behrend H, Giesinger K. Association of psychological status and patient-reported physical outcome measures in joint arthroplasty: a lack of divergent validity. Health Qual Life Outcomes. 2013;11:64. https://doi.org/10.1186/1477-7525-11-64.
2. Hirschmann MT, Testa E, Amsler F, Friederich NF. The unhappy total knee arthroplasty (TKA) patient: higher WOMAC and lower KSS in depressed patients prior and after TKA. Knee Surgery, Sport Traumatol Arthrosc. 2013; 21:2405–11. https://doi.org/10.1007/s00167-013-2409-z.
3. Feeney SL. The relationship between pain and negative affect in older adults: anxiety as a predictor of pain. J Anxiety Disord. 2004;18:733–44. https://doi.org/10.1016/j.janxdis.2001.04.001.
4. Brander VA, Stulberg SD, Adams AD, Harden RN, Bruehl S, Stanos SP, et al. Predicting total knee replacement pain: a prospective, observational study. Clin Orthop Relat Res. 2003:27–36. https://doi.org/10.1097/01.blo.0000092983.12414.e9.
5. Goubert L, Crombez G, Van Damme S. The role of neuroticism, pain catastrophizing and pain-related fear in vigilance to pain: a structural equations approach. Pain. 2004;107:234–41. https://doi.org/10.1016/j.pain.2003.11.005.
6. Edwards RR, Haythornthwaite JA, Smith MT, Klick B, Katz JN. Catastrophizing and depressive symptoms as prospective predictors of outcomes following total knee replacement. Pain Res Manag. 2009;14:307–11.
7. Filardo G, Merli G, Roffi A, Marcacci T, Berti Ceroni F, Raboni D, et al. Kinesiophobia and depression affect total knee arthroplasty outcome in a multivariate analysis of psychological and physical factors on 200 patients. Knee Surgery, Sport Traumatol Arthrosc. 2016; https://doi.org/10.1007/s00167-016-4201-3.
8. Johnston M, Vögele C. Benefits of psychological preparation for surgery: a meta-analysis. Ann Behav med a Publ Soc. Behav Med. 1993;15:245–56.
9. Nelson EA, Dowsey MM, Knowles SR, Castle DJ, Salzberg MR, Monshat K, et al. Systematic review of the efficacy of pre-surgical mind-body based therapies on post-operative outcome measures. Complement Ther Med. 2013;21:697–711. https://doi.org/10.1016/j.ctim.2013.08.020.
10. Devine EC. Effects of psycho- educational care for adult surgical patients: a meta-analysis of 191 studies. Patient Educ Couns. 1992;19:129–42. https://doi.org/10.1016/0738-3991(92)90193-M.
11. Singh JA, Lewallen DG. Time trends in the characteristics of patients undergoing primary total knee arthroplasty. Arthritis Care Res (Hoboken). 2014;66:897–906. https://doi.org/10.1002/acr.22233.
12. Hofmann SG, Asnaani A, Vonk IJJ, Sawyer AT, Fang A. The efficacy of cognitive behavioral therapy: a review of meta-analyses. Cogn Ther Res. 2012;36:427–40. https://doi.org/10.1007/s10608-012-9476-1.
13. Brewin CR. Understanding cognitive behaviour therapy: a retrieval competition account. Behav Res Ther. 2006;44:765–84. https://doi.org/10.1016/j.brat.2006.02.005.
14. Beck AT. Cognitive therapy: nature and relation to behavior therapy. Behav Ther. 1970;1:184–200. https://doi.org/10.1016/S0005-7894(70)80030-2.
15. Ellis A. Reason and emotion in psychotherapy. Commentary. 1962;11:442. https://doi.org/10.1002/jclp.20252.
16. Ellis A. The revised ABC's of rational-emotive therapy (RET). J Ration Cogn Ther. 1991;9:139–72. https://doi.org/10.1007/BF01061227.
17. Beck AT, Rush AJ, Shaw BF, Emery G. Cognitive therapy of depression. 1979.
18. Blagys MD, Hilsenroth MJ. Distinctive activities of cognitive–behavioral therapy. Clin Psychol Rev. 2002;22:671–706. https://doi.org/10.1016/S0272-7358(01)00117-9.
19. Goldman CR. Toward a definition of psychoeducation. Hosp Community Psychiatry. 1988;39:666–8. https://doi.org/10.1007/BF02648210.
20. Colom F. Keeping therapies simple: Psychoeducation in the prevention of relapse in affective disorders. Br J Psychiatry. 2011;198:338–40. https://doi.org/10.1192/bjp.bp.110.090209.

21. Hayes R, Gantt A. Patient psychoeducation: the therapeutic use of knowledge for the mentally ill. Soc Work Health Care. 1992;17:53–67. https://doi.org/10.1300/J010v17n01_04.
22. Freeman A. Encyclopedia of cognitive behavior therapy. New York, USA: springer science + business media; 2005.
23. Lukens EP, Mcfarlane WR. Psychoeducation as Evidence-Based Practice : Considerations for Practice, Research, and Policy 2004;4. doi:https://doi.org/10.1093/brief-treatment/mhh019.
24. Rollnick S, Miller WR. What is motivational interviewing? Behav Cogn Psychother. 1995;23:325–34. https://doi.org/10.1017/S135246580001643X.
25. Rollnick S, Allison J. Motivational Interviewing. In: Heather N, Stockwell T, editors. Essent. Handb. Treat. Prev. Alcohol Probl., West Sussex, England: John Wiley & Sons; 2004, p. 119–29.
26. Van Dixhoorn J, Duivenvoorden H. Effect of relaxation therapy on cardiac events after myocardial infarction: a 5-year follow-up study. J Cardpulm Rehabil. 1999;19:178–85. https://doi.org/10.1097/00008483-199905000-00005.
27. Van Dixhoorn J, White A. Relaxation therapy for rehabilitation and prevention in ischaemic heart disease: a systematic review and meta-analysis. Eur J Cardiovasc Prev Rehabil. 2005;12:193–202. https://doi.org/10.1097/00149831-200506000-00002.
28. Halpin LS, Speir AM, CapoBianco P, Barnett SD. Guided imagery in cardiac surgery. Outcomes Manag. 2002;6:132–7.
29. Giedt JF. Guided imagery: a psychoneuroimmunological intervention in holistic nursing practice. J Holist Nurs. 1997;15:112–27. https://doi.org/10.1177/089801019701500204.
30. Lewandowski W, Jacobson A. Bridging the gap between mind and body: a biobehavioral model of the effects of guided imagery on pain, pain disability, and depression. Pain Manag Nurs. 2013;14:368–78. https://doi.org/10.1016/j.pmn.2011.08.001.
31. The Cochrane Collaboration. The Cochrane Risk of Bias Tool 2017. http://methods.cochrane.org/bias/assessing-risk-bias-included-studies# The Cochrane Risk of Bias Tool (accessed February 1, 2017).
32. Berge DJ, Dolin SJ, Williams AC, Harman R. Pre-operative and post-operative effect of a pain management programme prior to total hip replacement: a randomized controlled trial. Pain. 2004;110:33–9. https://doi.org/10.1016/j.pain.2004.03.002.
33. Doering S, Katzlberger F, Rumpold G, Roessler S, Hofstoetter B, Schatz DS, et al. Videotape preparation of patients before hip replacement surgery reduces stress. Psychosom Med. 2000;62:365–73.
34. Frost KL. Influence of a motivational exercise counseling intervention on rehabilitation outcomes in individuals with arthritis who received total hip replacement: University of Pittsburgh; 2003.
35. McGregor AH, Rylands H, Owen A, Doré CJ, Hughes SPF. Does preoperative hip rehabilitation advice improve recovery and patient satisfaction? J Arthroplast. 2004;19:464–8. https://doi.org/10.1016/j.arth.2003.12.074.
36. Jacobson AF, Umberger WA, Palmieri PA, Alexander TS, Myerscough RP, Draucker CB, et al. Guided imagery for Total knee replacement: a randomized, placebo-controlled pilot study. J Altern Complement Med. 2016;22:563–75. https://doi.org/10.1089/acm.2016.0038.
37. Grossman LE. The effects of guided imagery and HRV biofeedback training on psychological variables and post-operative outcome measures of orthopaedic surgical patients: Florida State University; 2016.
38. Forward JB, Greuter NE. Effect of structured touch and guided imagery for pain and anxiety in elective joint replacement patients—a randomized controlled trial: M-TIJRP. Perm J. 2015;19:18–28. https://doi.org/10.7812/TPP/14-236.
39. Newman S, Mulligan K, Steed L. What is meant by self-management and how can its efficacy be established? Rheumatology (Oxford). 2001;40:1–4. https://doi.org/10.1093/rheumatology/40.1.1.
40. Herbert C. Giving information: usually necessary, but often insufficient to achieve behaviour change. Patient Educ Couns. 1996;29:229–30. https://doi.org/10.1016/S0738-3991(96)00983-4.
41. van de Mortel T. Faking it: social desirability response bias in self-report research report research. Aust J Adv Nurs. 2008;25:40–8.
42. Wylde V, Dieppe P, Hewlett S, Learmonth ID. Total knee replacement: is it really an effective procedure for all? Knee. 2007;14:417–23. https://doi.org/10.1016/j.knee.2007.06.001.
43. Forsythe ME, Dunbar MJ, Hennigar AW, Sullivan MJL, Gross M. Prospective relation between catastrophizing and residual pain following knee arthroplasty: two-year follow-up. Pain Res Manag. 2008;13:335–41. https://doi.org/10.1155/2008/730951.

15

Impact of a tailored activity counselling intervention during inpatient rehabilitation after knee and hip arthroplasty – an explorative RCT

Mirko Brandes[1*], Norman Wirsik[2], Hanna Niehoff[3], Jörg Heimsoth[4] and Bernd Möhring[4]

Abstract

Background: The aim of the study was to improve physical activity (PA), well-being and clinical outcome after total knee and hip arthroplasty through tailored activity counselling during inpatient rehabilitation.

Methods: 65 patients (aged 70.4 ± 7.3 years, BMI 28.5 ± 4.3) starting inpatient rehabilitation after primary knee or hip arthroplasty due to osteoarthritis were recruited and pseudo-randomized into an intervention (IG) and a control group (CG). Twice a week, the IG was encouraged to increase their daily step count by 5%. PA, e. g. number of steps, step frequency, or active minutes, was measured by step activity monitoring. Well-being and clinical outcome were assessed using the SF-36, Oxford Knee/Hip Score and Global rating of Change. Procedures were conducted at the onset of inpatient rehabilitation, and repeated one and 6 months after inpatient rehabilitation.

Results: Data sets were obtained from 49 patients (IG: $n = 23$, CG: $n = 26$). Both groups significantly increased their number of daily steps from the 1 month to the 6 months follow up after rehabilitation: CG: 9019 (95%CI: 7812, 10,226), IG: 9280 (7972, 10,588) and CG: 10921 (9571, 12,271), IG: 11326 (9862, 12,791) respectively. Additionally, well-being and clinical outcome improved significantly in both groups. No significant differences in physical activity, clinical outcome and well-being were found between the groups.

Conclusions: PA counselling during inpatient rehabilitation does not improve PA, well-being and clinical outcome in patients with primary knee or hip arthroplasty in addition to the rehabilitation program. PA interventions may be more effective after the completion of the inpatient rehabilitation phase.

Keywords: Physical activity, Well-being, Clinical outcome, Step counting, Oxford score

Background

Around 250 million people in the world experience pain, reduced physical function, and restricted well-being due to osteoarthritis (OA) of the knee or hip. In Germany, more than 40% of the population above 60 years of age is affected by OA [1]. Therefore, knee and hip OA represents one of the most common joint disorders, and is predicted to increase further due to the aging population and obesity epidemic [2, 3]. Despite the availability of conservative treatment, joint arthroplasty is a common treatment. Clinicians as well as patients expect the treatment to reduce pain, improve lower extremity function, enable a return to a physically active lifestyle comparable to that of healthy peers, and to improve the overall well-being of patients [4, 5].

Unfortunately, due to their walking disability, patients suffering from OA are more prone to cardiovascular diseases, leading to significantly increased mortality [6]. The health risks for OA patients regarding reduced physical activity (PA), (such as a higher prevalence of type II diabetes), as well as the positive aspects of being

* Correspondence: brandes@leibniz-bips.de
[1]Department of Prevention and Evaluation, Unit Applied Health Intervention Research, Leibniz Institute for Prevention Research and Epidemiology - BIPS GmbH, Achterstraße 30, 28359 Bremen, Germany
Full list of author information is available at the end of the article

physically active, (such as less prevalence of metabolic syndrome), were recently summarized in a vivid review by Paxton and colleagues [7]. However, several studies have demonstrated that PA after knee or hip arthroplasty is low, and that, although clinical outcomes and physical functioning appears to be good, patients do not meet current activity guidelines [8–11]. While a wide range in the amount of PA after knee and hip arthroplasty has been reported in previous research in Germany, in each study PA among patients was observed to be less compared to that of healthy peers [12–14]. Thus, the conclusion is that future research should implement PA interventions aiming to increase PA after knee and hip joint replacement. However, it is unclear at what point after joint arthroplasty PA interventions are most effective [7]. The inpatient rehabilitation is probably the earliest point at which a cost and time effective PA intervention can be delivered because hip and knee patients are then more condensed and approachable compared to immediately after surgery. In Germany, most people receive 3 weeks of rehabilitation after knee or hip replacement, starting a few days after surgery. Moreover, German patients can chose between outpatient and inpatient rehabilitation. We hypothesize that patients would benefit from additional PA interventions during inpatient rehabilitation. Therefore, the objective of the current explorative study was to implement a PA intervention after knee or hip joint replacement and to evaluate the effects of the PA interventions at one and 6 months after the inpatient rehabilitation.

Methods

Sixty five patients (aged 70.4 ± 7.3 years, BMI 28.5 ± 4.3, 35 females, 26 knee arthroplasties) were included in the study, which was approved by the Oldenburg University ethics committee. The inclusion criterion was primary, unilateral joint replacement due to OA of the knee or hip. Exclusion criteria were revision joint replacements, additional previous joint replacement in the knee or hip on either side, any comorbidities with severe impact on the ability to perform physical activity, such as COPD, walking with crutches, and metabolic syndrome. Patients were recruited from a single rehabilitation centre in Oldenburg, which has a large catchment area in Northwest Germany. After providing written informed consent, the patients were pseudo-randomized into an intervention group, (n = 28), receiving the standard rehabilitation program and the individualized activity counselling, and a control group, (n = 37), receiving the standard rehabilitation program only. Pseudo-randomization was performed by assigning a block of 10 patients to the intervention group and having them complete the inpatient rehabilitation. After the last of the intervention group patients left the institution, a block of 10 patients was assigned to the control group and also completed the inpatient rehabilitation. This procedure was repeated alternatively until the overall number of patients was enrolled into the study. Pseudo-randomization was favoured to avoid verbal exchange between intervention and control group. The patients as well as the scientific personnel were not blinded regarding patient allocation to the IG or CG. On average, the patients started the inpatient rehabilitation 13.4 ± 5.4 days after surgery and stayed 19.4 ± 1.4 days at the centre, including weekends. The standard program of the inpatient rehabilitation included mobility and strength training, hydrotherapy, wound care, and management of everyday tasks. Physical applications were accompanied by theoretical instructions, usually provided in classes. Timing, frequency and duration of the rehabilitation components were individualized due to patient characteristics. No rehabilitation was offered on weekends.

Study procedures

The study procedures were conducted at baseline, on the first day of arrival at the inpatient rehabilitation centre, and repeated one, and 6 months after completing the inpatient rehabilitation. A separate and quiet room in the rehabilitation centre was available for the study procedures. Physical activity was measured using the Step Activity Monitor (SAM; Step Activity Monitor 3.0, modus health, Washington, USA). The device, that has been described elsewhere [15–19], has proven excellent validity and reliability in measuring daily steps in populations with walking impairments and during inpatient treatment. According to the manufacturers' instructions, the device was mounted to the ankle of the opposite leg of the affected limb. Gait cycles were stored at one-minute intervals. The device does not give feedback to the patients and acts as a black box. Data were downloaded using the dedicated software (StepWatch 3.4, modus health, Washington, USA) and further processed with Microsoft Excel to calculate the number of steps (twice the number of gait cycles), and movement intensity (gait cycles per minute), as well as active minutes per day with at least 60 steps/min. The average number of daily steps was considered the primary outcome of the study. The baseline measurements covered the initial days of the inpatient rehabilitation (4.2 ± 1.7 days). At one and 6 months post rehabilitation, the patients were requested to wear the device for seven consecutive days including weekends. Before each measurement, the device was adjusted to the patients' gait characteristics (leg length and cadence).

As secondary outcomes, the valid and reliable Oxford Knee Score and the Oxford Hip Score were utilized to assess the clinical outcome in knee and hip patients, respectively [20, 21]. Patients had to answer 12 questions, each with 5 response options. The responses were valued as "4" for the best clinical option, to "0" for the worst clinical option. Thus, the outcome of the Oxford Score ranges from "0", reflecting the worst clinical outcome, to "48", reflecting the best clinical outcome. Well-being was estimated using the SF-36 questionnaire, a valid approach in knee and hip patients [22, 23]. The overall score as well as sub-scores for physical functioning, pain, role limitations due to physical health, and physical component score (PCS) and mental component score (MCS) were extracted. For both the clinical outcome and well-being, the data are expressed as a percentage of the maximum score, with 0% reflecting the worst clinical score or well-being, and 100% reflecting the best clinical score or well-being. Global rating of change compared to the pre-operation status was measured with a seven-point Likert-Scale ranging from 1 ("very much worse") to 7 ("very much better").

Physical activity counselling

The physical activity counselling was tailored following an adaptive approach by adding + 5% in daily steps compared to the previous days. This adaptive approach has been shown to be more effective in weight loss interventions [24] and cardiology [25] than rigid recommendations, such as to ambulate 10.000 steps per day. Further, the approach was favoured by the study team because it takes the individual capacities of the patients into account. Only patients assigned to the intervention group received the counselling twice a week, preferably on a Monday and Thursday. The patients wore the SAM continuously for the entire inpatient rehabilitation period. Two students, who were familiar with the rehabilitation centre and the rehabilitation programs, were trained to be counsellors and offered the PA counselling to the IG. The counsellors downloaded the data from the device and prepared graphical visualizations of the steps taken during the previous days that they showed to the patients. Visualization included a colour figure displaying the time of day on the x-axis, and the number of steps recorded minute-by-minute on the y-axis. Furthermore, the total number of steps was displayed in the figure. Therefore, patients and counsellors were able to identify periods of walking and to estimate the number of steps taken outside the rehabilitation program, for example while walking in the park. The current data of the previous 3 or 4 days were compared to the days before that. Finally, the counsellors encouraged the patients to increase their number of daily steps by 5% over the following days, and suggested walking tasks to help meet the goal. For example: "Your average number of steps for the last days was 3000 steps. Please note that your short walk in the park counted around 300 steps. If you just add half of the short walk, you will reach the goal for the next three days."

Because the main purpose of the counselling was to encourage the patients to make use of their restored walking capabilities, a strict adherence to increasing exactly + 5% in daily steps was less important. Consequently, regardless of whether patients increased or decreased their daily steps, they were encouraged to increase their activity with respect to the previous days by 5%. The duration of each counselling ranged from 10 to 20 min. Neither additional incentives for meeting the recommendations nor any penalties if the patients failed to increase their activity were instituted. The counselling was only provided during inpatient rehabilitation and stopped on the day of discharge from the centre.

Statistical analysis

Parameters at onset of inpatient rehabilitation were analysed with respect to significant differences between the control group and the intervention group using an independent t-test. Differences between occasions and between intervention and control group were investigated using multi-level linear models, adjusting for age, sex and repeated measurements. This procedure allowed for the inclusion of patients measured on at least two occasions (at baseline, one or 6 months post inpatient rehabilitation). The tests were performed at a significance level of $\alpha = 0.05$. All statistical analyses were performed using SAS 9.3 (SAS Institute Inc., Cary, NC, USA). We used PROC MIXED in SAS, which can handle unbalanced data and included only patients with at least 2 observations (baseline plus any follow-up examination).

Results

Sixteen patients that signed a written informed consent at baseline dropped out of the study until the one month follow-up due to medical reasons (such as implant loosening, infections, or wound healing disorders) or withdrawal of participation (Fig. 1). Consequently, 26 patients in the control group and 23 patients in the intervention group who had at least two measurement occasions were available for statistical analysis. In anthropometric data, no differences existed between the intervention group and the control group (Table 1). With respect to the outcome data, no significant differences were observed between the intervention and the control group, neither in physical activity, nor in clinical outcome or well-being, at any time. On average, the control group and the intervention group patients wore the SAM for 4.2 and 4.4 days respectively, with a minimum of 13 h/day during the initial days of inpatient rehabilitation. At one and 6 months after inpatient rehabilitation, the control group achieved an average of 5.9 and 6.8 valid days, respectively, while the

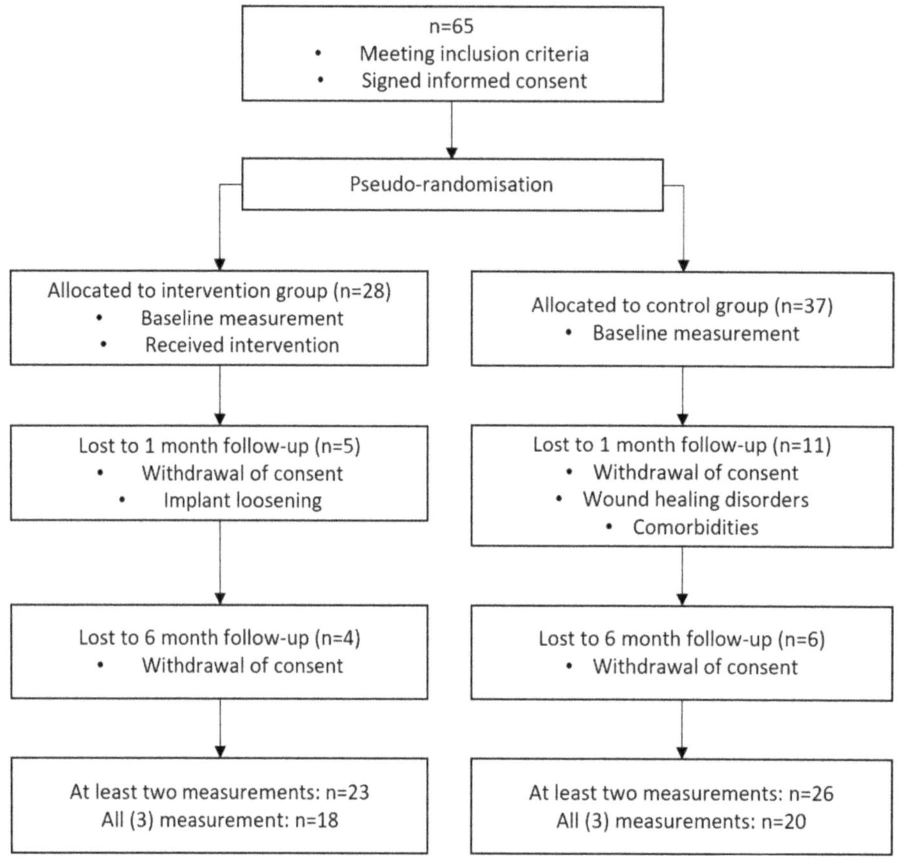

Fig. 1 Patient flow chart

intervention group reached 6.9 and 7.0 valid days for the respective time points. The control group increased their PA from 9519 steps/day at onset to 10,921 steps/day 6 months after rehabilitation, and the intervention group from 9513 to 11,326 steps/day over the same period (Fig. 2). The average duration of inactive bouts while wearing the device decreased from 13.3 min at baseline to 10.7 min at 6 months post rehabilitation in the control group, and from 14.8 to 12.8 min in the intervention group. Both groups accumulated more minutes with active walking (> 60 steps/minute) during inpatient rehabilitation (CG = 66.6 and IG = 64.5 min), compared to 1 month (CG = 35.6 and IG = 40.3 min) and 6 months (CG = 49.6 and IG = 50.7) after rehabilitation. Further details of PA parameters are given in Table 2.

The clinical outcome, measured using the Oxford Score, increased significantly in both groups from baseline to 6 months post rehabilitation. Furthermore, both

Table 1 Anthropometric data of control and intervention group at baseline. Data are given as mean values (95% confidence interval). IR = inpatient rehabilitation; convalescence = days between surgery and inpatient rehabilitation. Only patients considered for analysis (=at least two observations) are included

	Control group (n = 26)	Intervention group (n = 23)	p
Age (years)	69.9 (67.3, 72.5)	70.7 (68.0, 73.5)	0.61
Height (cm)	170.0 (166.3, 173.6)	171.6 (166.8, 176.4)	0.66
Weight (kg)	81.1 (76.0, 86.2)	82.2 (74.2, 90.2)	0.18
BMI	27.1 (24.1, 30.1)	27.5 (25.7, 29.3)	0.34
Hip replacements (n, %)	18 (69.2)	16 (69.6)	
Females (n, %)	14 (53.8)	12 (52.2)	
Convalescence (days)	12.3 (10.9, 13.7)	14.0 (10.9, 17.0)	0.09
Duration IR (days)	19.2 (18.6, 19.8)	19.9 (19.3, 20.5)	0.272

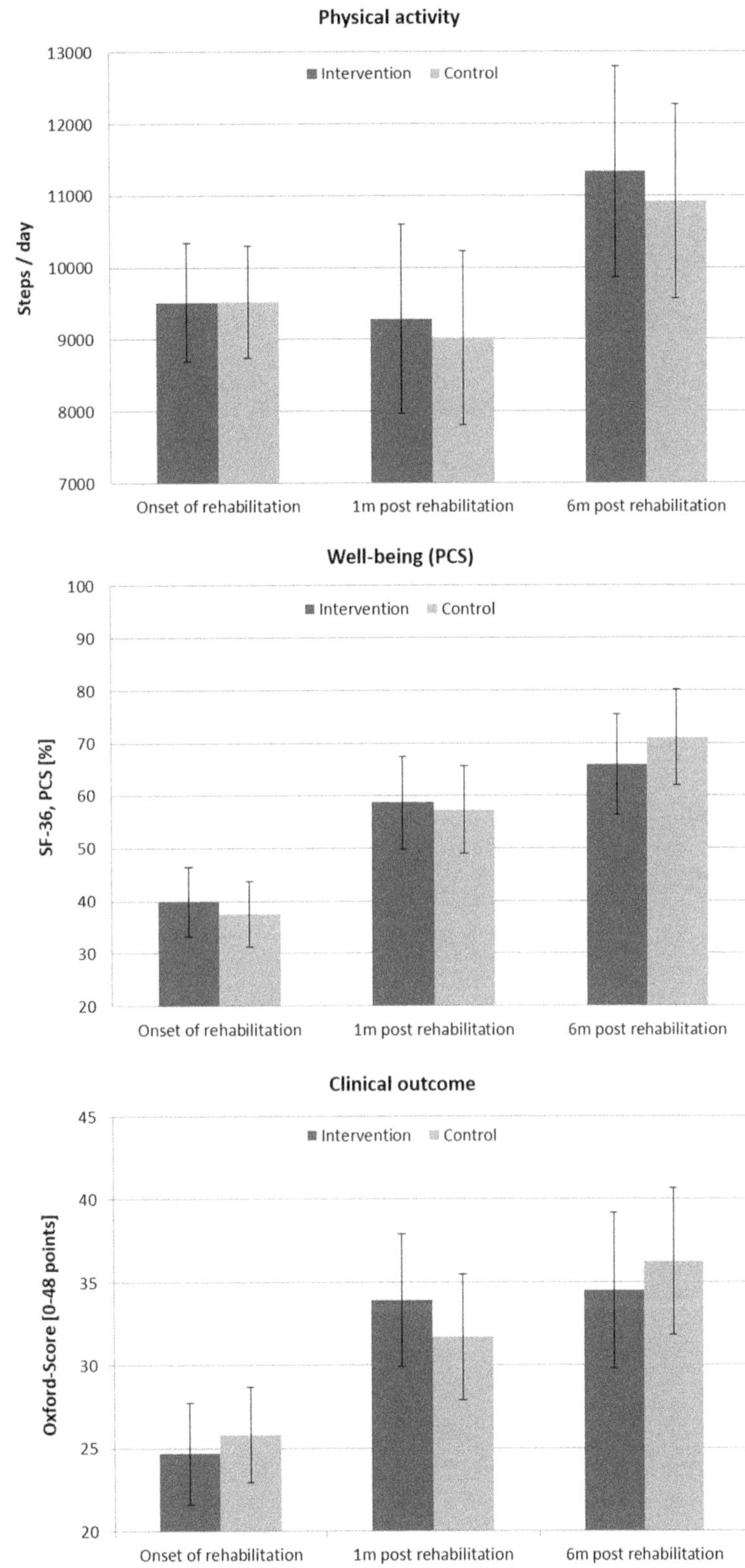

Fig. 2 Differences between intervention ($n = 23$) and control group ($n = 26$) in physical activity, well-being (physical component score) and clinical outcome (mean, 95% CI)

Table 2 Physical activity parameters for the control (CG) and intervention group (IG). Data are given as mean values (95% confidence interval).[1] = $p < 0.05$ compared to 1 m post rehabilitation, [O] = $p < 0.05$ compared to onset inpatient rehabilitation

	Onset inpatient rehabilitation		1 month post rehabilitation		6 month post rehabilitation	
	CG ($n = 26$)	IG ($n = 23$)	CG ($n = 26$)	IG ($n = 23$)	CG ($n = 20$)	IG ($n = 18$)
Steps/day	9519 (8737, 10,301)	9513 (8692, 10,335)	9019 (7812, 10,226)	9280 (7972, 10,588)	10,921 (9571, 12,271)[1]	11,326 (9862, 12,791)[1]
Active minutes (> 0 steps/min)	295.1 (272.9, 317.2)	294.2 (271.0, 317.5)	338.6 (304.7, 372.4)[O]	328.8 (292.1, 365.5)	363.3 (328.1, 398.5)[O]	376.4 (338.3, 414.6)[1,O]
Active minutes (> 60 steps/min)	66.6 (59.2, 74.1)	64.5 (56.7, 72.3)	35.6 (27.5, 43.6)[O]	40.3 (31.6, 49.0)[O]	49.6 (39.6, 59.6)[1,O]	50.7 (39.8, 61.5)
Mean step frequency (> 60 steps/min)	40.2 (39.1, 41.4)	40.9 (39.7, 42.1)	40.4 (38.8, 42.0)	40.5 (38.8, 42.2)	41.4 (39.7, 43.1)	40.5 (38.7, 42.4)
#min with 1–20 steps/min	147.7 (131.8, 163.6)	147.7 (131.0, 164.4)	171.7 (154.5, 188.9)	162.5 (143.8, 181.2)	170.4 (156.2, 184.7)	173.4 (157.9, 188.9)[O]
#min with 21–40 steps/min	51.9 (46.1, 57.8)	52.7 (46.6, 58.8)	89.4 (79.7, 99.1)[O]	84.7 (74.2, 95.2)[O]	97.9 (87.0, 108.9)[O]	101.2 (89.4, 113.1)[1,O]
#min with 41–60 steps/min	31.9 (28.2, 35.6)	32.4 (28.5, 36.3)	43.5 (36.2, 50.8)[O]	42.7 (34.9, 50.8)	50.2 (40.9, 59.6)[O]	56.9 (46.7, 67.0)[1,O]
#min with 61–80 steps/min	38.3 (31.8, 44.7)	34.3 (27.6, 41.1)	16.8 (13.0, 20.6)[O]	18.7 (14.6, 22.9)[O]	22.9 (17.4, 28.5)[O]	25.6 (19.6, 31.7)
#min with 81–100 steps/min	18.0 (12.7, 23.2)	19.6 (14.1, 25.1)	10.1 (6.3, 13.8)	12.2 (8.1, 16.2)	13.4 (9.7, 17.1)	13.6 (9.6, 17.6)
#min with > 100 steps/min	6.6 (4.2, 8.9)	7.6 (5.1, 10.0)	6.0 (3.2, 8.9)	6.7 (3.6, 9.8)	9.9 (5.9, 14.0)	7.6 (3.3, 12.0)
Mean duration of inactive bouts (min)	13.3 (11.0, 15.7)	14.8 (12.3, 17.4)	13.3 (11.0, 15.7)	13.6 (11.1, 16.1)	10.7 (8.2, 13.2)	12.8 (10.1, 15.4)
Max. duration of inactive bouts (min)	131.8 (108.0, 155.6)	134.4 (109.1, 159.7)	124.6 (104.3, 144.9)	117.0 (95.5, 138.6)	101.0 (81.5, 120.4)	106.0 (85.5, 126.6)
Total inactive time (9 am – 6 pm)	380.5 (364.0, 397.1)	393.0 (375.3, 410.6)	371.0 (352.8, 389.3)	383.0 (363.5, 402.5)	351.2 (328.5, 373.9)	339.0 (315.1, 363.0)[1,O]
Max. mean gait frequency for 5 min	60.0 (55.7, 64.2)	58.8 (54.3, 63.3)	50.7 (46.8, 54.5)[O]	54.0 (49.9, 58.1)	56.4 (52.9, 60.0)	56.3 (52.9, 59.9)
Max. mean gait frequency for 10 min	57.2 (52.6, 61.7)	56.0 (51.2, 60.8)	45.7 (41.1, 50.3)[O]	50.4 (45.6, 55.3)	51.8 (47.6, 55.9)	52.5 (47.6, 55.9)

Table 3 Clinical outcome (Oxford score) and well-being (SF-36) for the control (CG) and intervention group (IG). Data are given as mean values (95% confidence interval). PCS = physical component score; MCS = mental component score; PF = subscale physical functioning; PR = subscale for role limitations due to physical health; Pain = subscale pain; GRC = global rating of change. [1] = $p < 0.05$ compared to 1 m post rehabilitation, [O] = $p < 0.05$ compared to onset inpatient rehabilitation

		Onset inpatient rehabilitation		1 month post rehabilitation		6 month post rehabilitation	
		CG ($n = 26$)	IG ($n = 23$)	CG ($n = 26$)	IG ($n = 23$)	CG ($n = 20$)	IG ($n = 18$)
Clinical outcome		53.8 (47.8, 59.8)	51.4 (45.0, 57.8)	66.0 (58.1, 73.9)	70.6 (62.3, 78.9)[O]	75.5 (66.3, 84.7)[O]	71.8 (62.1, 81.6)[O]
Well-being	Overall	50.3 (43.3, 57.3)	54.2 (46.8, 61.6)	64.1 (56.2, 72.1)[O]	66.9 (58.6, 75.3)	74.7 (67.6, 81.9)[1,O]	72.1 (64.5, 79.7)[O]
	PCS	37.5 (31.3, 43.8)	39.8 (33.2, 46.5)	57.2 (48.9, 65.6)[O]	58.6 (49.8, 67.4)[O]	71.1 (62.0, 80.2)[1,O]	65.8 (56.2, 75.4)[O]
	MCS	63.2 (53.8, 72.6)	68.5 (58.5, 78.5)	68.7 (59.6, 77.8)	75.1 (65.3, 84.9)	77.1 (69.7, 84.4)	78.3 (70.4, 86.1)
	PF	35.4 (27.6, 43.2)	31.6 (23.4, 39.9)	58.3 (49.9, 66.8)[O]	62.9 (54.0, 71.8)[O]	74.2 (64.7, 83.7)[1,O]	67.8 (57.8, 77.8)[O]
	PR	23.4 (10.1, 36.8)	31.8 (17.6, 46.0)	39.2 (23.3, 55.1)	40.5 (23.9, 57.2)	64.1 (46.2, 82.1)[O]	59.6 (40.7, 78.6)
	Pain	25.0 (18.3, 31.7)	30.3 (23.3, 37.4)	64.0 (53.9, 74.0)[O]	64.9 (54.4, 75.5)[O]	77.1 (67.9, 86.2)[1,O]	74.0 (64.3, 83.6)[O]
GRC		4.9 (4.2, 5.5)	4.9 (4.2, 5.6)	5.8 (5.4, 6.3)[O]	5.9 (5.4, 6.4)[O]	6.2 (5.8, 6.6)[O]	6.2 (5.8, 6.6)[O]

groups showed superior clinical outcome 6 months post rehabilitation compared to 1 month post rehabilitation (Table 3). Regarding patients' well-being reported using the SF-36, most scores improved significantly from baseline to 6 months post rehabilitation. For both clinical score and well-being, no significant differences were observed between the control group and the intervention group at any time (Fig. 2, Table 3). Similarly, in both patient groups satisfaction with their global improvements increased significantly 1 month after rehabilitation, but not from 1 to 6 months post rehabilitation (Table 3).

Discussion

The aim of the present study was to evaluate an individualized physical activity counselling intervention during inpatient rehabilitation in patients having undergone primary knee or hip arthroplasty. Six months post rehabilitation, no differences were observed between the control group and the intervention group in any measure of PA, clinical outcome or well-being.

The intervention group as well as the control group of our study showed a fairly high activity level with respect to the number of steps per day, for example compared to observations made by Tsonga et al., who reported 3518 ± 1835 steps/day for Greek elderly women treated for knee arthroplasty. However, the population investigated by Tsonga et al. included several patients with contralateral pain and/or treatments, a higher BMI and less well-being 6 months after treatment, as demonstrated by an overall SF-36 score of 62.4 ± 2.7, a PCS of 56.7 ± 2.9 and a MCS of 68.1 ± 15.3 [8]. Knee and hip patients, investigated by Harding et al., showed statistically and clinically significant improvements in the Oxford Score and well-being 6 months postoperatively compared to the baseline values before surgery. In contrast to our study findings, these patients did not improve their PA, measured by accelerometry [9]. Notably, the study by Harding et al. included patients with a higher BMI compared to our patients and 2.6 comorbidities on average. On the other hand, in another study conducted in a south-eastern region of Germany involving knee patients with a slightly higher BMI compared to our sample, Lützner et al. reported a significant improvement in daily steps from preoperative to 1 year after knee arthroplasty to 6473 ± 3654, suggesting that a higher BMI does not prohibit an increase in daily PA after rehabilitation [12]. Our own findings from a previous study including knee patients from a southern region in Germany revealed an average of 10,992 ± 3938 steps per day, and scores in well-being very similar to the current study (e. g. SF-36 overall score: 76.6 ± 16.2) [13]. Consequently, we assume that in the recent study we included a rather active population of knee and hip patients with a relatively low BMI and less comorbidities compared to other knee patient populations. We therefore presume that adoption to a physical activity intervention in these patients would be less than in knee and hip patients with a considerably lower activity. However, the PA of our patients was remarkably lower compared to the count of ~ 13,300 steps per day observed in healthy control groups of similar age investigated in two other studies from Germany [12, 14]. Thus, the patients in our study ambulated less than their healthy peers at 6 months post operatively, implying that they might potentially benefit from PA interventions to achieve equity with their peers.

We did not observe any effects of the individualized activity counselling during inpatient rehabilitation in the intervention group. Although patients were satisfied with talking to the counsellor every 3 days and reflecting and discussing their PA, they were not able to systematically increase their daily PA. The daily PA measured during the inpatient rehabilitation showed rather random movement patterns, with a large day-to-day variability (data not shown). Therefore, we assume that the patients were not able to focus on their daily PA due to the rehabilitation program demands. Although patients agreed to aim for reaching 5% more steps than performed in the previous days, they often reported a need to recover from the standard rehabilitation program before they could start on their PA aims. This response is understandable as it is known that lack of energy is a common barrier to undertaking physical activity [26, 27]. Thus, we conclude that the PA counselling had no impact on objectively measured PA.

The decline in PA in contrast to an increase in clinical outcome and well-being from presurgery status to 1 to 3 months after rehabilitation, followed by a further increase in PA, clinical outcome and well-being from 3 to 6 months after rehabilitation has been observed in previous studies [8, 13]. However, in our study the baseline PA values do not represent presurgery status. Instead, the number of steps taken was influenced by the schedules and the program of the inpatient rehabilitation and does not represent habitual daily steps. Nevertheless, both the control group as well as the intervention group ambulated less when they returned home, compared to during the inpatient rehabilitation. We assume that after joint arthroplasty patients have to rearrange their daily life when returning home, and that this time is characterized by less continuous activity as reflected by the active minutes with a minimum step count of 60 steps per minute. Instead, patients show non-continuous walking patters as reflected by the active minutes without a minimum step count per minute. But 6 months after rehabilitation, patients were able to increase their overall daily PA. Both groups reduced the duration of inactive bouts and instead accumulated more active minutes as detected by the SAM. These active minutes are distributed well over the entire spectrum of walking frequency, but were pronounced in the moderate walking frequencies from 21 to 100 steps/min. However, the patients did not achieve the PA level of their healthy peers even 6 months after rehabilitation.

The clinical outcome and well-being significantly improved from the onset of inpatient rehabilitation until the 6 months follow up. Interestingly, the control group showed lower values 1 month after rehabilitation, but exceeded the clinical outcome and well-being of the intervention group 6 months after rehabilitation, except for the mental component score.

Some limitations concerning our study have to be addressed. Unfortunately, we lost 16 patients after successful baseline measurement. The remaining number of 49 patients included in our study might not have enough power to disclose any significant differences between the control and intervention group and between hip and knee patients. There was an additional medical reason why we chose the step activity monitor as the intervention tool, and not providing continuous feedback to the patients. Our intention was to avoid overexertion induced by a lower step count as well as inter-individual comparisons between patients. We are aware that this approach is rather conservative, and we hypothesize that, at least in some patients, a pedometer with continuous feedback would have increased their PA.

The fact that we did not have presurgery data for our patients limits our findings. The rehabilitation centre of Oldenburg, where the intervention took place, receives patients from a catchment area covering a large proportion of Northwest Germany. Furthermore, as most patients in Germany can choose the rehabilitation centre they want to go to, it is not possible to get prior information on which patients would chose the Oldenburg Centre for inpatient rehabilitation. Thus, we could not relate the physical activity of the patients included in our study to their pre-surgical physical activity. Moreover, our inclusion criteria led to a rather fit sample of knee patients. Consequently, our findings should be transferred to other patient populations, e. g. with severe comorbidities or higher BMI, with caution. Potentially, adoptions of PA interventions are expected to be higher when baseline PA level is lower. Therefore, we recommend that our study be repeated in different patient populations. We were also not able to measure daily PA during inpatient rehabilitation in the control groups, thus we have no information on whether the counselling in the intervention group altered PA during inpatient rehabilitation.

In this study, we utilized a step activity monitor blinded to the patients as it does not show the recorded number of steps to the patient. On the one hand, this limits the possibilities of the patients to check if they have reached the intended number of steps. On the other hand, patients were not able to compare their daily step counts with each other, reducing their chances of challenging each other to perform more steps. This could potentially lead to excessive demands or overloads being made on the joint treated.

Conclusions

The results of this study indicate that physical activity counselling, based on the daily number of steps during inpatient rehabilitation, does not lead to better outcomes after discharge. Consequently, we suggest that interventions aiming to improve daily PA should not be implemented during inpatient treatment in addition to the standard rehabilitation program because the physical capacities of knee and hip patients are fully claimed by the rehabilitation program. Due to the difference in PA between patients and their healthy peers, we recommend that the implementation of PA counselling during the period following inpatient rehabilitation, when patients resume their daily life at home, be further examined.

Acknowledgements
We thank Thore Linda for his outstanding help during data collection.

Authors' contributions
MB, JH and BM designed the study. NW and HN collected and analysed the data. MB and HN drafted the manuscript. All authors interpreted the data, read and approved the final manuscript.

Consent for publication
Not applicable.

Competing interests
The authors declare that they have no competing interests.

Author details
[1]Department of Prevention and Evaluation, Unit Applied Health Intervention Research, Leibniz Institute for Prevention Research and Epidemiology - BIPS GmbH, Achterstraße 30, 28359 Bremen, Germany. [2]Department of Biometry and Data Management, Unit Statistical Modelling of Primary Data, Leibniz Institute for Prevention Research and Epidemiology - BIPS GmbH, Bremen, Germany. [3]Institute of Sports Science, Oldenburg University, Oldenburg, Germany. [4]Orthopaedic Department, Rehabilitation Centre Oldenburg, Oldenburg, Germany.

References

1. Fuchs J, Rabenberg M, Scheidt-Nave C. Prevalence of selected musculoskeletal conditions in Germany: results of the German health interview and examination survey for adults (DEGS1). Bundesgesundheitsblatt Gesundheitsforschung Gesundheitsschutz. 2013; 56(5–6):678–86.
2. Vos T, Flaxman AD, Naghavi M, Lozano R, Michaud C, Ezzati M, Shibuya K, Salomon JA, Abdalla S, Aboyans V, et al. Years lived with disability (YLDs) for 1160 sequelae of 289 diseases and injuries 1990-2010: a systematic analysis for the global burden of disease study 2010. Lancet. 2012;380(9859):2163–96.
3. Woolf AD, Erwin J, March L. The need to address the burden of musculoskeletal conditions. Best Pract Res Clin Rheumatol. 2012;26(2):183–224.

4. Ethgen O, Bruyere O, Richy F, Dardennes C, Reginster JY. Health-related quality of life in total hip and total knee arthroplasty. A qualitative and systematic review of the literature. J Bone Joint Surg Am. 2004;86-A(5):963–74.
5. Nilsdotter AK, Toksvig-Larsen S, Roos EM. Knee arthroplasty: are patients' expectations fulfilled? A prospective study of pain and function in 102 patients with 5-year follow-up. Acta Orthop. 2009;80(1):55–61.
6. Nuesch E, Dieppe P, Reichenbach S, Williams S, Iff S, Juni P. All cause and disease specific mortality in patients with knee or hip osteoarthritis: population based cohort study. Bmj. 2011;342:d1165.
7. Paxton RJ, Melanson EL, Stevens-Lapsley JE, Christiansen CL. Physical activity after total knee arthroplasty: a critical review. World J Orthop. 2015;6(8):614–22.
8. Tsonga T, Kapetanakis S, Papadopoulos C, Papathanasiou J, Mourgias N, Georgiou N, Fiska A, Kazakos K. Evaluation of improvement in quality of life and physical activity after total knee arthroplasty in greek elderly women. Open Orthopaedics J. 2011;5:343–7.
9. Harding P, Holland AE, Delany C, Hinman RS. Do activity levels increase after total hip and knee arthroplasty? Clin Orthop Relat Res. 2014;472(5):1502–11.
10. de Groot IB, Bussmann HJ, Stam HJ, Verhaar JA. Small increase of actual physical activity 6 months after total hip or knee arthroplasty. Clin Orthop Relat Res. 2008;466(9):2201–8.
11. Arnold JB, Walters JL, Ferrar KE. Does physical activity increase after Total hip or knee arthroplasty for osteoarthritis? A systematic review. J Orthop Sports Phys Ther. 2016;46(6):431–42.
12. Lutzner C, Kirschner S, Lutzner J. Patient activity after TKA depends on patient-specific parameters. Clin Orthop Relat Res. 2014;472(12):3933–40.
13. Brandes M, Ringling M, Winter C, Hillmann A, Rosenbaum D. Changes in physical activity and health-related quality of life during the first year after total knee arthroplasty. Arthritis Care Res (Hoboken). 2011;63(3):328–34.
14. Brandes M, Schomaker R, Mollenhoff G, Rosenbaum D. Quantity versus quality of gait and quality of life in patients with osteoarthritis. Gait Posture. 2008;28(1):74–9.
15. Gundle KR, Punt SE, Conrad Iii EU. Assessment of objective ambulation in lower extremity sarcoma patients with a continuous activity monitor: rationale and validation. Sarcoma. 2014;2014:947082.
16. Schmidt AL, Pennypacker ML, Thrush AH, Leiper CI, Craik RL. Validity of the StepWatch step activity monitor: preliminary findings for use in persons with Parkinson disease and multiple sclerosis. J Geriatr Phys Ther. 2011;34(1):41–5.
17. Macko RF, Haeuber E, Shaughnessy M, Coleman KL, Boone DA, Smith GV, Silver KH. Microprocessor-based ambulatory activity monitoring in stroke patients. Med Sci Sports Exerc. 2002;34(3):394–9.
18. Resnick B, Nahm ES, Orwig D, Zimmerman SS, Magaziner J. Measurement of activity in older adults: reliability and validity of the step activity monitor. J Nurs Meas. 2001;9(3):275–90.
19. Treacy D, Hassett L, Schurr K, Chagpar S, Paul SS, Sherrington C. Validity of different activity monitors to count steps in an inpatient rehabilitation setting. Phys Ther. 2017;97(5):581–8. https://doi.org/10.1093/ptj/pzx010.
20. Naal FD, Impellizzeri FM, Sieverding M, Loibl M, von Knoch F, Mannion AF, Leunig M, Munzinger U. The 12-item Oxford knee score: cross-cultural adaptation into German and assessment of its psychometric properties in patients with osteoarthritis of the knee. Osteoarthr Cartil. 2009;17(1):49–52.
21. Naal FD, Sieverding M, Impellizzeri FM, von Knoch F, Mannion AF, Leunig M. Reliability and validity of the cross-culturally adapted German Oxford hip score. Clin Orthop Relat Res. 2009;467(4):952–7.
22. Bullinger M, Alonso J, Apolone G, Leplege A, Sullivan M, Wood-Dauphinee S, Gandek B, Wagner A, Aaronson N, Bech P, et al. Translating health status questionnaires and evaluating their quality: the IQOLA Project approach International Quality of Life Assessment. J Clin Epidemiol. 1998;51(11):913–23.
23. da Silva RR, Santos AA, de Sampaio Carvalho Junior J, Matos MA. Quality of life after total knee arthroplasty: systematic review. Rev Bras Ortop. 2014; 49(5):520–7.
24. Adams MA, Sallis JF, Norman GJ, Hovell MF, Hekler EB, Perata E. An adaptive physical activity intervention for overweight adults: a randomized controlled trial. PLoS One. 2013;8(12):e82901.
25. Kaminsky LA, Jones J, Riggin K, Strath SJ. A pedometer-based physical activity intervention for patients entering a maintenance cardiac rehabilitation program: a pilot study. Cardiovasc Diagnosis Ther. 2013; 3(2):73–9.
26. Ellingson LD, Kuffel AE, Vack NJ, Cook DB. Active and sedentary behaviors influence feelings of energy and fatigue in women. Med Sci Sports Exerc. 2014;46(1):192–200.
27. Ward-Ritacco CL, Adrian AL, O'Connor PJ, Binkowski JA, Rogers LQ, Johnson MA, Evans EM. Feelings of energy are associated with physical activity and sleep quality, but not adiposity, in middle-aged postmenopausal women. Menopause. 2015;22(3):304–11.

Psychosocial predictors for outcome after total joint arthroplasty: a prospective comparison of hip and knee arthroplasty

Marion Lindner[1*], Olaf Nosseir[2], Anett Keller-Pliessnig[1], Per Teigelack[1], Martin Teufel[1] and Sefik Tagay[1]

Abstract

Background: As findings regarding predictors for good outcome after total joint arthroplasty are highly inconsistent, aim of this study was to investigate the influence of the psychosocial variables sense of coherence and social support as well as mental distress on physical outcome after surgery. It should be investigated if different predictors are important in patients after total hip arthroplasty (THA) compared to patients after total knee arthroplasty (TKA).

Methods: In a prospective design, 44 patients undergoing THA and 61 patients undergoing TKA were examined presurgery and 6 and 12 weeks after surgery using WOMAC (disease-specific outcome), SF-36 (health-related quality of life), BSI (psychological distress), SOC-13 (sense of coherence), and F-SozU (social support). Changes over time were calculated by analyses of variance with repeated measures. Stepwise multiple linear regression analyses were computed for each group to predict scores of WOMAC total and all WOMAC subscales 12 weeks postoperatively.

Results: THA as well as TKA patients experienced improvements in all parameters (effect sizes for WOMAC scores between $\eta^2 = .387$ and $\eta^2 = .631$) with THA patients showing even better results than TKA patients. WOMAC scores 12 weeks after surgery were predicted predominantly by WOMAC baseline scores in TKA with an amount of explained variance between 9.6 and 19.5%. In THA, 12-weeks WOMAC scores were predicted by baseline measures of psychosocial aspects (anxiety, sense of coherence, social support). In this group, predictors accounted for 17.1 to 31.6% of the variance.

Conclusions: Different predictors for outcome after total joint arthroplasty were obtained for THA and TKA patients. Although psychosocial aspects seemed to be less important in TKA patients, preoperatively, distressed patients of both groups should be offered interventions to reduce psychological distress to obtain better outcomes after surgery.

Keywords: Total hip arthroplasty, Total knee arthroplasty, Health-related quality of life, Psychological distress, Psychosocial resources

Background

Besides objective medical parameters like mortality, prosthesis survival or range of motion, health-related quality of life (HRQoL) is an important outcome of surgical interventions. A large number of studies investigated HRQoL after total knee (TKA) or total hip (THA) arthroplasty and reported impressing results with highly significant increases in general HRQoL as well as in disease-specific outcome [1–6]. Nevertheless, a small proportion of patients do only reach poor or no improvement, raising the question which determinants could have an impact on joint replacement outcome. For this reason, sociodemographic and psychosocial variables have been taken into account, investigating their potential contribution to HRQoL after TKA or THA. For example, educational status, social support, depression [7] and mental distress [2] have been found to influence follow-up pain and physical function scores. As another widely used psychological parameter, sense of coherence (SOC) was shown to play an important role in perceived health and HRQoL of individuals with and without physical or mental illness, independent of age, sex, nationality and ethnicity [8, 9]. SOC, proclaimed by Antonovsky [10], describes "a global orientation that expresses the extent to which one has a

* Correspondence: marion.lindner@lvr.de
[1]Department of Psychosomatic Medicine and Psychotherapy, University of Duisburg-Essen, Virchowstraße 174, 45147 Essen, Germany
Full list of author information is available at the end of the article

pervasive, enduring though dynamic feeling of confidence" (p. 19), and consists of the three components comprehensibility, manageability and meaningfulness. In patients with osteoarthritis, a high baseline SOC was associated with a better mental as well as physical HRQoL after THA [11], yet SOC is generally stronger related to mental aspects of health [8, 9, 12].

Results of studies which evaluated THA and TKA patients separately suggest that patients´ benefit after THA is even greater with respect to pain, HRQoL, function and satisfaction than after TKA [3, 6, 13–15], but there are also different findings [16]. A review investigating psychological factors affecting the outcome of total joint arthroplasty [17] summarized that evidence is strong regarding TKA whereas results for THA are limited and conflicting.

Against this background, the purpose of this study is to examine the influence of the psychosocial resources SOC and social support as well as of mental distress on outcome separately in patients after THA and TKA to define different predictors in these two patient groups.

Methods

Study design

Over a period of 1 year, patients with either osteoarthritis of the hip or with osteoarthritis of the knee were consecutively recruited in the surgical ward of a German hospital. Patients had been diagnosed by clinical and radiological examinations, and total replacement of hip or knee was indicated. All knee arthroplasties were performed with cemented technique, hip arthroplasties were performed with uncemented technique whenever possible due to bone quality. Surgeries were predominantly performed by the second author. At the day of admission to the hospital, patients were asked for study participation. Inclusion criteria were indication of total joint arthroplasty due to either coxarthrosis or gonarthrosis, sufficient knowledge of German language to complete the questionnaires and voluntary study participation. Exclusion criteria were osteoarthritis of both hip and knee, contralateral arthroplasty or another joint arthroplasty, any neurological diseases like muscle weakness, Parkinson's disease or (suspected) dementia, movement restrictions caused by any other reason than osteoarthritis, joint infections, fractures and prosthesis replacements. After confirming written informed consent, patients filled in a questionnaire collecting sociodemographic data as well as the self-rating instruments WOMAC (disease-specific outcome), SF-36 (health-related quality of life), BSI (psychological distress), SOC-13 (sense of coherence), and F-SozU (social support) the first time (t0). Hospital length of stay was 12 days. Subsequently, all patients were referred to a rehabilitation clinic for treatment between 3 and 4 weeks. Six weeks (t1) as well as 12 weeks (t2) after surgery, patients returned to hospital for medical check-up and completed the same questionnaires again. The study was approved by the hospital's ethics committee.

Instruments

Western Ontario and Mac Master Universities Osteoarthritis Index (WOMAC) [18, 19]

The WOMAC is an internationally widely used reliable and valid instrument that measures disease-specific dimensions in patients with osteoarthritis in lower limb. It consists of 24 items which are grouped into the subscales pain, stiffness and functional limitations (function), altogether building the total score. The items are answered on an 11-point Likert-scale. A high value suggests a high degree of symptoms. At t0, the subscale pain showed an internal consistency of $\alpha = .88$, stiffness of $\alpha = .82$, function of $\alpha = .95$ and the total score of $\alpha = .96$.

Short Form-36 Health Survey (SF-36) [20, 21]

SF-36 is a psychometrically proven questionnaire for the assessment of general HRQoL. The 36 items are divided into eight subscales and a physical (PCS) as well as a mental (MCS) component summary score can be computed. A high value suggests a high HRQoL. In this study, the internal consistency of the subscales ranged from $\alpha = .61$ to $\alpha = .93$ at t0.

Brief Symptom Inventory (BSI) [22]

The BSI, a short form of the SCL-90-R, measures the subjective disturbance by physical and mental symptoms. The 53 items are summed up to nine subscales and three global values. In this study, the subscales anxiety and depression as well as the global severity index (GSI) were analyzed. High values suggest high psychological distress. At t0, the internal consistency for depression was $\alpha = .88$, for anxiety $\alpha = .78$ and for the whole questionnaire $\alpha = .96$.

Sense of coherence scale-13 (SOC-13) [23]

The SOC-13, a short form of the SOC-29, measures the extent of the sense of coherence as proclaimed by Antonovsky [10]. The 13 items are answered on a 7-point Likert-scale. A high value suggests a high sense of coherence. At t0, the SOC-13 showed an internal consistency of $\alpha = .74$.

Questionnaire for social support (F-SozU) [24]

F-SozU is used for the assessment of subjectively perceived social support. The short form consists of 22 items, which are answered on a 5-point Likert-scale. A high value suggests high social support. The internal consistency of this questionnaire was $\alpha = .92$ at t0.

Statistical analysis

Data were analyzed using the software SPSS 22.0 for Microsoft Windows®. For descriptive analyses, data were expressed as mean values (M) and standard deviation (SD). Mean differences of variables between THA and TKA patients were investigated by t-tests for independent samples and Chi-square-tests. Scores of all instruments except of WOMAC were compared with healthy reference groups of the questionnaire's manuals or from the literature by use of one sample t-tests (SF-36: n = 2773, healthy adults; BSI: n = 600, healthy adults; SOC-13: n = 1944, representative German sample; F-SozU: n = 2179, representative German sample). Analyses of variance with repeated measures were calculated to find changes over time, group effects (THA vs. TKA) and interaction effects between time and group. As measure for the effect size, eta-squared (η^2) was used. Values of eta-squared are interpreted as follows: $\eta^2 = 0.01$: small, $\eta^2 = 0.09$: medium, $\eta^2 = 0.25$: large. With stepwise multiple linear regression analyses the relative contribution of possible predictors to the outcome parameters WOMAC pain, WOMAC stiffness, WOMAC function and WOMAC total have been investigated for each group separately. As independent variables the baseline scores of BSI anxiety, BSI depression, SOC-13, F-SozU and of each model's dependent variable have been included. As there was no significant correlation between age and the outcome parameters and because no differences were found between males and females regarding the WOMAC scales, age and gender were not included as independent variables in the regression models. For comparisons with reference samples, α-level was corrected for multiple testing (2 groups × 3 time points: $\alpha = .05/6 = .008$). For all other tests, a significance level of $\alpha \leq .05$ was predetermined.

Results

Sample

Overall, 119 consecutive TKA and THA patients were screened for eligibility and asked for participation in the study. Seven patients (5.9%) declined participation and two patients (1.7%) did not meet inclusion criteria, thus 110 patients (92.4%) were included. During the study period, two patients rejected participation (1.8%), one patient (0.9%) could not continue because of health reasons independently of joint arthroplasty and two patients (1.8%) lacked to complete the questionnaires so that 105 data sets were analyzed.

Of the patients, 41.9% had osteoarthritis of the hip, in the other 58.1%, the knee was affected. Mean age was 67.4 years (SD = 10.3) for THA and 66.4 years (SD = 10.6) for TKA patients. In the THA sample, 52.3% were female, in the TKA sample 60.7%. Both groups only differed significantly from each other regarding the marital status ($\chi^2 = 8.499$; $p = .037$). Table 1 shows the sociodemographic data separately for THA and for TKA patients.

With respect to psychometric instruments, patient groups showed no significant differences in all WOMAC scales, SF-36 PCS, BSI anxiety and depression, SOC-13, and F-SozU before surgery. However, THA patients showed higher SF-36 MCS ($t = 2.43$; $p = .017$) and lower BSI GSI scores ($t = -2.03$; $p = .046$) than TKA patients.

Changes in disease-specific dimensions

Changes in all WOMAC scales for THA and TKA patients are presented separately in Fig. 1(a) and (b). There was a significant main effect for the factor time, showing an improvement of the total score and all WOMAC subscales from t0 to t2 with large effect sizes (pain: $F(1.72) = 172.42$; $p = <.001$; $\eta^2 = .631$; stiffness: $F(1.59) = 63.75$; $p < .001$; $\eta^2 = .387$; function: $F(1.57) = 131.79$; $p < .001$; $\eta^2 = .566$; total: $F(1.57) = 156.90$; $p < .001$; $\eta^2 = .608$). Also significant main effects for the factor group (THA vs. TKA) were detected for the subscales pain ($F(1) = 7.12$; $p = .009$; $\eta^2 = .066$) and stiffness ($F(1) = 5.02$; $p = .027$; $\eta^2 = .047$), with TKA patients having worse values at all time points on both scales. Furthermore, there were significant interactions between time and group for the subscales pain ($F(1.72) = 5.61$; $p = .006$; $\eta^2 = .053$) and stiffness ($F(1.59) = 4.94$; $p = .014$; $\eta^2 = .047$) as well as for the total score ($F(1.57) = 4.23$; $p = .024$; $\eta^2 = .040$). On the subscale pain, THA patients improved significantly from t0 to t1 ($p = <.001$) and from t1 to t2 ($p = .030$), whereas scores of TKA patients decreased significantly from t0 to t1 ($p = <.001$) but remained stable from t1 to t2 ($p = .741$). Regarding stiffness, THA as well as TKA patients showed significant improvements from t0 to t1 (THA: $p < .001$; TKA: $p = .001$) but did not change from t1 to t2 (THA: $p = 1.00$; TKA: $p = .054$). On the total score, again both groups improved significantly from t0 to t1 (both: $p < .001$), but from t1 to t2, scores further decreased for THA patients ($p = .021$) but not for TKA patients ($p = .069$). For both groups, the improvement in all three scales from t0 to t2 was highly significant (all: $p < .001$).

Changes in general HRQoL

A significant main effect for the factor time was found for PCS ($F(1.83) = 16.37$; $p < .001$; $\eta^2 = .142$) as well as for MCS scores ($F(1.80) = 4.39$; $p = .017$; $\eta^2 = .042$) (Fig. 1(c)), demonstrating increasing values over time. For neither of the scales, the analyses revealed a significant main effect for the factor group. The interaction between time and group was significant only for MCS ($F(1.80) = 5.67$; $p = .006$; $\eta^2 = .054$). In THA patients, MCS did not change from t0 to t1 ($p = 1.00$), but increased significantly from t1 to t2 ($p = .039$), whereas in TKA patients, the trend was contrary (t0 to t1: $p = .001$; t1 to t2: $p = .264$). Changes resulted in an overall improvement of MCS from t0 to t2 in TKA patients ($p = .036$) but not in the THA group ($p = .502$).

The comparisons of THA and TKA patients to a healthy reference group [20] can be seen in Fig. 1(c).

Table 1 Sociodemographic data of THA and TKA patients

	THA: $n = 44$ (41.9%)	TKA: $n = 61$ (58.1%)	
Age	M = 67.4 (SD = 10.3)	M = 66.4 (SD = 10.6)	$t = 0.479$; $p = .633$
Sex			$X^2 = 0.734$; $p = .392$
Male	21 (47.7%)	24 (39.3%)	
Female	23 (52.3%)	37 (60.7%)	
Marital status			$X^2 = 8.499$; $p = .037$
Single	1 (2.3%)	8 (13.1%)	
Married	39 (88.6%)	40 (65.6%)	
Separated/divorced	0	3 (4.9%)	
Widowed	4 (9.1%)	10 (16.4%)	
Living situation			$X^2 = 5.459$; $p = .243$
Alone	3 (6.8%)	10 (16.4%)	
With partner	29 (65.9%)	37 (60.7%)	
With children	1 (2.3%)	4 (6.6%)	
With partner and children	10 (22.7%)	7 (11.5%)	
Others	1 (2.3%)	3 (4.9%)	
Partnership			$X^2 = 3.032$; $p = .082$
Yes	39 (88.6%)	45 (73.8%)	
No	4 (9.1%)	13 (21.3%)	
Unknown	1 (2.3%)	3 (4.9%)	
Education			$X^2 = 5.406$; $p = .248$
No certificate	2 (4.5%)	6 (9.8%)	
Certificate of secondary education	26 (59.1%)	40 (65.6%)	
General certificate of secondary education	9 (20.5%)	12 (19.7%)	
University certification	1 (2.3%)	1 (1.6%)	
College degree	5 (11.4%)	1 (1.6%)	
Unknown	1 (2.3%)	1 (1.6%)	
Employment status			$X^2 = 4.002$; $p = .549$
Employed	10 (22.7%)	17 (27.8%)	
Housewife/–husband	11 (25.0%)	15 (24.6%)	
Retired	23 (52.3%)	27 (44.3%)	
Unknown	0	2 (3.3%)	

Legend: *THA* total hip arthroplasty, *TKA* total knee arthroplasty, *M* mean value, *SD* standard deviation

Changes in psychological distress

The anxiety (F(1.09) = 10.31; $p < .001$; $\eta^2 = .093$) and the depression subscale (F(1.92) = 3.97; $p = .022$; $\eta^2 = .039$) as well as the GSI (F(1.91) = 9.963; $p < .001$; $\eta^2 = .089$) demonstrated significant main effects for the factor time, indicating improvements from t0 to t2 on all three scales (Fig. 1(d)). Neither significant main effects for the factor group nor significant interactions between time and group could be detected for any of the scales.

Figure 1(d) presents the comparisons to a healthy reference sample [22].

Changes in sense of coherence

The analyses showed a significant main effect for the factor time (F(1.93) = 6.271; $p = .003$; $\eta^2 = .064$) as SOC-13 scores increased from t0 to t2. No significant main effect of the factor group and no interaction between time and group have been found.

At t0, scores of THA ($t = 1.68$; $p = .101$) as well as TKA patients ($t = 1.014$; $p = .315$) were comparable to a representative reference sample [25], whereas at t1 and t2, both groups showed significantly higher scores (t1: THA ($t = 3.43$; $p = .001$), TKA ($t = 2.90$; $p = .005$); t2: THA ($t = 3.56$; $p = .001$), TKA ($t = 3.76$; $p < .001$)).

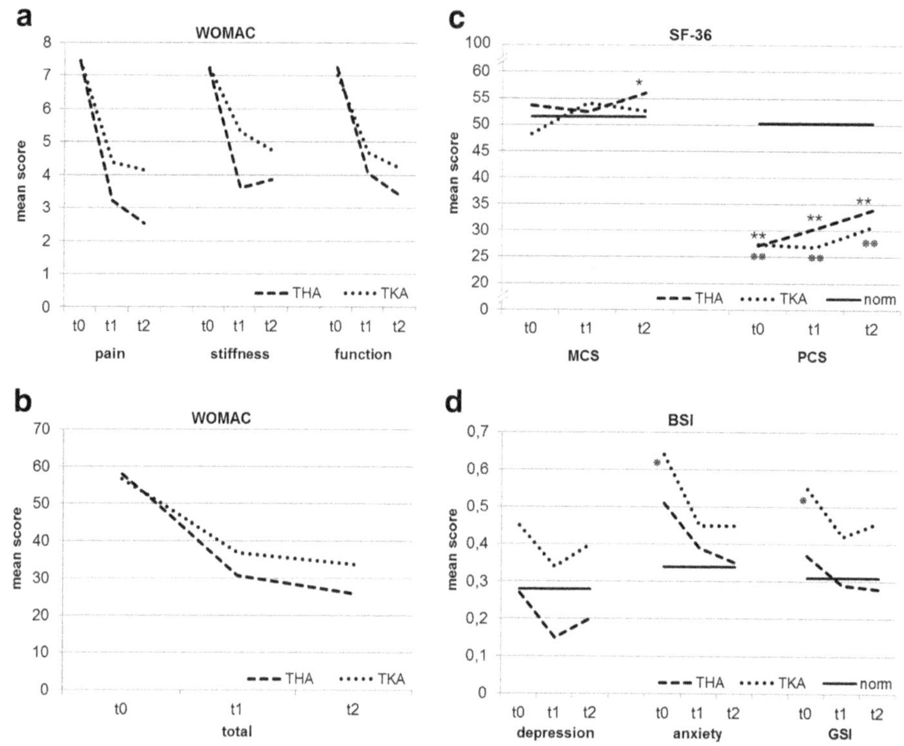

Fig. 1 Changes in THA and TKA patients over 12 weeks and comparisons with healthy reference groups. **a** THA and TKA patients show improvements on all WOMAC subscales. **b** THA and TKA patients show improvements on the WOMAC total score. **c** Mental HRQoL (MCS) showed an overall improvement in TKA but not in THA patients. Physical HRQoL (PCS) improved in both groups. **d** THA and TKA patients improved on all three BSI scales. BSI=Brief Symptom Inventory, GSI = global severity index, HRQoL = Health-related quality of life, MCS = mental component summary, PCS = physical component summary, SF-36 = Short Form-36 Health Survey, THA = total hip arthroplasty, TKA = total knee arthroplasty, WOMAC=Western Ontario and Mac Master Universities Osteoarthritis Index, norm: healthy reference group. t0: 1 day pre surgery, t1: 6 weeks post surgery, t2: 12 weeks post surgery, THA vs. norm: * $p \leq .008$, ** $p \leq .001$. TKA vs. norm: • $p \leq .008$, •• $p \leq .001$

Changes in social support

A significant main effect for the factor time was found, indicating an increase of social support over time ($F(1.48) = 4.07$; $p = .030$; $\eta^2 = .038$). Neither a significant main effect for the factor group nor an interaction between time and group could be detected.

THA as well as TKA patients exhibited significantly higher scores than a representative reference sample [24] at all three time points (t0: THA ($t = 4.30$; $p < .001$), TKA ($t = 3.57$; $p = .001$); t1: THA ($t = 6.97$; $p < .001$), TKA ($t = 6.01$; $p < .001$); t2: THA ($t = 7.25$; $p < .001$), TKA ($t = 5.46$; $p < .001$)).

Identification of predictors

For THA and TKA patients, separate regression analyses have been calculated for t2-scores of WOMAC total as well as all WOMAC subscales. As possible predictors, baseline BSI anxiety, BSI depression, SOC-13, F-SozU and the baseline score of each model's dependent variable have been included. Results of the regression analyses are shown in Table 2.

Regarding THA patients, the only significant predictor for WOMAC pain was anxiety, showing a positive relationship. WOMAC stiffness was predicted by the baseline score in a positive direction as well as by SOC-13 in a negative direction. Significant predictors for WOMAC function were anxiety and social support. Higher functional limitations were predicted by higher anxiety and less social support. The same two predictors, in the same directions, revealed significant for WOMAC total.

In the group of TKA patients, for the WOMAC subscales pain and function as well as for the total score the respective baseline scores revealed as only significant predictors. Each outcome variable was positively correlated to its baseline score. WOMAC stiffness was predicted by anxiety, showing a positive relationship. For all outcome parameters in both groups, the amount of explained variance ranged between 9.6 and 31.6%.

Discussion

This study compared in a prospective design outcomes of patients after THA with those after TKA and investigated which psychosocial parameters had an influence on outcomes in each group. To our knowledge, it is the

Table 2 Regression analyses for THA and TKA patients

	Dependent variable	R^2 corrected	Significant predictors	B	SE B	β	t	p
THA	t2 WOMAC pain	.171	t0 BSI anxiety	1.52	0.49	.44	3.11	.003
	t2 WOMAC stiffness	.214	t0 WOMAC stiffness	0.32	0.11	.38	2.78	.008
			t0 SOC-13	−0.82	0.35	−.32	−2.32	.026
	t2 WOMAC function	.316	t0 BSI anxiety	1.89	0.51	.48	3.69	.001
			t0 F-SozU	−0.72	0.35	−.27	−2.08	.044
	t2 WOMAC total	.305	t0 BSI anxiety	14.06	3.91	.47	3.60	.001
			t0 F-SozU	−5.38	2.64	−.27	−2.04	.048
TKA	t2 WOMAC pain	.137	t0 WOMAC pain	0.36	0.12	.39	3.13	.003
	t2 WOMAC stiffness	.096	t0 BSI anxiety	1.17	0.45	.34	2.61	.012
	t2 WOMAC function	.183	t0 WOMAC function	0.45	0.12	.45	3.65	.001
	t2 WOMAC total	.195	t0 WOMAC total	0.46	0.12	.46	3.79	<.001

Legend: *THA* total hip arthroplasty, *TKA* total knee arthroplasty, *WOMAC* Western Ontario and Mac Master Universities Osteoarthritis Index, *BSI* Brief Symptom Inventory, *SOC-13* Sense of coherence scale-13, *F-SozU* questionnaire of social support
Independent variables in the regression model: t0 BSI anxiety, t0 BSI depression, t0 SOC-13, t0 F-SozU, t0-score of the model's dependent variable

first study to define predictors for each procedure separately and to contrast them.

As expected, THA as well as TKA patients showed high improvements in disease-specific variables and in general HRQoL after surgery, consistent with the existing literature. Because most variables did not differ between patient groups before surgery, comparability of changes was warranted. Overall, in our study the improvements seen in the WOMAC scores were even stronger for the THA than for the TKA group, which replicates the results of other studies regarding joint-specific instruments [3, 6, 14, 15]. Beyond that, in both patient groups we saw a reduction of psychological distress as measured by the three BSI scales and an increase in psychosocial resources, namely sense of coherence and social support. Whereas the decrease in anxiety and depression is in line with the literature [7, 11, 16, 26, 27] a change in SOC or social support has rarely been investigated [7]. The strong relationship of SOC to perceived health has widely been proven [8] and social support has shown to be an essential protective factor against psychological strain for example after traumatic experiences [28]. So it was our goal to examine the role of these two important constructs in the context of total joint arthroplasty. We know only one study which investigated SOC as predictor after surgery and this was restricted to THA, not including TKA patients [11]. Social support has been studied in different investigations but with conflicting results [4, 7, 29, 30].

Our main finding, which adds to the existing literature, was the difference between THA and TKA patients regarding the relationship of WOMAC with psychosocial variables. With one exception (stiffness baseline score predicted stiffness at 12 weeks), in THA, the regression analyses with all WOMAC scales as dependent variables solely revealed psychosocial parameters as significant predictors and WOMAC baseline scores seemed to be negligible. In contrast, in TKA patients, almost all scales were predicted by the baseline scores of the corresponding scales and with one exception (anxiety as predictor for stiffness) psychosocial variables did not play a role in predicting disease-specific outcome. This suggests that the relationship between physical and psychological aspects is much greater in THA patients. Maybe, the different results for the stiffness scale are due to its lower reliability compared to the pain and function scales because it only consists of two items.

The literature regarding psychosocial variables as predictors for physical outcome after THA or TKA is highly inconsistent. For this reason, we aimed to provide more evidence concerning this topic. In TKA patients, the results of other studies are heterogeneous. Desmeules et al. [31] found psychological distress (anxiety and depression) to influence SF-36 physical functioning but not WOMAC pain and function. Social support did not predict either of the scales. A review by Lewis et al. [32] identified depression, anxiety and social support as predictors for pain. In a study by Lopez-Olivo et al. [7] depression and one form of social support influenced WOMAC function but not WOMAC pain. Anxiety did not reveal as predictor for function or pain in this study. Depression predicted neither WOMAC function nor WOMAC pain in a study by Sullivan et al. [33]. Beyond anxiety, depression and social support, which were also investigated in our study, different coping styles, locus of control [7], (pain) catastrophizing [32, 33] and mental health [32] revealed as predictors for some physical variables but not for others in different investigations. However, despite all these conflicting findings, the baseline score of a particular physical variable nearly always predicted the outcome score after TKA [16, 31–33], which confirms the result of our study. With respect to

THA, we found only few studies investigating the influence of psychosocial variables on physical outcome after surgery. Quintana et al. [30] found baseline scores and mental health but not social support to influence WOMAC and SF-36 scores. Sense of coherence, anxiety as a trait and neuroticism but not anxiety as a state, depression or extraversion predicted SF-36 PCS and MCS in a study by Badura-Brzoza et al. [11]. Only partially in accordance with that, we identified anxiety, social support and sense of coherence as predictors for the different WOMAC scales in our study. But as all these investigations show significant methodical differences they are difficult to compare.

As mentioned above, in TKA, the influence of physical baseline scores on the corresponding outcome is the most consistent finding [31]. From our results we conclude, that they even have the strongest effect on physical outcome after surgery. In contrast, the impact of psychosocial variables seems to be much weaker in this group. Even if we had detected additional psychosocial predictors with a larger sample size, physical baseline scores still would seem to play the most important role. It is the strength of our study that we investigated TKA as well as THA patients, so we found out that in THA, the results are contrary. In this group we saw a stronger influence of presurgery psychosocial parameters than of physical baseline scores on the physical outcome.

These findings could possibly be explained by the differences in recovery after both procedures. Several studies pointed out that in both groups the greatest improvements occur in the first 3 to 6 months after surgery followed by slighter improvements thereafter [6, 13, 16, 34]. But even if THA and TKA patients lastly reached a similar level of specific or general HRQoL, THA patients showed faster recovery than TKA patients [3, 6, 34]. Dailiana et al. [16] reported the same trend for WOMAC pain and stiffness but not for WOMAC function and total score, in which the TKA group showed higher improvements (on both scales, TKA patients already exhibited better baseline scores). Furthermore, patients who underwent both, THA and TKA, reported more postoperative pain, lower improvements in range of movement and in quality of life, longer time before they felt physically better than they had before surgery and more required physiotherapy after TKA than after THA. THA was only rated inferior to TKA regarding the longer acute hospital length of stay [15]. So, patients after THA were more overall satisfied than TKA patients [3, 15, 34, 35] and more willing to undergo another total joint arthroplasty [15, 35]. It can therefore be concluded that TKA is a more difficult procedure than THA with a longer and more complicated recovery process. This could be the reason why a better physical status presurgery constituted a predictive factor for a better physical outcome after surgery in this group. Possibly, psychosocial factors also had an influence in TKA, but this was overlapped by the high impact of WOMAC baseline scores. Instead, in THA, results seem to be more independent from baseline physical conditions, at least in the early recovery process, so psychosocial parameters′ effects are more evident. Indeed, TKA patients showed psychological distress as indicated by significantly higher BSI GSI scores compared to the THA group, both before and after surgery. The worse prognosis and concerns of possible complications might have been the reason for higher distress in this group already prior to operation. Maybe patients informed themselves about the planned intervention and TKA patients found more discouraging information than THA patients. After arthroplasty, the higher distress presumably was related to the inferior physical condition.

As the follow-up period in our study took no more than 3 months, patients experienced a critical phase in recovery. If we had investigated our sample 6 or 12 months later, it could have been possible that the observed differences between THA and TKA patients regarding predictors for physical outcome scores no longer would have been found. Suggestive of this possibility are the results of two studies which investigated THA and TKA patients together. Serra-Sutton et al. [4] found that THA as well as TKA patients with low baseline scores in the SF-36 subscale mental health presented worse values in all SF-36 and all WOMAC scales 1 year after surgery. In the study by Dailiana et al. [16], in both patient groups predictive variables for changes in WOMAC scales 12 months after surgery were the corresponding baseline scores (with the exception of stiffness in TKA), whereas none of the investigated sociodemographic variables had an influence.

Overall, in our study, from all psychosocial variables tested, anxiety most often revealed as a significant predictor and showed elevated preoperative levels at least in the TKA group. So in preparing for total joint arthroplasty, distressed patients should be offered interventions for minimizing anxiety (for example psychosomatic contacts) to reveal a better outcome after surgery. Also, to a lesser extent, social support and sense of coherence influenced outcome in the THA group. In our study, the patients showed average or even above average scores in both parameters, but other patients could have a need to improve sense of coherence before surgery or could benefit from contacts to social services.

A limitation of our study is the relatively short follow-up period of 12 weeks. A longer follow-up period would have provided the opportunity to analyze if the identified differences between THA and TKA patients will maintain over time or maybe decrease. However, as mentioned above, the most significant changes occur shortly after surgery, so this was the phase we were primarily interested in. Furthermore, we did not investigate possible confounders like comorbidities or BMI. So other studies with greater sample sizes and controlling for different confounders are needed to further test our hypothesis.

Conclusions

To our knowledge, this is the first study to contrast predictors of physical outcome after surgery in THA vs. TKA patients. Our results suggest that although disease-specific dimensions and general HRQoL as well as psychological distress and psychosocial resources show great improvements after a total joint arthroplasty, the improvements in physical outcome are predicted by different variables in THA and TKA in the early recovery process. Whereas in the first 3 months after surgery physical outcome seems to be stronger influenced by physical baseline scores in TKA patients, in THA patients it seems to be stronger influenced by psychosocial aspects. However, TKA patients also reported mental distress before and after surgery, so patients in both groups, who exhibit a respective need, should be offered interventions to reduce psychological distress.

Abbreviations

BSI: Brief Symptom Inventory; F-SozU: Questionnaire for social support; GSI: Global severity index; HRQoL: Health-related quality of life; M: Mean; MCS: Mental component summary; PCS: Physical component summary; SD: Standard deviation; SF-36: Short Form-36 Health Survey; SOC: Sense of coherence; SOC-13: Sense of coherence scale-13; THA: Total hip arthroplasty; TKA: Total knee arthroplasty; WOMAC: Western Ontario and Mac Master Universities Osteoarthritis Index

Funding

This research did not receive any specific grant from funding agencies in the public, commercial, or not-for-profit sectors.

Authors' contributions

ML analyzed and interpreted the data and was a major contributor in writing the manuscript. ON made substantial contributions to conception and design of the study and performed the arthroplasties. AK, PT and MT were involved in interpretation of data and in writing the manuscript. ST made substantial contributions to conception and design of the study and was involved in interpretation of data and in writing the manuscript. All authors read and approved the final manuscript.

Competing interests

The authors declare that they have no competing interests.

Author details

[1]Department of Psychosomatic Medicine and Psychotherapy, University of Duisburg-Essen, Virchowstraße 174, 45147 Essen, Germany. [2]Department of General, Orthopedic and Accident Surgery, Sankt Josef-Hospital GmbH, In der Hees 4, 46509 Xanten, Germany.

References

1. Gandhi R, Davey JR, Mahomed NN. Predicting patient dissatisfaction following joint replacement surgery. J Rheumatol. 2008;35:2415–8.
2. Lingard EA, Riddle DL. Impact of psychological distress on pain and function following knee arthroplasty. J Bone Joint Surg Am. 2007;89:1161 9.
3. Hamilton D, Henderson GR, Gaston P, MacDonald D, Howie C, Simpson AHRW. Comparative outcomes of total hip and knee arthroplasty: a prospective cohort study. Postgrad Med J. 2012;88:627–31.
4. Serra-Sutton V, Allepuz A, Martínez O, Espallargues M. En nombre del Grupo de Trabajo de Evaluación de las Artroplastias en Cataluña. Quality of life-associated factors at one year after total hip and knee replacement: a multicentre study in Catalonia. Rev Esp Cir Ortop Traumatol. 2013;57:254–62.
5. Shan L, Shan B, Suzuki A, Nouh F, Saxena A. Intermediate and long-term quality of life after total knee replacement: a systematic review and meta-analysis. J Bone Joint Surg Am. 2015;97:156–68.
6. Bachmeier CJM, March LM, Cross MJ, Lapsley HM, Tribe KL, Courtenay BG, et al. A comparison of outcomes in osteoarthritis patients undergoing total hip and knee replacement surgery. Osteoarthr Cartil. 2001;9:137–46.
7. Lopez-Olivo MA, Landon GC, Siff SJ, Edelstein D, Pak C, Kallen MA, et al. Psychosocial determinants of outcomes in knee replacement. Ann Rheum Dis. 2011;70:1775–81.
8. Eriksson M, Lindström B. Antonovsky's sense of coherence scale and the relation with health: a systematic review. J Epidemiol Community Health. 2006;60:376–81.
9. Tan KK, Vehviläinen-Julkunen K, Chan SWC. Integrative review: salutogenesis and health in older people over 65 years old. J Adv Nurs. 2014;70:497–510.
10. Antonovsky A. Unraveling the mystery of health. San Francisco: Jossey-Bass; 1987.
11. Badura-Brzoza K, Zajac P, Brzoza Z, Kasperska-Zajac A, Matysiakiewicz J, Piegza M, et al. Psychological and psychiatric factors related to health-related quality of life after total hip replacement - preliminary report. Eur Psychiatry. 2009;24:119–24.
12. Benz T, Angst F, Lehmann S, Aeschlimann A. Association of the sense of coherence with physical and psychosocial health in the rehabilitation of osteoarthritis of the hip and knee: a prospective cohort study. BMC Musculoskelet Disord. 2013;14:159.
13. Kiebzak GM, Campbell M, Mauerhan DR. The SF-36 general health status survey documents the burden of osteoarthritis and the benefits of total joint arthroplasty: but why should we use it? Am J Manag Care. 2002;8:463–74.
14. Wylde V, Blom AW, Whitehouse SL, Taylor AH, Pattison GT, Bannister GC. Patient-reported outcomes after total hip and knee arthroplasty: comparison of midterm results. J Arthroplast. 2009;24:210–6.
15. De Beer J, Petruccelli D, Adili A, Piccirillo L, Wismer D, Winemaker M. Patient perspective survey of total hip vs total knee arthroplasty surgery. J Arthroplasty. 2012;27:865–9. e1–5
16. Dailiana ZH, Papakostidou I, Varitimidis S, Liaropoulos L, Zintzaras E, Karachalios T, et al. Patient-reported quality of life after primary major joint arthroplasty: a prospective comparison of hip and knee arthroplasty. BMC Musculoskelet Disord. 2015;16:366.
17. Vissers MM, Bussmann JB, Verhaar JAN, Busschbach JJV, Bierma-Zeinstra SMA, Reijman M. Psychological factors affecting the outcome of total hip and knee arthroplasty: a systematic review. Semin Arthritis Rheum. 2012;41: 576–88.
18. Bellamy N, Buchanan WW, Goldsmith CH, Campbell J, Stitt LW. Validation study of WOMAC: a health status instrument for measuring clinically important patient relevant outcomes to antirheumatic drug therapy in patients with osteoarthritis of the hip or knee. J Rheumatol. 1988;15:1833–40.
19. Stucki G, Meier D, Stucki S, Michel BA, Tyndall AG, Dick W, et al. Evaluation of a German version of WOMAC (western Ontario and McMaster universities) arthrosis index. Z Rheumatol. 1996;55:40–9. German
20. Bullinger M, Kirchberger I. The SF-36 questionnaire to assess health status. A manual. Göttingen: Hogrefe; 1998. German
21. Ware JE Jr, Sherbourne CD. The MOS 36-item short-form health survey (SF-36). I. Conceptual framework and item selection. Med Care. 1992;30:473–83.
22. Derogatis LR. Brief symptom inventory (BSI): administration, scoring, and procedures manual. 3rd ed. Minneapolis: NCS Pearson, Inc.; 1993.
23. Antonovsky A. The structure and properties of the sense of coherence scale. Soc Sci Med. 1993;36:725–33.
24. Fydrich T, Sommer G, Brähler E. Questionnaire of social support (F-SozU). Manual. Göttingen: Hogrefe; 2007. German
25. Schumacher J, Wilz G, Gunzelmann T, Brähler E. The Antonovsky sense of coherence scale. Test statistical evaluation of a representative population sample and construction of a brief scale. Psychother Psychosom Med Psychol. 2000;50:472–82.
26. Caracciolo B, Giaquinto S. Self-perceived distress and self-perceived functional recovery after recent total hip and knee arthroplasty. Arch Gerontol Geriatr. 2005;41:177–81.

27. Pérez-Prieto D, Gil-González S, Pelfort X, Leal-Blanquet J, Puig-Verdié L, Hinarejos P. Influence of depression on total knee arthroplasty outcomes. J Arthroplast. 2014;29:44–7.
28. Brewin CR, Andrews B, Valentine JD. Meta-analysis of risk factors for posttraumatic stress disorder in trauma-exposed adults. J Consult Clin Psychol. 2000;68:748–66.
29. Lungu E, Desmeules F, Dionne CE, Belzile ÉL, Vendittoli PA. Prediction of poor outcomes six months following total knee arthroplasty in patients awaiting surgery. BMC Musculoskelet Disord. 2014;15:299.
30. Quintana JM, Escobar A, Aguirre U, Lafuente I, Arenaza JC. Predictors of health-related quality-of-life change after total hip arthroplasty. Clin Orthop Relat Res. 2009;467:2886–94.
31. Desmeules F, Dionne CE, Belzile ÉL, Bourbonnais R, Champagne F, Frémont P. Determinants of pain, functional limitations and health-related quality of life six months after total knee arthroplasty: results from a prospective cohort study. BMC Sports Sci Med Rehabil. 2013;5:2.
32. Lewis GN, Rice DA, McNair PJ, Kluger M. Predictors of persistent pain after total knee arthroplasty: a systematic review and meta-analysis. Br J Anaesth. 2015;114:551–61.
33. Sullivan M, Tanzer M, Stanish W, Fallaha M, Keefe FJ, Simmonds M, et al. Psychological determinants of problematic outcomes following total knee arthroplasty. Pain. 2009;143:123–9.
34. Naal FD, Impellizzeri FM, Lenze U, Wellauer V, von Eisenhart-Rothe R, Leunig M. Clinical improvement and satisfaction after total joint replacement: a prospective 12-month evaluation on the patients' perspective. Qual Life Res. 2015;24:2917–25.
35. Bourne RB, Chesworth B, Davis A, Mahomed N, Charron K. Comparing patient outcomes after THA and TKA: is there a difference? Clin Orthop Relat Res. 2010;468:542–6.

17

Model-based roentgen stereophotogrammetric analysis using elementary geometrical shape models: 10 years results of an uncemented acetabular cup component

Anne Jacobsen[1], Frank Seehaus[1], Yutong Hong[1], Han Cao[1], Alexander Schuh[2], Raimund Forst[1] and Stefan Sesselmann[1,3*]

Abstract

Background: Non-cemented acetabular cup components demonstrated different clinical performance depending on their surface texture or bearing couple. However, clinical osseointegration needs to be proved for each total joint arthroplasty (TJA) design. Aim of this study was to detect the in vivo migration pattern of a non-cemented cup design, using model-based roentgen stereophotogrammetric analysis with elementary geometrical shape models (EGS-RSA) to calculate early cup migration.

Methods: Interchangeable applicability of the model-based EGS-RSA method next to gold standard marker-based RSA method was assessed by clinical radiographs. Afterwards, in vivo acetabular cup migration for 39 patients in a maximum follow up of 120 months (10 years) was calculated using model-based EGS-RSA.

Results: For the axes with the best predictive capability for acetabular cup loosening, mean (±SD) values were calculated for migration and rotation of the cup. The cup migrated 0.16 (±0.22) mm along the cranio-caudal axis after 24 months and 0.36 (±0.72) mm after 120 months, respectively. It rotated − 0.61 (±0.57) deg. about the medio-lateral axis after 24 months and − 0.53 (±0.67) deg. after 120 months, respectively.

Conclusions: Interchangeable applicability of model-based EGS-RSA next to gold standard marker-based RSA method could be shown. Model-based EGS-RSA enables an in vivo migration measurement without the necessity of TJA specific surface models. Migration of the investigated acetabular cup component indicates significant migration values along all the three axes. However, migration values after the second postoperative year were within the thresholds reported in literature, indicating no risk for later aseptic component loosening of this TJA design.

Keywords: Total hip replacement, Acetabular cup, Implant migration, Roentgen stereophotogrammetric analysis, RSA, Elementary geometrical shapes

* Correspondence: s.sesselmann@oth-aw.de
[1]Department of Orthopaedic Surgery, Friedrich-Alexander-Universität Erlangen-Nürnberg (FAU), Rathsberger Str. 57, 91054 Erlangen, Germany
[3]Institute for Medical Technology, Ostbayerische Technische Hochschule Amberg-Weiden, Hetzenrichter Weg 15, 92637 Weiden, Germany
Full list of author information is available at the end of the article

Background

The medical intervention for hip osteoarthritis finally ends with a surgical treatment of the affected joint by total hip arthroplasty (THA) [1]. Forecasts for primary and revision THA procedures predict an increasing case number [2]. However, THA presents an established orthopaedic intervention with a reported survivorship greater than 95% at 10-year and 80% at 25-year follow-up [3]. National registries [4] and clinical studies [5, 6] indicate that THA survivorship is affected by several factors like total joint arthroplasty (TJA) design, bearing couple or surface texture of non-cemented designs. In summary, THA failure most often is caused by aseptic loosening [3, 4, 7] and periprosthetic joint infection [8, 9], both associated with an important economic impact [10].

According THA, the interpretation of survivorship rates must be performed separately for femoral stem and acetabular cup components. For instance Hallan et al. [11] reported a good survivorship at 15-years follow-up for non-cemented femoral stems, whereas non-cemented metal-backed acetabular cup components revealed poor clinical outcome in comparison to cemented all-polyethylene components. Non-cemented metal backed cups showed different clinical outcomes, i.e. grit-blasted and hydroxyapatite-coated acetabular cups indicate a three times higher risk of revision than hydroxyapatite-coated, threaded acetabular cups in cause of aseptic loosening [11]. Palomäki et al. [12] reported data for uncemented cups of the second generation, collected within the Finnish Arthroplasty Register, showing survival rates similar to cemented treatment. However, these results based on mid-term data, longtime data for these cups were still necessary.

The clinical performance of non-cemented coated TJA components in general depends on several factors predicting the bony osseointegration: (*i*) properties of the implant surface likewise surface texture, coating layer thickness and applied pore size, (*ii*) host bone quality, (*iii*) surgical site preparation, (*iv*) preoperative loading conditions and (*v*) preventing initial and chronic infections [13, 14].

If the bony osseointegration of a TJA design fails, loosening of the implant will occur. Gold standard method to assess the in vivo fixation of TJA components presents Roentgen Stereophotogrammetric Analysis (RSA) [15, 16]. It is important to monitor TJA fixation within preclinical trials using gold standard methods, since worst case scenarios of clinical TJA failure – likewise the Boneloc cement disaster within the early 1990s – could be avoided [17–20] and the migration pattern of TJA is affected by the implant design and its fixation philosophy [21, 22]. Using RSA, early implant migration within the first two postoperative years could be detected, which has been shown to correlate well with later aseptic loosening of femoral stems [23] and acetabular cups [24, 25].

Several variations of RSA exist, i.e. using markers attached to the implant (marker-based RSA) or a surface model of the investigated TJA components (model-based RSA) to calculate early implant migration [20, 26]. The interchangeable applicability of the both methods has been demonstrated [27–29]. Model-based RSA using elementary geometrical shape (EGS-RSA) is an approach which uses geometrical bodies likewise spheres or cylinders to calculate migration by rigid body kinematics instead of implant specific surface models [30–33].

Nieuwenhuijse et al. [24] identified thresholds for micromotion of a cemented acetabular cup to distinguish between safe or at risk implants. This research group found cranial migration > 1.76 mm or sagittal rotational migration > 2.53 deg. within the first two postoperative years to be risk factors for subsequent aseptic component failure of acetabular cups. Although a cemented cup was investigated, the authors state that the results of their study should be independent of the fixation method [24]. In accordance with this statement, Pijls et al. [25] reported in a systematic review a similar threshold for cemented as well as uncemented cups. A mean cranial migration of 0.2 mm or less was classified as acceptable, with revision rates of < 5% after 10 years.

Aim of this study is to determine the in vivo migration behavior of a non-cemented titanium cup (*Phoenix cup*; Peter Brehm GmbH, Weisendorf, Germany) for 10 years, using model-based EGS-RSA. The authors hypothesize that no translational migration > 1.7 mm in cranial direction or rotational migration > 2.5 deg. around anterior-posterior axis is detectable within a two-year follow-up. Thus, the authors expect good ten-year performance of the cup with a revision rate of less than 5% caused by aseptic implant failure.

Methods

Retrospectively, out of a former classical marker-based RSA study of 50 patients (Fig. 1a), RSA radiographs were analysed using model-based RSA approach with a hemisphere elementary geometrical shape surface model (Fig. 1b). Marker-based migration calculation was not possible due to implant-marker occlusion problems (in 43 of 50 cases) within the RSA radiographs (Fig. 1c, d). But using a model-based RSA approach with EGS models, migration calculation was possible in 39 of 50 cases.

Surgical treatment

All included patients showed clinical signs of hip osteoarthritis and were treated by primary THA with a non-cemented titanium acetabular cup component (*Phoenix cup*, Peter Brehm GmbH, Weisendorf, Germany) (Fig. 1a). The *Phoenix cup* is a hemispherical press-fit cup with a titanium rough coating and a surface roughness of Rz 100–150 μm. A single well

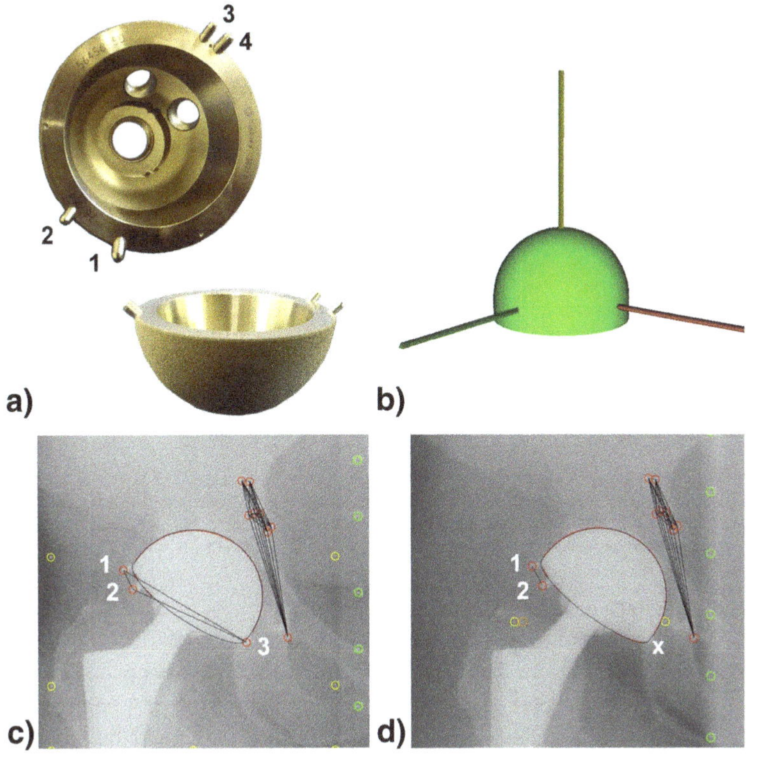

Fig. 1 a Non-cemented titanium ($TiAl_6V_4$) acetabular cup component, composed of a cylinder attached to the rim of a spherical segment, covered by TiRC coating (Titan Rough Coating) with a surface layer thickness of approximately 300 µm, a surface roughness of R_z = 100–150 µm and four additional attached and pairwise-arranged tantalum markers for marker-based RSA measurements. This special RSA cup was in accordance with legal rules. **b** For model-based EGS-RSA approach, a hemisphere model with a curvature radius and implant height according to the technical drawings of the investigated cup component was generated. The local EGS model coordinate system was set to the centre of gravity. All axes were aligned perpendicular to each other. **c** Left image of an RSA reference radiographic image pair with three of four visible implant markers. Implant marker no. 4 occluded by the implant itself within the RSA image. **d** Occluded implant marker problem for marker-based RSA approach. Left image out of the same patient follow up series, with occluded implant markers no. 3 (x) and 4. As at least three implant markers were necessary for marker-based RSA approach, for this RSA image pair a migration calculation was not possible

skilled surgeon performed all the surgeries, using a direct lateral approach. For each patient six to eight CE-certified tantalum markers (diameter: 1.0 mm) were inserted during surgery to the implant surrounding acetabular bone.

RSA measurement setup

A uniplanar RSA setup consisting of two x-ray tubes (*Multix RD 82477–01 Vertix ACS* and *Mobilett Plus*; Siemens, Berlin, Germany) was used. Both x-ray tubes were positioned at an angle of 40 deg. in relation to each other and 1.40 m above the calibration cage (*Umea Cage 43 calibration cage*, RSA BioMedical Innovations AB, Umea, Sweden). The THA treated hip joints of the supine patients were arranged within the intersection of the two x-ray pathways. Accuracy of this RSA setup was determined using a custom made phantom model (Table 1), as double examinations were declined by the ethical committee to minimize x-ray exposure of the patients.

Measurement protocol

Reference RSA image pairs were taken within the first two postoperative days before load bearing of the treated hip joint. Follow-up examinations were performed at six, 12 weeks, six, 12, 24, 60 and 120 months postoperatively.

The RSA image pairs of all patients ($n = 50$) were analysed using model-based RSA software package (*MBRSA 3.4*, MEDIS specials, Leiden, Netherlands) and custom made EGS models of the investigated acetabular cup component (Fig. 1b). Standard thresholds were applied to verify the quality of the calibration procedure and the rigid body error of the detected bone markers of the acetabular bone [34–36]. If all quality criteria were fulfilled in the image pairs, these datasets were included for statistical analysis, indicating that no artefacts or analysis errors were present. Only patients with at least one follow-up at 2 years, 5 years or 10 years were included.

RSA image analyses were performed in accordance with the recommendations of the RSA ISO standard

Table 1 Accuracy of the investigated acetabular cup component within a phantom-model and a performed relative motion protocol

	RSA Translation [mm]			EGS Translation [mm]			set-point [mm]
	x	y	z	x	y	z	
mean	0.50	0.48	0.51	0.49	0.48	0.44	0.5
SD	0.03	0.05	0.08	0.03	0.05	0.18	
bias	0.00	−0.02	0.01	−0.01	− 0.02	− 0.06	
95% CI (↓)	−0.05	− 0.08	− 0.12	−0.04	− 0.08	−0.27	
95% CI (↑)	0.08	0.13	0.20	0.06	0.13	0.43	
mean	1.49	1.47	1.52	1.49	1.47	1.49	1.5
SD	0.02	0.06	0.05	0.04	0.06	0.25	
bias	−0.01	−0.03	0.02	−0.01	−0.03	−0.01	
95% CI (↓)	−0.01	0.00	−0.02	−0.02	− 0.03	−0.12	
95% CI (↑)	0.08	0.22	0.17	0.15	0.20	0.86	

After taking RSA image pairs of the reference setup, using a spring-loaded micrometer, stepwise increments of 0.5 up to 1.5 mm (set-point value for single translation along each axis) of the cup along the x-, y- and z-axis was performed. At each step a RSA image pair was taken. This protocol was repeated $n = 8$ times. RSA image pairs were analysed by marker-based RSA and model-based EGS-RSA

SD standard deviation, *bias* difference between mean value and set point value, *CI* confidence interval with upper (↑) and lower (↓) limit

16,087:2013(E) [36] and the guidelines proposed by Valstar et al. [34]. All patients gave their written informed consent to study participation and to data publication. The Ethics Committee of Friedrich-Alexander-Universität Erlangen-Nürnberg approved the study (registration no. 1.077).

Statistics

Calculated migrations of clinical data were presented as mean (±SD). An analysis of variance including Bonferroni correction was used to prove significant changes of migration values between the follow-ups. The level of significance was set to $p < 0.05$. Statistical analyses were performed using SPSS 24.0 (*SPSS Inc.*, Chicago, Illinois, USA).

Results

Patient cohort

Within this retrospective analysis, 11 patients of the entire patient cohort ($n = 50$) had to be excluded due to technical errors (e.g. high rigid body error of the bone markers at the postoperative) ($n = 4$), death ($n = 1$), study exclusion for reasons unrelated to the implant ($n = 4$) or for unknown reasons ($n = 2$). In summary radiographs for 39 patients, which completely fulfilled analysis criteria for model-based EGS-RSA measurement were included. After the 2-years follow-up, 16 patients dropped out of the study for infirmity not related to the implant ($n = 8$) or for unknown reasons ($n = 8$), as it was not possible to contact the latter patients. After the 5-years follow-up, again five more patients got lost to the study for unknown reasons (Fig. 2).

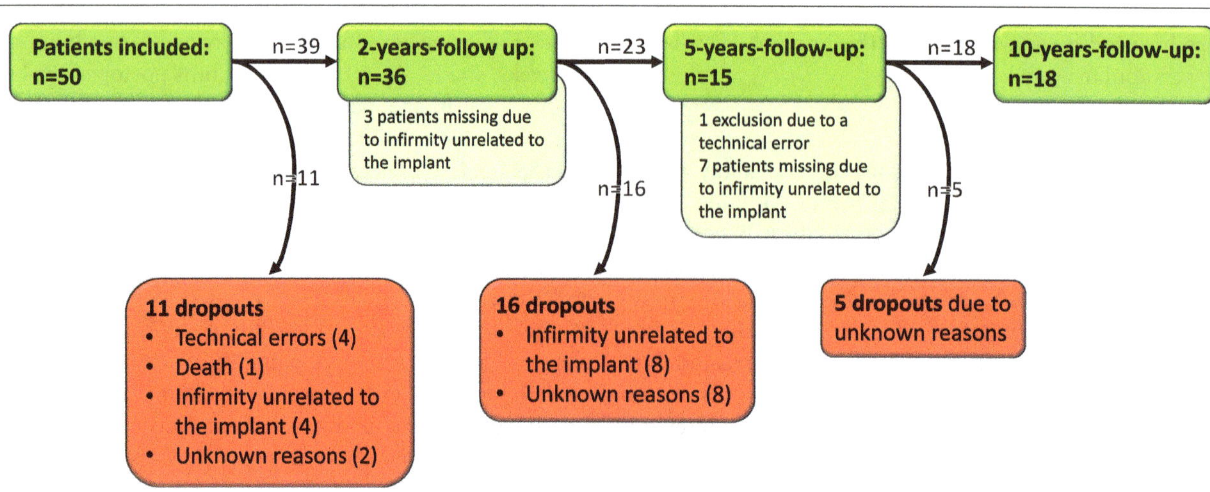

Fig. 2 Flowchart of dropouts and missing patients. Green boxes: attending patients on follow-up. Pale green boxes: patients missing the correspondent follow-up. Red boxes: final dropouts

The entire patient cohort ($n = 39$) consisted of 24 women and 15 men (18 left and 21 right hip replacements). The mean age of the patients at time of surgery was 67.2 (±9.5) years, ranging from 35.8 to 79.6 years.

Experimental accuracy of marker- and model-based EGS-RSA for the investigated cup component

Maximum bias (±SD) for marker-based RSA was – 0.03 (±0.06) mm (95% CI between < 0.01 and 0.22 mm) in cranio-caudal direction (y-axis), for model-based EGS-RSA, it was – 0.06 (±0.18) mm (95% CI between – 0.27 and 0.43 mm) along anterior-posterior direction (z-axis), for the both investigated relative motion set points of 0.5 mm and 1.5 mm (Table 1).

Clinical cup migration data

Highest mean (±SD) migrations were observable along medio-lateral direction (x-axis) with 0.29 (±0.52) mm at 60 months and along cranio-caudal direction (y-axis) with 0.36 (±0.27) mm at 120 months (Table 2). Rotational migration about the y-axis was not calculated according to axi-symmetric implant geometry. For the remaining axes the highest rotation occurred around medio-lateral direction of – 0.61 (±0.57) deg. at 24 months follow-up (Table 2).

For the most predictable axis of acetabular cup loosening, migration along cranio-caudal axis increased continuously from 0.11 (±0.22) mm at 6 weeks up to 0.36 (±0.27) mm at 120 months.

In cranio-caudal direction significant migration values according to the reference follow-up examination were observable for the 6 months follow-up ($p = 0.029$), 12 months follow-up ($p = 0.029$), 24 months follow-up ($p = 0.017$) and 120 months follow-up ($p < 0.001$). However, for the 60 months follow-up ($p = 0.114$) no significant difference to the reference follow-up could be observed (Fig. 3a, Table 2). For rotation about medio-lateral axis a significant different mean ($p = 0.034$) compared to the reference follow up was observable at 24 months (Fig. 3b, Table 2). For remaining migrations and rotations, significance criteria were not fulfilled.

Table 2 Non-cemented titanium acetabular cup component migration – mean and standard deviation values at 6, 12 weeks, 6, 12, 24, 60 and 120 months follow-up using model-based EGS are presented. According to axis-symmetric implant design of the cup component, Ry migration values are not given

Follow-up	Translation [mm]			Rotation [deg]			Cases [n]
	x	*y*	*z*	*Rx*	*Ry*	*Rz*	
Reference							
mean	0.00	0.00	0.00	0.00	–	0.00	39
SD	0.00	0.00	0.00	0.00	–	0.00	
6 weeks							
mean	0.20	0.11	−0.04	−0.17	–	−0.10	32
SD	0.41	0.22	0.33	0.96	–	0.72	
12 weeks							
mean	0.16	0.14	−0.06	−0.12	–	−0.08	33
SD	0.44	0.23	0.39	0.86	–	0.80	
6 months							
mean	0.22	***0.16**	0.03	−0.27	–	0.05	37
SD	0.45	0.25	0.42	0.95	–	0.76	
12 months							
mean	0.23	***0.16**	0.07	−0.30	–	−0.19	39
SD	0.44	0.22	0.38	0.91	–	0.67	
24 months							
mean	0.28	***0.17**	0.02	***-0.61**	–	0.00	36
SD	0.46	0.24	0.50	0.57	–	1.03	
60 months							
mean	0.29	0.19	−0.02	−0.21	–	– 0.07	15
SD	0.52	0.27	0.43	1.24	–	0.47	
120 months							
mean	0.19	***0.36**	−0.04	– 0.53	–	0.22	18
SD	0.69	0.27	0.35	0.67	–	1.21	

SD standard deviation

*mean value significant different ($p < 0.05$) to reference results

Discussion

Accuracy determined by using a phantom investigation showed better values for the marker-based RSA than for the model-based EGS-RSA method. However, both methods provided results within the range of RSA accuracy reported by Kärrholm [37], which is between 0.05 and 0.5 mm for translational migration. Thus, we consider that the loss of accuracy from using model-based EGS-RSA is acceptable for a clinical application of the methodology.

The clinical outcome of the investigated cup component indicates statistically significant migration according to the reference examination along the cranio-caudal axis at the 6 months (0.16 mm; $p = 0.029$), 12 months (0.16 mm; $p = 0.029$) and 24 months follow-up (0.17 mm; $p = 0.017$). At 120 months follow up, migration of the cup component increased significantly up to 0.36 (±0.27) mm ($p < 0.001$). It is important to note that in the first 24 months the observable maximum mean migration in cranial (0.11 mm) direction occurred within the first 6 weeks after surgery (Table 2). Afterwards a steady state mode of the detected migration was observable for the upcoming follow-up intervals within the first 5 years. Between five and 10 years the cup continued to migrate in cranial direction again by another 0.17 mm.

The only observable significant different rotation occurred around the medio-lateral axis at the 24 months follow-up (– 0.61 deg.; $p = 0.034$).

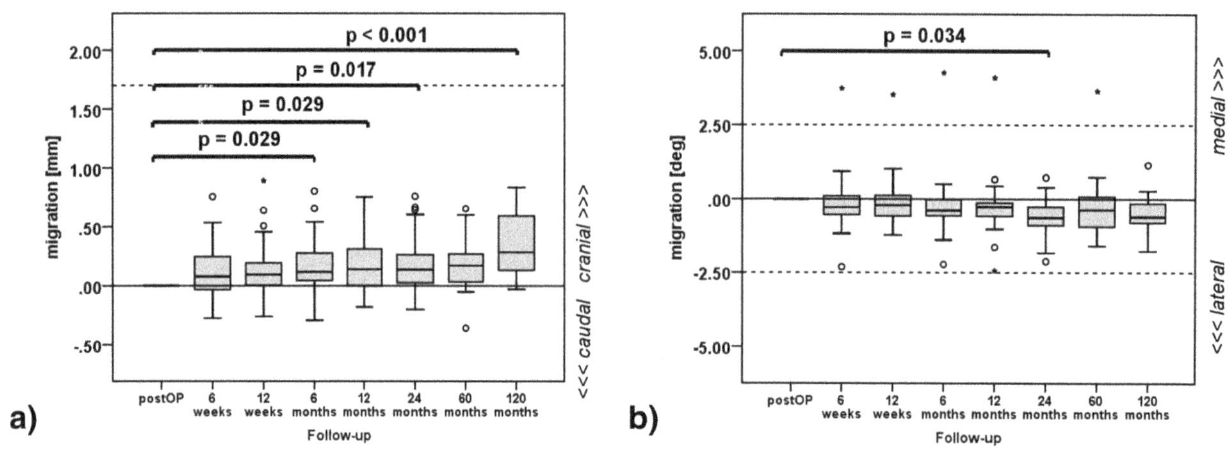

Fig. 3 Calculated acetabular cup migration (**a**) along cranio-caudal direction [mm] and (**b**) about medio-lateral direction [deg] at six, 12 weeks, six, 12, 24, 60 and 120 months follow-up. The boxes represent 50% of included data (bound the 25th to 75th percentile) with the median (horizontal line), smallest and largest value (whisker bars) as well as outliers (circles) and extreme values (stars). Dotted horizontal lines indicate threshold for cranial (> 1.76 mm) acetabular cup migration according to Nieuwenhuijse et al. [24]

Two patients showed especially noticeable migration greater than 1.0 mm in the medial direction (Pat 1; 1.7 mm) and of approximately 1.0 mm in lateral direction (Pat 2) within the first 6 weeks, after which the cup appeared to stabilise up to the 24 months follow up (Fig. 4a). However, Pat 2 cup starts to migrate again in lateral direction after 24 months follow up. Conventional anterior-posterior radiographs indicate no clinical signs of loosening (e.g. radiolucent lines).

Some patients ($n = 13$ at 24 months; $n = 11$ at 120 months, including Pat 1) showed migration between 0.2 mm and 1.0 mm in cranial direction (Fig. 4b), however no cups were identified to migrate more than 1.0 mm. The maximum cranial migration value was observable after 6 weeks with 0.76 mm (Pat 1), which remained unchanged for this patient during the next follow-up investigations. Thus, this cup seems to have stabilised with no further migration in this direction.

In anterior-posterior direction one patient (Pat 3) had a migration value of − 1.28 mm at 6 weeks follow-up, which increased to > − 2.0 mm at the 24 months follow up (Fig. 4c).

Cranial migration is seen as a relevant predictive value for late aseptic loosening of acetabular cup components [24, 25, 38, 39]. In a systematic review, Pijls et al. [25] reported an average increase of 10% in the 10-year revision rate for every millimetre of cranial migration of an acetabular cup component. The authors suggested that inferior components could be identified by RSA within the first two postoperative years, thereby avoiding their widespread implementation. Furthermore, they provided proximal migration thresholds for acetabular cups, whereas cups with a mean cranial migration of 0.2 mm or less were classified as acceptable, with revision rates of < 5% after 10 years. In contrast, cups with a mean cranial migration of 1.0 mm or more were classified as unacceptable, with a > 5% risk for 10-year revision.

For the investigated cup component, a mean proximal migration of 0.17 mm occurred after two postoperative years ($n = 36$ patients at 24 months), which is less than the proposed threshold of 0.2 mm suggested by Pijls et al. [25]. In summary, 13 patients at 24 months were classified at risk (migration between 0.2 mm and 1.0 mm), no patient could be classified as unacceptable (migration > 1.0 mm). These results indicate good performance for the investigated cup component, according to suggestion of Pijls et al. [25]. As none of the followed implants had to be revised after 10 years, this study verifies the suggestions of Pijls et al. [25].

One limitation of this study was the absence of rotational measurements about the cranio-caudal axis. Due to technical restrictions of EGS-RSA, analysis of this rotational migration could not be conducted as the cup has an axis-symmetrical design. This is a well-known problem in model-based RSA [40]. Nonetheless, migration in cranial direction and rotation about the anterior-posterior axis could be calculated, which are the essential movements to predict later cup loosening [24, 25]. Current studies evaluate computed tomography (CT) as an alternative measurement tool to RSA to analyze implant migration. They describe comparable accuracy and precision values for CT-based methods, especially in experimental settings [41–44]. Moreover, CT-based migration measurement could handle some disadvantages of RSA: CT is available in almost every hospital, picture acquisition does not require a special setup or briefed personnel, migration in all directions can be calculated, and there is no problem of marker occlusion by the implant [45]. On

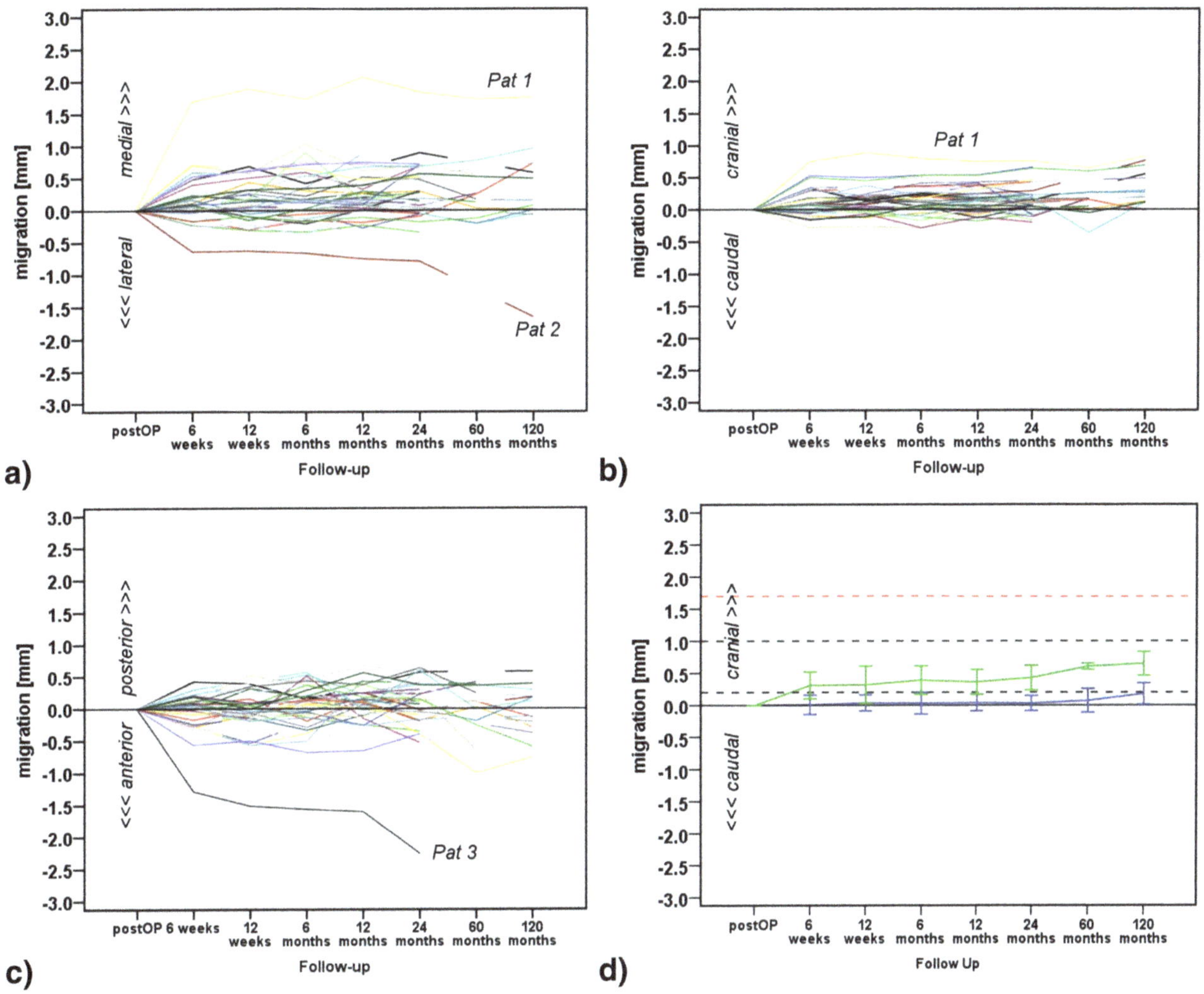

Fig. 4 Calculated acetabular cup migration [mm] at six, 12 weeks, six, 12, 24, 60 and 120 months follow-up along (**a**) medio-lateral, **b** cranio-caudal and (**c**) anterior-posterior direction. **d** Mean ± SD value for each patient, classified at 24 months follow up according to Pijls et al. [25] as an acceptable cup (blue graph; migration < 0.2 mm represented by black dotted line) and cup at risk (green graph; migration between 0.2 mm and 1.0 mm represented by black dotted line). Red dotted line indicates threshold (> 1.76 mm) for cranial acetabular cups migration at risk according to Nieuwenhuijse et al. [24]

the other hand, conventional CT examinations expose patients to higher radiation doses than stereoradiographs, but there is some evidence that a reduction of CT radiation dose does not impair the accuracy of migration analysis [42, 43]. However, there is still a lack of clinical trials and long-term examinations evaluating CT-based migration measurement. Besides, there are still some problems to deal with, as for example artifacts of metallic implants, the influence of soft tissue or the immobilization of patients during CT scanning [44]. In summary, CT-based methods need further validation before they can be considered as an alternative to gold standard RSA.

Another limitation of this study is the number of drop-outs. However, the drop-out rate is comparable to those of other RSA studies [23, 24, 46–48]. During the crucial period of the first 2 years, that are relevant for RSA-prognosis, eleven patients had to be excluded. The remaining number of 39 patients also complies with the RSA guidelines proposed by Valstar et al., who recommend a number of 15–25 patients for the special case of RSA studies [34].

Unfortunately, it is not possible to define prognostic migration thresholds out of the results, as there was no implant failure observable in 10 years of follow-up. However, the results confirm the above-mentioned thresholds of previous studies.

The migration pattern of the investigated acetabular cup component showed migration along all the three axes, particularly in medio-lateral and cranio-caudal direction. Migration along the latter mentioned direction is considered to be the most important prognostic factor for a later aseptic loosening but was still within acceptable limits according to Pijls et al. [25]. It would be interesting to follow the patients for a longer period in order to evaluate how the migration pattern of all axes will influence the long-term stability of the investigated non-cemented acetabular cup.

Conclusions

Model-based EGS-RSA enables an in vivo migration measurement of TJA components without the necessity of TJA specific surface models. The investigated acetabular cup component demonstrates significant differences for calculated migration values along the most predictable axis of acetabular cup loosening, migration along cranio-caudal axis with 0.17 (±0.24) mm at 24 months. However, the measured in vivo cup migration at 2 years of follow-up were within the acceptable thresholds reported in literature [24, 25]. For the cranio-caudal axis, migration continuously increased up to 0.36 (±0.27) mm at 120 months follow-up but is still within above mentioned thresholds. However, performed migration measurement by model-based EGS-RSA within this study highlights the importance and benefit of RSA for the evaluation of implants. There may be other possible applications in the future, such as the early detection of septic loosening of joint implants [49].

Abbreviations

EGS - RSA: Roentgen stereophotogrammetric analysis using elementary geometrical shape models; CT: Computed tomography; EGS: Elementary geometrical shapes; RSA: Roentgen stereophotogrammetric analysis; SD: Standard deviation; THA: Total hip arthroplasty; TJA: Total joint arthroplasty

Acknowledgements

The present work was performed in partial fulfilment of the requirements for obtaining the degree "Dr. med." (AJ). None of the data is published yet.

Funding

We thank the public research funding organization Deutsche Arthrose-Hilfe e.V. (Frankfurt am Main, Germany) for the financial support to realize this study. The funding body had no influence on the design of the study.

Authors' contributions

Each of the authors (AJ, FS, YH, HC, AS, RF, SS) has read and concurs with the content in the final manuscript. The following authors have designed the study (SS), gathered and analysed the data (AJ, FS, YH, HC, SS), written the initial draft, and ensured the accuracy of the data and analysis (AJ, FS, YH, HC, AS, RF, SS).

Consent for publication

Not applicable.

Competing interests

The authors declare that they have no competing interests.

Author details

[1]Department of Orthopaedic Surgery, Friedrich-Alexander-Universität Erlangen-Nürnberg (FAU), Rathsberger Str. 57, 91054 Erlangen, Germany. [2]Muskuloskelettales Zentrum, Klinikum Neumarkt, Nürnberger Str. 12, 92318 Neumarkt i. d. OPf, Germany. [3]Institute for Medical Technology, Ostbayerische Technische Hochschule Amberg-Weiden, Hetzenrichter Weg 15, 92637 Weiden, Germany.

References

1. Hochberg MC, Altman RD, Brandt KD, Clark BM, Dieppe PA, Griffin MR, Moskowitz RW, Schnitzer TJ. Guidelines for the medical management of osteoarthritis. Part I Osteoarthritis of the hip American College of Rheumatology. Arthritis Rheum. 1995;38(11):1535–40.
2. Kurtz S, Ong K, Lau E, Mowat F, Halpern M. Projections of primary and revision hip and knee arthroplasty in the United States from 2005 to 2030. J Bone Joint Surg Am. 2007;89(4):780–5.
3. Pivec R, Johnson AJ, Mears SC, Mont MA. Hip arthroplasty. Lancet. 2012; 380(9855):1768–77.
4. Registry AOANJR: Annual Report 2016. 2016, 2017(11.04.2017).
5. Pakvis D, Luites J, van Hellemondt G, Spruit M. A cementless, elastic press-fit socket with and without screws. Acta Orthop. 2012;83(5):481–7.
6. Strom H, Kolstad K, Mallmin H, Sahlstedt B, Milbrink J. Comparison of the uncemented cone and the cemented Bimetric hip prosthesis in young patients with osteoarthritis: an RSA, clinical and radiographic study. Acta Orthop. 2006;77(1):71–8.
7. Chalmers PN, Sporer SM, Levine BR. Correlation of aspiration results with aseptic loosening in total hip arthroplasty. J Arthroplast. 2013;28(9):1671–6.
8. Portillo ME, Salvado M, Alier A, Sorli L, Martinez S, Horcajada JP, Puig L. Prosthesis failure within 2 years of implantation is highly predictive of infection. Clin Orthop Relat Res. 2013;471(11):3672–8.
9. Trampuz A, Zimmerli W. Prosthetic joint infections: update in diagnosis and treatment. Swiss Med Wkly. 2005;135(17–18):243–51.
10. Kurtz SM, Ong KL, Schmier J, Mowat F, Saleh K, Dybvik E, Karrholm J, Garellick G, Havelin LI, Furnes O, et al. Future clinical and economic impact of revision total hip and knee arthroplasty. J Bone Joint Surg Am. 2007; 89(Suppl 3):144–51.
11. Hallan G, Dybvik E, Furnes O, Havelin LI. Metal-backed acetabular components with conventional polyethylene: a review of 9113 primary components with a follow-up of 20 years. J Bone Joint Surg Br. 2010;92(2): 196–201.
12. Palomaki A, Lempainen L, Matilainen M, Eskelinen A, Remes V, Virolainen P, Makela KT. Survival of uncemented cups from a single manufacturer implanted from 1985 to 2013: Finnish arthroplasty register data. Arch Orthop Trauma Surg. 2017;137(3):311–20.
13. Muschler GF, Nakamoto C, Griffith LG. Engineering principles of clinical cell-based tissue engineering. J Bone Joint Surg Am. 2004;86-A(7):1541–58.
14. Isaacson BM, Jeyapalina S. Osseointegration: a review of the fundamentals for assuring cementless skeletal fixation. Orthop Res Rev. 2014;6:55–65.
15. Sundfeldt M, Carlsson LV, Johansson CB, Thomsen P, Gretzer C. Aseptic loosening, not only a question of wear: a review of different theories. Acta Orthop. 2006;77(2):177–97.
16. Valstar ER, HS Gill R. Radiostereometric analysis in orthopaedic surgery: editorial comment. Clin Orthop Relat Res. 2006;448:2.
17. Gebuhr P, Stentzer K, Thomsen F, Levi N. Failure of total hip arthroplasty with Boneloc bone cement. Acta Orthop Belg. 2000;66(5):472–6.
18. Furnes O, Lie SA, Havelin LI, Vollset SE, Engesaeter LB. Exeter and charnley arthroplasties with Boneloc or high viscosity cement. Comparison of 1,127 arthroplasties followed for 5 years in the Norwegian arthroplasty register. Acta Orthop Scand. 1997;68(6):515–20.
19. Riegels-Nielsen P, Sorensen L, Andersen HM, Lindequist S. Boneloc cemented total hip prostheses. Loosening in 28/43 cases after 3-38 months. Acta Orthop Scand. 1995;66(3):215–7.
20. Karrholm J, Gill RH, Valstar ER. The history and future of radiostereometric analysis. Clin Orthop Relat Res. 2006;448:10–21.
21. Acklin YP, Jenni R, Bereiter H, Thalmann C, Stoffel K. Prospective clinical and radiostereometric analysis of the Fitmore short-stem total hip arthroplasty. Arch Orthop Trauma Surg. 2016;136(2):277–84.
22. Kutzner KP, Freitag T, Donner S, Kovacevic MP, Bieger R. Outcome of extensive varus and valgus stem alignment in short-stem THA: clinical and radiological analysis using EBRA-FCA. Arch Orthop Trauma Surg. 2017;137(3):431–9.

23. Karrholm J, Borssen B, Lowenhielm G, Snorrason F. Does early micromotion of femoral stem prostheses matter? 4-7-year stereoradiographic follow-up of 84 cemented prostheses. J Bone Joint Surg Br. 1994;76(6):912–7.
24. Nieuwenhuijse MJ, Valstar ER, Kaptein BL, Nelissen RG. Good diagnostic performance of early migration as a predictor of late aseptic loosening of acetabular cups: results from ten years of follow-up with roentgen stereophotogrammetric analysis (RSA). J Bone Joint Surg Am. 2012;94(10): 874–80.
25. Pijls BG, Nieuwenhuijse MJ, Fiocco M, Plevier JW, Middeldorp S, Nelissen RG, Valstar ER. Early proximal migration of cups is associated with late revision in THA: a systematic review and meta-analysis of 26 RSA studies and 49 survivalstudies. Acta Orthop. 2012;83(6):583–91.
26. Valstar ER, de Jong FW, Vrooman HA, Rozing PM, Reiber JH. Model-based roentgen stereophotogrammetry of orthopaedic implants. J Biomech. 2001; 34(6):715–22.
27. Kaptein BL, Valstar ER, Stoel BC, Reiber HC, Nelissen RG. Clinical validation of model-based RSA for a total knee prosthesis. Clin Orthop Relat Res. 2007; 464:205–9.
28. Hurschler C, Seehaus F, Emmerich J, Kaptein BL, Windhagen H. Comparison of the model-based and marker-based roentgen stereophotogrammetry methods in a typical clinical setting. J Arthroplast. 2009;24(4):594–606.
29. Seehaus F, Emmerich J, Kaptein BL, Windhagen H, Hurschler C. Experimental analysis of model-based roentgen Stereophotogrammetric analysis (MBRSA) on four typical prosthesis components. J Biomech Eng. 2009;131(4):041004.
30. Kaptein BL, Valstar ER, Spoor CW, Stoel BC, Rozing PM. Model-based RSA of a femoral hip stem using surface and geometrical shape models. Clin Orthop Relat Res. 2006;448:92–7.
31. Prins AH, Kaptein BL, Stoel BC, Nelissen RG, Reiber JH, Valstar ER. Handling modular hip implants in model-based RSA: combined stem-head models. J Biomech. 2008;41(14):2912–7.
32. Borlin N, Rohrl SM, Bragdon CR. RSA wear measurements with or without markers in total hip arthroplasty. J Biomech. 2006;39(9):1641–50.
33. Valstar ER, Spoor CW, Nelissen RG, Rozing PM. Roentgen stereophotogrammetric analysis of metal-backed hemispherical cups without attached markers. J Orthop Res. 1997;15(6):869–73.
34. Valstar ER, Gill R, Ryd L, Flivik G, Borlin N, Karrholm J. Guidelines for standardization of radiostereometry (RSA) of implants. Acta Orthop. 2005; 76(4):563–72.
35. Soderkvist I, Wedin PA. Determining the movements of the skeleton using well-configured markers. J Biomech. 1993;26(12):1473–7.
36. Standardization IOf: International Standard ISO 16087:2013(E). Implants for surgery – Roentegen stereophotogrammetric analysis for the assessment of migration of orthopaedic implants. 2013, ISO 16087:2013(E).
37. Karrholm J. Roentgen stereophotogrammetry. Review of orthopedic applications. Acta Orthop Scand. 1989;60(4):491–503.
38. Karrholm J, Herberts P, Hultmark P, Malchau H, Nivbrant B, Thanner J. Radiostereometry of hip prostheses. Review of methodology and clinical results. Clin Orthop Relat Res. 1997;344:94–110.
39. Klerken T, Mohaddes M, Nemes S, Karrholm J. High early migration of the revised acetabular component is a predictor of late cup loosening: 312 cup revisions followed with radiostereometric analysis for 2-20 years. Hip Int. 2015;25(5):471–6.
40. Seehaus FEJ, Kaptein BL, Windhagen H, Hurschler C. Applicability of model-based RSA for an axis symmetric hip resurfacing prosthesis design. J Biomech. 2008;41:S38.
41. Boettner F, Sculco P, Lipman J, Renner L, Faschingbauer M. A novel method to measure femoral component migration by computed tomography: a cadaver study. Arch Orthop Trauma Surg. 2016;136(6):857–63.
42. Boettner F, Sculco PK, Lipman J, Saboeiro G, Renner L, Faschingbauer M. The effect of a low radiation CT protocol on accuracy of CT guided implant migration measurement: a cadaver study. J Orthop Res. 2016;34(4):725–8.
43. Broden C, Olivecrona H, Maguire GQ Jr, Noz ME, Zeleznik MP, Skoldenberg O. Accuracy and precision of three-dimensional low dose CT compared to standard RSA in acetabular cups: an experimental study. Biomed Res Int. 2016;2016:5909741.
44. Scheerlinck T, Polfliet M, Deklerck R, Van Gompel G, Buls N, Vandemeulebroucke J. Development and validation of an automated and marker-free CT-based spatial analysis method (CTSA) for assessment of femoral hip implant migration: in vitro accuracy and precision comparable to that of radiostereometric analysis (RSA). Acta Orthop. 2016;87(2):139–45.
45. Otten V, Maguire GQ Jr, Noz ME, Zeleznik MP, Nilsson KG, Olivecrona H. Are CT scans a satisfactory substitute for the follow-up of RSA migration studies of Uncemented cups? A comparison of RSA double examinations and CT datasets of 46 Total hip arthroplasties. Biomed Res Int. 2017;2017:3681458.
46. Wolf O, Mattsson P, Milbrink J, Larsson S, Mallmin H. The effects of different weight-bearing regimes on press-fit cup stability: a randomised study with five years of follow-up using radiostereometry. Int Orthop. 2012;36(4):735–40.
47. Budde S, Seehaus F, Schwarze M, Hurschler C, Floerkemeier T, Windhagen H, Noll Y, Ettinger M, Thorey F. Analysis of migration of the Nanos(R) short-stem hip implant within two years after surgery. Int Orthop. 2016;40(8):1607–14.
48. Nilsson KG, Theodoulou A, Mercer G, Quinn SJ, Krishnan J. Mid-term migration of a cementless, porous acetabular cup: a 5 year Radiostereometric analysis. J Orthop. 2017;14(4):454–60.
49. Sesselmann S, Hausotte T, Timmermann M, Liebsch G, Forst R, Trampuz A, Jacobsen A. Radiostereometric analysis as a need for early detection of septic loosening. EC Orthopaedics. 2015;2(3):87–94.

18

Simplified Chinese version of hip and knee replacement expectations surveys in patients with osteoarthritis and ankylosing spondylitis: cross-cultural adaptation, validation and reliability

Chen Wang[†], Chen Zhang[†], De-Lin Liu[†], Wen-Wen Tong, Chong-Ru He, Xuan Huang[*] and Wei-Dong Xu[*]

Abstract

Background: The Hospital for Special Surgery Hip Replacement Expectations Survey (HSS-THRES) and Knee Replacement Expectations Survey (HSS-TKRES) are widely used tools developed to assess patients' preoperative expectations for total hip and knee arthroplasty. This study aimed to translate and adapt the HSS-THRES and HSS-TKRES into Chinese versions (SC-THRES/TKRES) and evaluate their psychometric properties in patients with osteoarthritis (OA) and ankylosing spondylitis (AS).

Methods: Patients scheduled for total hip (104 hip OA and 51 AS) or knee replacements (101 knee OA) were recruited in this study. Confirmatory Factor Analysis (CFA) was used to evaluate structural validity. The internal consistency was assessed by the Cronbach's α coefficient. The intraclass correlation coefficient (ICC) was used to assess test-retest reliability. The construct validity was analyzed by evaluating the correlations between SC-THRES/TKRES and the Expectation WOMAC. The correlations with the Expectation WOMAC were tested against our hypotheses. We additionally compared preoperative expectations of AS patients to those of hip OA patients.

Results: The results of CFA for the SC-THRES and SC-TKRES demonstrated good fit. The results for the SC-THRES/TKRES revealed good test-retest reliability and good internal consistency (AS: ICC = 0.893, Cronbach's α = 0.815; hip OA: ICC = 0.878, Cronbach's α = 0.814; knee OA: ICC = 0.806, Cronbach's α = 0.808). The correlations between the SC-THRES/TKRES and the Expectation WOMAC were moderate (0.541 for AS, 0.490 for hip OA and 0.465 for knee OA), which were consistent with the hypotheses.

Conclusion: The SC-THRES/TKRES are reliable, valid for the evaluation of Chinese patients with OA and AS undergoing total hip and knee arthroplasty. The surveys can be used as part of preoperative assessments. Meanwhile, additional research is needed to replicate these findings and to assess the content validity in a larger sample.

Keywords: Preoperative expectation, Questionnaire, Simplified Chinese version, Hip and knee arthroplasty, Reliability, Validity

* Correspondence: 11791709@qq.com; xuwdshanghaichyy@126.com
[†]Chen Wang, Chen Zhang and De-Lin Liu contributed equally to this work.
Department of Orthopedics, Changhai Hospital, Second Military Medical University, No. 168, Changhai Road, Shanghai 200433, China

Background

Total joint arthroplasties (TJAs) have proven to be effective surgical interventions for patients with moderate to severe hip or knee disorders [1]. The number of TJA procedures has doubled over recent decades and is expected to increase over the coming two decades [2]. Total hip arthroplasty (THA) and total knee arthroplasty (TKA) are extremely effective in reducing pain and restoring function in patients with end-stage osteoarthritis (OA) and ankylosing spondylitis (AS) [3–5].

More recently, increasing emphasis is focused on patient satisfaction and patient-reported outcomes of the surgery [6, 7]. Previous researches have indicated that fulfillment of preoperative expectations was one of the most important factors affecting satisfaction and was a large contributor to functional outcomes [8–13]. Fulfilled expectations correlate with increased patient compliance with postoperative recommendations, follow-up care and monitoring [14–17]. Several studies have shown that compared with the actual ability after surgery, preoperative expectations were higher [11, 18]. There was a large discrepancy between what patients expected and what they truly achieved. Additionally, more disabled patients often have higher preoperative expectations than their surgeons [19, 20]. Unrealistically high expectations may weaken the doctor-patient trust and cause patients to be discouraged after surgery [21]. Nowadays, as a consequence of the complexity of the healthcare environment, the doctor-patient relationship is increasingly tensional in China [22, 23]. Patients requiring TJA often have overly optimistic preoperative expectations, and many of them do not trust their surgeons. Thus, it is of great significance to investigate patients' expectations before surgery. Currently there are no standard methods to assess expectations based on patient-derived measures.

Recent surveys have been developed and validated to capture patients' expectations before THA or TKA [24–27]. The Hospital for Special Surgery Total Hip Replacement Expectations Survey (HSS-THRES) [27] and the Hospital for Special Surgery Total Knee Replacement Expectations Survey (HSS-TKRES) [25] are patient-reported surveys assessing patients' preoperative expectations successfully, which have also been cross-culturally adapted to Dutch [28], French [29] and German [30]. To our knowledge, the HSS-THRES and the HSS-TKRES are the first two questionnaires developed to assess preoperative expectations for patients undergoing TJA. However, a Chinese version has yet to be developed. In addition, no study has proven to be a reliable and valid assessment of the HSS-THRES for patients with AS undergoing THA.

Therefore, the aims of this study were (1) to translate the original version of the HSS-THRES and the HSS-TKRES into Chinese, and (2) to evaluate the psychometric properties of the translated surveys in patients with AS and OA. We additionally compared preoperative expectations of AS patients to those of OA patients undergoing THA.

Methods

Patients

All 270 patients on the waiting list for primary THA/TKA from the orthopedic department of our hospital between November 2015 and July 2017 were invited to participate in this study. The major criteria for inclusion were as follows: (1) native Chinese speakers aged at least 18 years, (2) able to complete the questionnaire independently, (3) OA patients fulfilled the criteria of the American College of Rheumatology [31] with operative indications and willing to receive THA/TKA for the first time. (4) AS patients with hip ankylosis fulfilled the modified New York criteria [32], with operative indications and willing to receive THA for the first time. Subjects with (1) symptomatic OA in other joints, (2) a history of lower limb or spine surgery, (3) severe systematic illnesses were excluded from the study. The sample size was consistent with the study recommended by Terwee et al. [33]. Detailed information was recorded, including gender, age, body mass index (BMI), educational level and living situation. All the participants signed informed consent and the study was approved by the ethics committee of our university (No.CHEC2017–163).

Translation and cross-cultural adaptation

First of all, the developer of the original questionnaires was informed of the purposes of the study and gave consent to a simplified Chinese translation of the HSS-THRES and HSS-TKRES (Carol Mancuso, MD, Hospital for Special Surgery, New York, USA, personal communication).

Based on the previously published guidelines [34], we carried out the cross-cultural adaptation and translation in five stages.

Stage I - forward translation

Three bilingual translators (mother-tongue Chinese and fluent in English) translated the questionnaire into simplified Chinese independently. Two of them are orthopedic surgeons in our hospital; the other one is a professional translator without any medical background who is unaware of the purpose of this study.

Stage II – Synthesis

The first synthetic version of the questionnaire was obtained by discussion of the three translators in order to resolve the discrepancies.

Stage III - back translation

The back translation of the first synthesis was completed separately by three native English speakers fluent in

Chinese, totally blind to the original English version, and with no medical background.

Stage IV - expert committee review

The composition of the expert committee included the six translators from stage I and III, a linguist, a methodologist and two experts in orthopedics. Then the committee reviewed all the translations to resolve any discrepancies and drafted the pre-final version of the questionnaire.

Stage V – Pretesting

Twenty patients (more details were shown in Additional file 1) who were ready to undergo THA/TKA in our hospital were recruited to fill in the pre-final version. The final simplified Chinese version (SC-THRES/TKRES) was generated after the committee had resolved all the problems recognized in the pre-testing.

Instruments

Hospital for Special Surgery Total hip Replacement Expectations Survey (HSS-THRES)

The HSS-THRES is designed by Mancuso et al. to investigate patients' expectations before hip arthroplasty [27]. It is a self-reported questionnaire composed of 18 items relating to pain, physical activity, social activity and psychological well-being. Patients were asked how much improvement or relief they expect for each item followed by THA. The response format used in the questionnaire was as follows: 'back to normal or completely improvement, 'a lot of improvement', 'a moderate amount of improvement', 'a little improvement' or 'this expectation does not apply to me or I do not have this expectation'. The total score ranging from 0 to 72 was adapted into a 100-point scale, with a higher score representing higher expectations. The original English version showed good reliability and construct validity [27, 35].

Hospital for Special Surgery Total Knee Replacement Expectations Survey (HSS-TKRES)

Similarly, the HSS-TKRES is a 19-item questionnaire developed by Mancuso et al. [25]. The response format was similar to the one used in HSS-THRES. The total score was normalized to values between 0 (no expectation) and 100 (highest expectation). The initial English-language survey showed good reliability and construct validity [25, 35].

Expectation WOMAC

To determine construct validity, we compared the SC-THRES/TKRES with the Expectation WOMAC (Western Ontario and Mc Master Universities Osteoarthritis index). The Expectation WOMAC was adapted from the original version of the WOMAC [36]. The WOMAC is a 24-item index including three subscales: pain (five items), stiffness (two items) and functional disability (17 items). With excellent validity and reliability, it has already been successfully translated into Chinese [37, 38]. The Expectation WOMAC consisted of accurately the same domains of the WOMAC. Since the goal was to assess the patient's expectation after surgery, we made a slight modification to the initial wording of the questions: we employed the question "How do you expect to feel six months after the arthroplasty?" rather than "How much pain or stiffness and how many limitations are you experiencing currently?" A five-point Likert scale was adopted the same as in the original WOMAC. Every single item was counted on a scale of 0 (extreme) - 4 (none). The total score ranged from 0 to 96. The higher the score is, the higher the expectations are.

Study design

In the orthopedics outpatient department of our hospital, participants were asked to complete the SC-THRES/TKRES and the Expectation WOMAC within 10 min, respectively. Demographic variables were collected. Two weeks later, prior to surgery, they were asked to complete the surveys for the second time. Patients were excluded if they had experienced any new treatments since the completion of the first interview.

Structural validity and reliability

The dimensionality of the original English version has been determined [25, 27]. In this study, the Confirmatory Factor Analysis (CFA) was used to test a priori construct of several dimensions identical to the original English version. It was suggested that the values of the two indexes, the comparative fit index (CFI) and goodness-of-fit index (GFI), greater than roughly 0.90 may indicate reasonably good fit of the model [39]. Furthermore, the root mean square error of approximation (RMSEA) was considered as a measure of fit. The criterion of judgment was as follows: RMSEA≤0.05, close approximate fit; RMSEA between 0.05 and 0.08, reasonable error of approximation; RMSEA≥0.10, poor fit.

The internal consistency and test-retest reliability were used to evaluate the reliability. The Cronbach's alpha coefficient (α) was used to assess the internal consistency, where a value greater than 0.7 was considered adequate [33]. The test-retest reliability was measured by intraclass correlation coefficient (ICC, two-way random effects model, absolute agreement). The values of ICC were reported with 95% confidence internals (CIs). When ICC was above 0.80, the result was considered as good reproducibility [40]. To determine agreement, the Bland-Altman plots were made, in which the mean difference (d) between the first and second measurements with corresponding 95% CI and the 95% Limits Of Agreement (LOA) were presented ($d \pm t_{n-1} \times SD_d$) [41]. A Bland-Altman plot not only described the mean score of the two measurements and the difference between them, but also was used to assess whether there was a systematic bias between the test and retest of the SC-THRES/TKRES.

Construct validity

Good convergent validity indicates good correlations between the questionnaire and other measures of similar concepts. Convergent validity was obtained by calculating the Pearson's correlation coefficients (r) between the total scores of the SC-THRES/TKRES and the Expectation WOMAC. The criterion of judgment was as follows: $r = 0–0.20$, poor; $r = 0.21–0.40$, fair; $r = 0.41–0.60$, moderate; $r = 0.61–0.80$, good; $r = 0.81–1.0$, excellent [42]. Convergent construct validity of SC-THRES/TKRES was tested using a hypothesis. We hypothesized the Expectation WOMAC would have moderate to strong correlations (0.40–0.80) with the SC-THRES/TKRES. Moreover, Bland-Altman analyses were performed to determine whether bias occurred.

Floor and ceiling effects

We conducted this analysis by calculating the percentage frequency of the highest or lowest score achieved by subjects, which a value higher than 15% was considered to be significant.

Statistical analysis

Statistical analysis was performed by using SPSS version 19.0 (SPSS, Chicago, USA) and the Medcalc software version 16.4 (Medcalc, Ostend, BEL). Means and standard deviation (SD) were applied for the patient characteristics and scores of the questionnaires. P values less than 0.05 were considered statistically significant.

Results

Cross-cultural adaption

As a result of the distance measure of "one block" is not popular in China, so is "mile", the expert committees discussed and decided to use "100 m" instead if "one block", "1500 m" instead of "one mile". According to the situation in China, the expert committee specified the "exercise or participate in sports" with "brisk walking or jogging" in our study.

Sociodemographic and clinical characteristics

In total, 270 patients were recruited into the registry. A total of 14 patients (5.2%) who met the exclusion criteria were not included in the analysis. Finally, a total of 256 eligible patients (104 hip OA, 51 AS, 101 knee OA) were enrolled in the research. Females of hip OA group, Knee OA group and AS group numbered 55 (52.4%), 68 (67.3%) and 5 (9.8%), respectively. All the patients completed the questionnaires without any difficulties. Of the 256 patients, 202 patients (86 hip OA, 42 AS, 74 knee OA) were included in the test–retest reliability. More clinical characteristics and the distribution of the scores were shown in Table 1.

Floor and ceiling effects

The lowest score of HSS-THRES/TKRES was not observed in any participant. While the highest score was observed in two AS patients (3.92%).

Simplified Chinese hip replacement expectations survey

Structural validity

In this present study, the CFA was used to test the structural validity. The results of CFA revealed good fit ($\chi^2 = 272.35$, CFI = 0.933, GFI = 0.915, RMSEA = 0.052, more details were shown in Additional file 2).

Reliability

The SC-THRES showed good test-retest reliability, both in hip OA and AS groups. In hip OA group, the mean score of the retest (73.9 ± 9.6) was similar to the first test (75.3 ± 12.7). The ICC between the two sessions was 0.878 (95% CI, 0.818–0.920). In AS group, the mean score of the second test (78.4 ± 11.3) was similar to the former result (79.5 ± 12.9). ICC for the test-retest was 0.893 (95% CI, 0.801–0.942). The internal consistency was good. The Cronbach's α values were 0.814 and 0.815

Table 1 Patient characteristics and mean total scores of the questionnaires

Characteristics[a]	OA		AS
	Hip	Knee	
Number	104	101	51
Gender			
female	55 (52.4)	68 (67.3)	5 (9.8)
Age in years	63.8 ± 9.4	65.1 ± 8.4	41.3 ± 12.1
Body mass index in kg/m^2	24.9 ± 3.1	26 ± 2.2	21.7 ± 2.0
Education			
Low	63 (60.6)	65 (64.4)	18 (35.3)
Medium	29 (27.9)	26 (25.7)	27 (52.9)
High	12 (11.5)	10 (9.9)	6 (11.8)
Living situation			
Living alone	20 (19.2)	24 (23.1)	8 (15.7)
Living with partner and/or children	84 (80.8)	77 (76.2)	43 (84.3)
Expectation Score A	75.3 ± 12.7	72.6 ± 11.1	79.5 ± 12.9
Expectation Score B	73.9 ± 9.6	71.9 ± 8.3	78.4 ± 11.3
Expectation WOMAC Score	88.1 ± 9.9	84.9 ± 10.8	91.1 ± 9.6

OA osteoarthritis, *AS* ankylosing spondylitis, *WOMAC* Western Ontario and Mc Master Universities Osteoarthritis index

[a]Quantitative variables: mean standard deviation; categorical variables: frequency (percentage)

for hip OA group and AS group, respectively (Table 2). As for the agreement, the Bland-Altman plots of the two groups showed that zero lies within the 95% CI of the mean difference (d) between the first and second measurement of the SC-THRES, indicating no bias (Fig. 1a, b). The 95% LOA were 0.54 ± 13.85 (hip OA group) and − 0.23 ± 14.53 (AS group).

Validity

Pearson's coefficients were shown in Table 3. The result demonstrated that the correlations between the SC-THRES and the Expectation WOMAC (0.490, $p < 0.01$; 0.541, $p < 0.01$) were moderate for hip OA group and AS group, respectively. This was in line with our hypotheses. The Bland-Altman plots (Fig. 2a, b) showed that the 95% LOA were − 12.85 ± 22.85 (hip OA group) and − 11.51 ± 21.83 (AS group). The mean SC-THRES score of hip OA group was 12.72 points lower than the mean Expectation WOMAC score. And the mean SC-THRES score of AS group was 11.51 points lower than that of the Expectation WOMAC. Systematic bias could be found in the two groups since zero was not in the 95% CI of mean difference (d).

Comparison between hip OA group and AS group

Average scores for each item of the SC-THRES were presented in Fig. 3. The most important expectation cited by patients was item 3 (improving walking), both in hip OA and AS group. The least important expectations cited were item 12 (be employed for monetary reimbursement) in hip OA group and item 2 (relieve pain that interferences with sleep) in AS group. Compared to hip OA group, the mean score of AS group for every individual item was mostly higher except for item 1 (relieve daytime pain), 2 (relieve pain that interferences with sleep) and 11 (eliminate the need for medications). There were significant differences between hip OA group and AS group in item 1 (relieve daytime pain, hip OA: 3.519, AS: 2.569; $p = 0.009$), 6 (remove need for cane, hip OA: 2.538, AS: 3; $p = 0.018$), 12 (be employed for monetary reimbursement, hip OA: 1.808, AS: 3.373; $p<0.001$), 13 (sexual activity, hip OA: 1.904, AS: 2.686; $p = 0.012$), 14 (improve ability to exercise/play sports, hip OA: 2.760, AS: 3.176; $p = 0.008$) and 15 (improve social activities, hip OA: 2.885, AS: 3.353; $p = 0.004$).

Table 2 Internal consistency and reliability of the SC-THRES/TKRES

Scale	Cronbach's α coefficient	ICC (95% CIs)
Hip Replacement Expectations Score		
OA group	0.814	0.878 (0.818–0.920)
AS group	0.815	0.893 (0.801–0.942)
Knee Replacement Expectations Score	0.808	0.806 (0.693–0.878)

SC-THRES Simplified Chinese Total Hip Replacement Expectations Survey, *SC-TKRES* Simplified Chinese Total Knee Replacement Expectations Survey, *ICC* intraclass correlation coefficient, *CIs* confidence internals, *OA* osteoarthritis, *AS* ankylosing spondylitis

Simplified Chinese knee replacement expectations survey

Structural validity

Also the results of CFA demonstrated good fit (χ^2 = 302.10, CFI = 0.929, GFI = 0.927, RMSEA = 0.054, more details were shown in Additional file 2).

Reliability

The mean score of the retest was 71.9 ± 8.3, which was similar to the first result (72.6 ± 11.1). The ICC between the first and second assessment was 0.806 (95% CI 0.693–0.878), which indicated good test-retest reliability. The internal consistency result was good as well. The Cronbach'α was 0.808 for the overall SC-TKRES (Table 2). In addition, the Bland-Altman plot (Fig. 1c) showed no systematic bias, in which zero lies within the 95% CI of the mean difference (d) between the measurements of the SC-TKRES in the two sessions. The 95% LOA were 0.05 ± 14.24.

Validity

As shown in Table 3, the result indicated good convergent validity. The correlation between the SC-TKRES score (first assessment) and the Expectation WOMAC total score (0.465, $p<0.01$) was moderate, which conformed to the hypotheses. The Bland-Altman plot showed the 95% LOA were − 12.09 ± 22.24 (Fig. 2c). Total score of the Expectation WOMAC was 12.09 points higher than that of the SC-TKRES and different from zero significantly, which indicated systematic bias.

Discussion

OA is a highly prevalent disease in the older population [43]. Although the prevalence of AS is lower than OA, the amount of patients with AS is also considerable because of the huge population of China, which lead to a heavy burden. TJA is an effective way in reducing pain and improving function in patients with end-stage OA and AS. As the demand for TJA continues to grow, understanding the factors associated with the outcomes of this procedure has become even more important. Nowadays clinical surgeons are placing more emphasis on self-reported outcome assessment. But patients' preoperative expectations have seldom been studied. Analyzing patients' expectations may help surgeons to understand better what is important for their patients and therefore enhance patients' satisfaction and the doctor–patient relationship. In addition, the differences of age and state between AS and OA may result in discrepancies of expectation, of which may be unrealistic and need to be educated before surgery. The HSS-THRES and the HSS-TKRES are widely used for

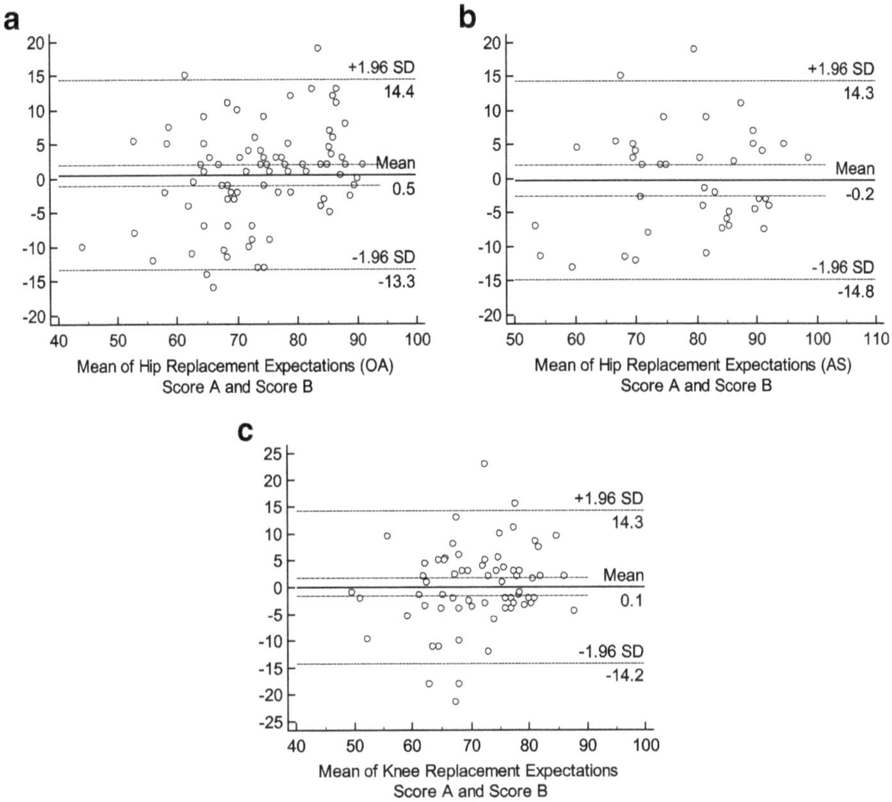

Fig. 1 Bland–Altman plots of test–retest reliability of the SC-THRES/TKRES. The plots are for the (**a**) hip OA group, (**b**) AS group and (**c**) knee OA group. Each data point indicates how the difference between the two test sessions for an individual patient compares to the mean of the two sessions for scores of the SC-THRES/TKRES. The long dashed line shows the 95% (±1.96 SD) limits of agreement. SD, standard deviation; SC-THRES, simplified Chinese total hip replacement expectations survey; SC-TKRES, simplified Chinese total knee replacement expectations survey

patients undergoing TJA, but to our knowledge, these widely used tools have not been validated in a Chinese population. So it is greatly meaningful to translate the questionnaires into Chinese. The translation process was nicely developed. All patients completed the questionnaires without any difficulties, which meant the translated questionnaires had good cultural acceptability. No significant floor and ceiling effects were observed in our study.

The interval time was two weeks between the first and second test in our study. It was appropriate to assess the test-retest reliability for the reason that the interval was

Table 3 Construct validity[a] of the SC-THRES/TKRES

	expectation WOMAC score
Hip Replacement Expectations Score	
OA	0.490 ($P < 0.01$)
AS	0.541 ($P < 0.01$)
Knee Replacement Expectations Score	0.465 ($P < 0.01$)

SC-THRES Simplified Chinese Total Hip Replacement Expectations Survey, *SC-TKRES* Simplified Chinese Total Knee Replacement Expectations Survey, *OA* osteoarthritis, *AS* ankylosing spondylitis, *WOMAC* Western Ontario and Mc Master Universities Osteoarthritis index

[a]Calculated by Pearson's correlation of the SC-THRES/TKRES with expectation WOMAC score in different groups

long enough to keep patients from completing the questionnaires from memory, and short enough to prevent dramatic changes in expectations. According to the results, both simplified Chinese surveys showed good test-retest reliability. The ICCs for the total scores (0.878, 0.893 and 0.806 for hip OA group, AS group and knee OA group, respectively) were all higher than the minimum criterion of 0.80 recommended by Fleiss et al. [40], similar to the results of validated Dutch [28] and French [29] versions. As a result of no available information regarding the reliability of the original tool, we did not compare our results with the English version. In addition, no bias between measurements of the two sessions was observed in the Bland-Altman analysis, which was in accordance with other cross-cultural adapted studies [28, 29]. Determined by Cronbach's α, the internal consistency of the simplified Chinese surveys were all good (0.814, 0.815 and 0.808 for hip OA group, AS group and knee OA group, respectively), which was also conformed with the criterion suggested by Terwee et al. [33]. With respect to surveys applied in patients with hip OA, the Cronbach's α (0.814) was above the original English version (0.77) [27] and the French version (0.72) [29], but slightly lower than the Dutch version (0.86) [28].

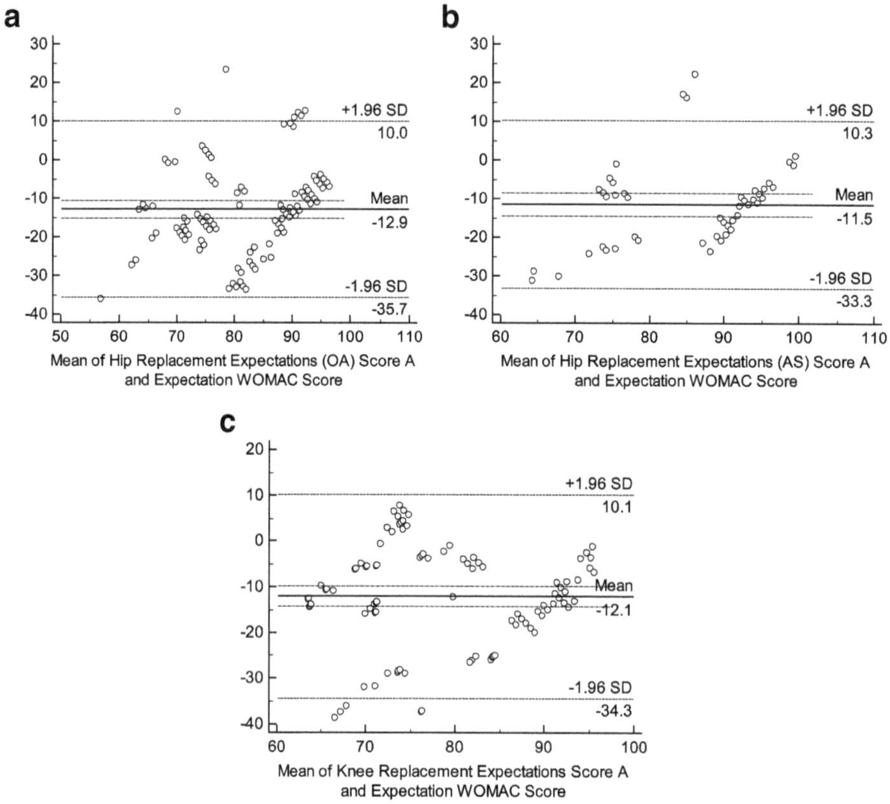

Fig. 2 Bland–Altman plots of concurrent validity of the SC-THRES/TKRES. The plots are for the (**a**) hip OA group, (**b**) AS group and (**c**) knee OA group. Each data point indicates how the difference between the two test sessions for an individual patient compares to the mean of the two sessions for scores of the SC-THRES/TKRES. The long dashed line shows the 95% (±1.96 SD) limits of agreement. SD, standard deviation; SC-THRES, simplified Chinese total hip replacement expectations survey; SC-TKRES, simplified Chinese total knee replacement expectations survey

As for the knee OA group, present value (0.808) was in line with the original version (0.79) [27] and the French version (0.82) [29], but lower than the Dutch version (0.91) [28].

Construct validity was demonstrated by assessing the correlation between the SC-THRES/TKRES scores and Expectation WOMAC scores. Until now, no so-called "gold standard" can be used to optimally evaluate patients' expectations. We employed the Expectation WOMAC for the reason that (1) it had been first presented and demonstrated by Haddad et al. [26] and had been used in other studies [28, 29]; (2) the Chinese WOMAC is proved to be reliable and valid [37, 38]. And we made a slight modification to result in the Expectation WOMAC. On the basis of the criterion, the Pearson's correlations between the SC-THRES/TKRES and Expectation WOMAC were moderate (0.49 for hip OA, 0.541 for hip AS and 0.465 for knee OA). Despite this moderate result, we found a systematic bias in the Bland-Altman analysis. Compared to the SC-THRES/TKRES, the mean scores of the Expectation WOMAC were higher. However, the same trend was found in the Dutch and French version [28, 29]. Van et al. [28] thought that the way the Expectation WOMAC was adapted from the original WOMAC resulted in answers whereby the patients also considered the current status. However, Neuprez et al. [29] believed that the response's categories and codification of the two measures were different. Our view was different from theirs. The subscales of Expectation WOMAC included pain, stiffness and functional disability. These were the main symptoms which patients wanted to get rid of as soon as possible. In addition to the items related to these symptoms, the THRES/TKRES also included psychological well-being, sexual activity and employment, which were not that important for patients. These sections may lower the mean scores of the THRES/TKRES.

The mean total score of AS group was higher both in the Expectation WOMAC and the SC-THRES. The majority of the mean score for an individual item revealed the same trend. It was suggested that item was of some importance to patients when the average score was ≥2 points. The majority of the average scores were over 2.5 and some were even over 3, indicating they were important to patients. Patients with AS undergoing THA were of worse functional status and had higher expectations

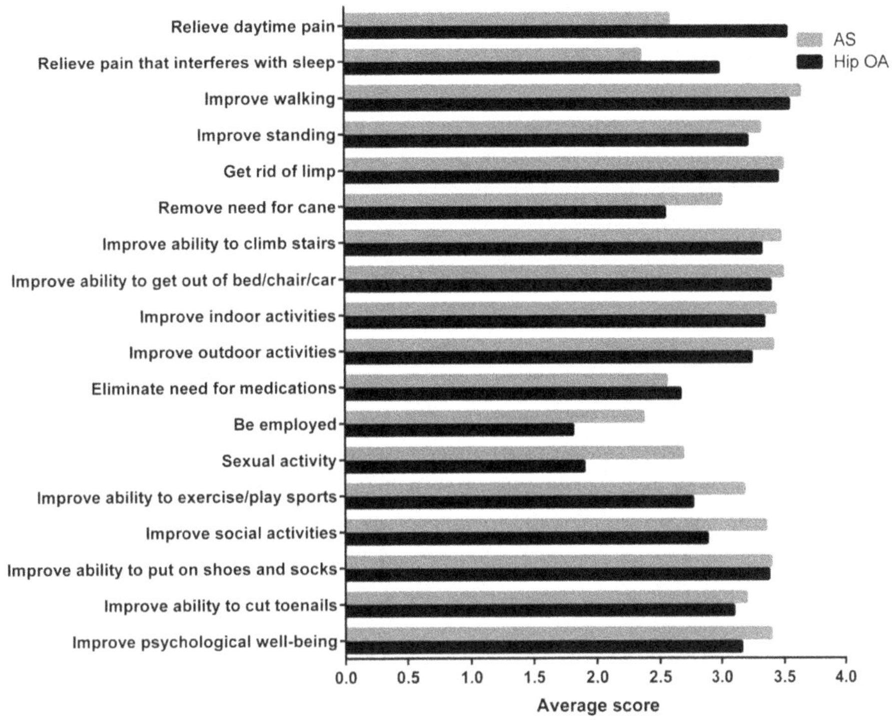

Fig. 3 Total hip replacement patients' responses to SC-THRES. OA, osteoarthritis; AS, ankylosing spondylitis; SC-THRES, simplified Chinese total hip replacement expectations survey

than those with hip OA [44]. Not only hip OA patients, but also AS patients showed the highest expectations to improve walking. This was because patients in both groups were almost end-staged with severe pain and dysfunction in the hips, which limited their abilities to walk. Patients with hip OA showed higher expectations for pain relief during daytime than those with AS. This can be explained because many patients in AS group were bony ankylosis with less pain currently. The mean age of hip OA group and AS group were 63.8 ± 9.4 and 41.3 ± 12.1, respectively. The majority of patients in hip OA group were retired from work and they showed lower expectations to be employed. However, patients with AS were always younger, and they were unable to work because of their physical disabilities. They were expected to be endorsed by family and society through rehabilitation. Similarly, patients with AS had more expectations in sexual activity than those with hip OA.

There were two strengths of our study. First, all the patients completed the questionnaires in the outpatient room of our hospital to avoid missing values. Second, to our knowledge, it was the first time that the surveys were validated in patients with AS.

With no doubt, there were some limitations in the current study that should be considered. First, considering the absence of validated tools assessing preoperative expectations, studying such questionnaire remains difficult. Although the Chinese WOMAC is reliable and valid, the psychometric properties of the Chinese version Expectation WOMAC are unknown. Without a doubt, this may result in some issues. For example, patients may take this adapted WOMAC as the original and consider the current state. Taking the expectations of orthopedic surgeons as reference would be an alternative way [28]. However, this is doubtful owing to the discrepancies between the expectations of orthopedic surgeons and those of patients [19, 20]. Thus we took the closest tool as a reference to evaluate the validity in our study. Second, the sample was limited in size, which may not be representative of the whole Chinese population. It was noteworthy that the sample of AS was too small for assessing the structural validity, we conducted this assessment among the OA and AS sample together. Last but not least, we translated the surveys into Mandarin, the official language of China, but traditional Chinese languages are still widely used in several areas of China. So it will be necessary to translate the surveys into traditional Chinese languages in the future.

Conclusion

In summary, the HSS-THRES and HSS-TKRES have been nicely adapted into Chinese versions with good psychometric properties. As self-reported questionnaires, the SC-THRES and SC-TKRES are reliable and valid for a Chinese population with OA or AS undergoing TJAs. Therefore, we suggest that the two questionnaires can be used to investigate patients' expectations before surgeries. And patients' expectations should be part of preoperative assessments. Future studies would be conducted to assess the content validity, cross-cultural validity and responsiveness of these two questionnaires.

Abbreviations

AS: Ankylosing spondylitis; CFA: Confirmatory Factor Analysis; CFI: Comparative fit index; CIs: Confidence internals; GFI: Goodness-of-fit index; HSS-THRES: Hospital for Special Surgery Total Hip Replacement Expectations Survey; HSS-TKRES: Hospital for Special Surgery Total Knee Replacement Expectations Survey; ICC: Intraclass correlation coefficient; LOA: Limits Of Agreement; OA: Osteoarthritis; RMSEA: Root mean square error of approximation; SC-THRES: Simplified Chinese Total Hip Replacement Expectations Survey; SC-TKRES: Simplified Chinese Total Knee Replacement Expectations Survey; SD: Standard deviation; THA: Total hip arthroplasty; TJAs: Total joint arthroplasties; TKA: Total knee arthroplasty; WOMAC: Western Ontario and Mc Master Universities Osteoarthritis index

Acknowledgements

We thank the staff from our outpatient clinics and the patients participating in the study. We are grateful for the help of three international medical students for the translation.

Authors' contributions

The following authors have made substantial contributions to the following: (1) the conception and design of the study (WC, ZC, LDL, HX, and XWD), acquisition of data (WC, ZC, TWW, and HCR), analysis and interpretation of data (WC, ZC, LDL, TWW, and HCR), (2) drafting the article (WC and ZC), revising critical for important intellectual content (WC, ZC, LDL, HX, and XWD), (3) All of the authors approved the final version of the manuscript.

Consent for publication

Not applicable.

Competing interests

The authors declare that they have no competing interests.

References

1. Singh JA. Epidemiology of knee and hip arthroplasty: a systematic review. Open Orthop J. 2011;5:80–5.
2. Kurtz S, Ong K, Lau E, Mowat F, Halpern M. Projections of primary and revision hip and knee arthroplasty in the United States from 2005 to 2030. J Bone Joint Surg Am. 2007;89(4):780–5.
3. Braun J, van den Berg R, Baraliakos X, Boehm H, Burgos-Vargas R, Collantes-Estevez E, Dagfinrud H, Dijkmans B, Dougados M, Emery P, et al. 2010 update of the ASAS/EULAR recommendations for the management of ankylosing spondylitis. Ann Rheum Dis. 2011;70(6):896–904.
4. Pivec R, Johnson AJ, Mears SC, Mont MA. Hip arthroplasty. Lancet. 2012; 380(9855):1768–77.
5. Carr AJ, Robertsson O, Graves S, Price AJ, Arden NK, Judge A, Beard DJ. Knee replacement. Lancet. 2012;379(9823):1331–40.
6. Stratford PW, Kennedy DM. Performance measures were necessary to obtain a complete picture of osteoarthritic patients. J Clin Epidemiol. 2006;59(2): 160–7.
7. Mizner RL, Petterson SC, Clements KE, Zeni JA Jr, Irrgang JJ, Snyder-Mackler L. Measuring functional improvement after total knee arthroplasty requires both performance-based and patient-report assessments: a longitudinal analysis of outcomes. J Arthroplasty. 2011;26(5):728–37.
8. Flood AB, Lorence DP, Ding J, McPherson K, Black NA. The role of expectations in patients' reports of post-operative outcomes and improvement following therapy. Med Care. 1993;31(11):1043–56.
9. Jain D, Nguyen LL, Bendich I, Nguyen LL, Lewis CG, Huddleston JI, Duwelius PJ, Feeley BT, Bozic KJ. Higher patient expectations predict higher patient-reported outcomes, but not satisfaction, in Total knee arthroplasty patients: a prospective multicenter study. J Arthroplast. 2017;32(9S):S166–70.
10. Hamilton DF, Lane JV, Gaston P, Patton JT, Macdonald D, Simpson AH, Howie CR. What determines patient satisfaction with surgery? A prospective cohort study of 4709 patients following total joint replacement. BMJ Open. 2013;3(4)
11. Nilsdotter AK, Toksvig-Larsen S, Roos EM. Knee arthroplasty: are patients' expectations fulfilled? A prospective study of pain and function in 102 patients with 5-year follow-up. Acta Orthop. 2009;80(1):55–61.
12. Noble PC, Conditt MA, Cook KF, Mathis KB. The John Insall award: patient expectations affect satisfaction with total knee arthroplasty. Clin Orthop Relat Res. 2006;452:35–43.
13. Bourne RB, Chesworth BM, Davis AM, Mahomed NN, Charron KD. Patient satisfaction after total knee arthroplasty: who is satisfied and who is not? Clin Orthop Relat Res. 2010;468(1):57–63.
14. Neuprez A, Delcour JP, Fatemi F, Gillet P, Crielaard JM, Bruyere O, Reginster JY. Patients' expectations impact their satisfaction following Total hip or knee arthroplasty. PLoS One. 2016;11(12):e0167911.
15. Dyck BA, Zywiel MG, Mahomed A, Gandhi R, Perruccio AV, Mahomed NN. Associations between patient expectations of joint arthroplasty surgery and pre- and post-operative clinical status. Expert Rev Med Devices. 2014;11(4): 403–15.
16. Palazzo C, Jourdan C, Descamps S, Nizard R, Hamadouche M, Anract P, Boisgard S, Galvin M, Ravaud P, Poiraudeau S. Determinants of satisfaction 1 year after total hip arthroplasty: the role of expectations fulfilment. BMC Musculoskelet Disord. 2014;15:53.
17. Mancuso CA, Jout J, Salvati EA, Sculco TP. Fulfillment of patients' expectations for total hip arthroplasty. J Bone Joint Surg Am. 2009;91(9):2073–8.
18. Koenen P, Bathis H, Schneider MM, Frohlich M, Bouillon B, Shafizadeh S. How do we face patients' expectations in joint arthroplasty? Arch Orthop Trauma Surg. 2014;134(7):925–31.
19. Jourdan C, Poiraudeau S, Descamps S, Nizard R, Hamadouche M, Anract P, Boisgard S, Galvin M, Ravaud P. Comparison of patient and surgeon expectations of total hip arthroplasty. PLoS One. 2012;7(1):e30195.
20. Ghomrawi HM, Franco Ferrando N, Mandl LA, Do H, Noor N, Gonzalez Della Valle A. How often are patient and surgeon recovery expectations for Total joint arthroplasty aligned? Results of a pilot study. HSS J. 2011;7(3):229–34.
21. Tilbury C, Haanstra TM, Leichtenberg CS, Verdegaal SH, Ostelo RW, de Vet HC, Nelissen RG, Vliet Vlieland TP. Unfulfilled expectations after Total hip and knee arthroplasty surgery: there is a need for better preoperative patient information and education. J Arthroplast. 2016;31(10):2139–45.
22. Jing W, Otten H, Sullivan L, Lovell-Simons L, Granek-Catarivas M, Fritzsche K. Improving the doctor-patient relationship in China: the role of balint groups. Int J Psychiatry Med. 2013;46(4):417–27.
23. Zhang X, Sleeboom-Faulkner M. Tensions between medical professionals and patients in mainland China. Camb Q Healthc Ethics. 2011;20(3):458–65.
24. Mancuso CA, Wentzel CH, Ghomrawi HMK, Kelly BT. Hip preservation surgery expectations survey: a new method to measure Patients' preoperative expectations. Arthroscopy. 2017;33(5):959–68.
25. Mancuso CA, Sculco TP, Wickiewicz TL, Jones EC, Robbins L, Warren RF, Williams-Russo P. Patients' expectations of knee surgery. J Bone Joint Surg Am. 2001;83-A(7):1005–12.
26. Haddad FS, Garbuz DS, Chambers GK, Jagpal TJ, Masri BA, Duncan CP. The expectations of patients undergoing revision hip arthroplasty. J Arthroplast. 2001;16(1):87–91.
27. Mancuso CA, Salvati EA, Johanson NA, Peterson MG, Charlson ME. Patients' expectations and satisfaction with total hip arthroplasty. J Arthroplast. 1997;12(4):387–96.
28. van den Akker-Scheek I, van Raay JJ, Reininga IH, Bulstra SK, Zijlstra W, Stevens M. Reliability and concurrent validity of the Dutch hip and knee replacement expectations surveys. BMC Musculoskelet Disord. 2010;11:242.
29. Neuprez A, Delcour JP, Fatemi F, Gillet P, Mawet M, Francois G, Bruyere O, Crielaard JM, Gosset C, Reginster JY. Development and validation of the French version of a tool assessing patient's expectations in lower limb osteoarthritis. J Orthop. 2015;12(1):46–57.

30. Balck F, Kirschner S, Jeszenszky C, Lippmann M, Gunther KP. Validity and reliability of the German version of the HSS expectation questionnaire on hip joint replacement. Z Orthop Unfall. 2016;154(6):606–11.
31. Altman R, Alarcon G, Appelrouth D, Bloch D, Borenstein D, Brandt K, Brown C, Cooke TD, Daniel W, Feldman D, et al. The American College of Rheumatology criteria for the classification and reporting of osteoarthritis of the hip. Arthritis Rheum. 1991;34(5):505–14.
32. van der Linden S, Valkenburg HA, Cats A. Evaluation of diagnostic criteria for ankylosing spondylitis. A proposal for modification of the New York criteria Arthritis Rheum. 1984;27(4):361–8.
33. Terwee CB, Bot SD, de Boer MR, van der Windt DA, Knol DL, Dekker J, Bouter LM, de Vet HC. Quality criteria were proposed for measurement properties of health status questionnaires. J Clin Epidemiol. 2007;60(1):34–42.
34. Beaton DE, Bombardier C, Guillemin F, Ferraz MB. Guidelines for the process of cross-cultural adaptation of self-report measures. Spine (Phila Pa 1976). 2000;25(24):3186–91.
35. Mancuso CA, Graziano S, Briskie LM, Peterson MG, Pellicci PM, Salvati EA, Sculco TP. Randomized trials to modify patients' preoperative expectations of hip and knee arthroplasties. Clin Orthop Relat Res. 2008;466(2):424–31.
36. Bellamy N, Buchanan WW, Goldsmith CH, Campbell J, Stitt LW. Validation study of WOMAC: a health status instrument for measuring clinically important patient relevant outcomes to antirheumatic drug therapy in patients with osteoarthritis of the hip or knee. J Rheumatol. 1988;15(12):1833–40.
37. Xie F, Li SC, Goeree R, Tarride JE, O'Reilly D, Lo NN, Yeo SJ, Yang KY, Thumboo J. Validation of Chinese western Ontario and McMaster universities osteoarthritis index (WOMAC) in patients scheduled for total knee replacement. Qual Life Res. 2008;17(4):595–601.
38. Symonds T, Hughes B, Liao S, Ang Q, Bellamy N. Validation of the Chinese western Ontario and McMaster universities osteoarthritis index in patients from mainland China with osteoarthritis of the knee. Arthritis Care Res (Hoboken). 2015;67(11):1553–60.
39. Lt H, Bentler PM. Cutoff criteria for fit indexes in covariance structure analysis: conventional criteria versus new alternatives. Struct Equ Model. 1999;6(1):1–55.
40. Fleiss JL, Shrout PE. The effects of measurement errors on some multivariate procedures. Am J Public Health. 1977;67(12):1188–91.
41. Bland JM, Altman DG. Statistical methods for assessing agreement between two methods of clinical measurement. Lancet. 1986;1(8476):307–10.
42. Zheng W, Li J, Zhao J, Liu D, Xu W. Development of a valid simplified Chinese version of the Oxford hip score in patients with hip osteoarthritis. Clin Orthop Relat Res. 2014;472(5):1545–51.
43. Quintana JM, Arostegui I, Escobar A, Azkarate J, Goenaga JI, Lafuente I. Prevalence of knee and hip osteoarthritis and the appropriateness of joint replacement in an older population. Arch Intern Med. 2008;168(14):1576–84.
44. Mancuso CA, Sculco TP, Salvati EA. Patients with poor preoperative functional status have high expectations of total hip arthroplasty. J Arthroplast. 2003;18(7): 872–8.

19

Efficacy and safety of oral compared with intravenous tranexamic acid in reducing blood loss after primary total knee and hip arthroplasty

Xiaozhen Han[1†], Guiqing Gong[1†], Naili Han[2] and Mei Liu[3*]

Abstract

Background: Tranexamic acid (TXA) is an anti-fibrinolytic agent successfully preventing blood loss when using intravenously (IV) in total hip arthroplasty (THA) and total knee arthroplasty (TKA). An oral administration, which is available on blood sparing, has been reported exhibit profound cost-saving benefits. The aim of this meta-analysis is to investigate whether the administration of oral and intravenous tranexamic acid postoperatively has equivalent blood-sparing properties in these patients.

Methods: The online electronic databases were searched for eligible literatures updated on September 2018. Studies assessing the effect between oral TXA and intravenous TXA (IV-TXA) in those undergoing TKA or THA were included. All the data were pooled with the corresponding 95% confidence interval (CI) using RevMan software. Based on the heterogeneity, we performed a systematic analysis to explore the overall results across the included studies.

Results: Nine studies met our inclusion criteria. No significant differences were identified with regard to the Hb drop (SMD = – 0.03,95%CI = – 0.18–0.12, $P = 0.67$), total Hb loss (SMD = 0.10,95%CI = – 0.06–0.26, $P = 0.24$), total blood loss (SMD = – 0.00,95%CI = – 0.20–0.20, $P = 1.00$), transfusion rate (OR = 0.77,95%CI = 0.54–1.10, $P = 0.14$), DVT rate (OR = 0.58,95%CI = 0.19–1.75, $P = 0.33$), and length of hospital stay (SMD = – 0.05,95%CI = – 0.28–0.17, $P = 0.63$) between the oral groups and intravenous group.

Conclusion: The blood-sparing efficacy of oral TXA is similar to that of the intravenous forms in the setting of THA and TKA. Considering the cost-benefit superiority and ease of administration of oral TXA, further studies and clinical trials are required to further identify the optimal administration for THA and TKA.

Keywords: Tranexamic acid, Total hip arthroplasty, Total knee arthroplasty, Meta-analysis

Background

Patients who suffer from osteoarthritis, rheumatoid arthritis, fractures, or the knee or hip cancer often need total knee and hip arthroplasty (TKA and THA) [1]. Although TKA and THA have been identified as an effective management in improving physical function and relieving pain, these procedures can result in high risk of perioperative anemia, which can be associated with increasing morbidity and cost. Thus, a considerable number of patients require blood transfusions to prevent anemia [2, 3].

Finding effective methods for minimizing the risk of transfusion and perioperative blood loss have been a goal for surgeons to perform total TKA and THA [3, 4]. Surgeons have implemented numerous methods to achieve this goal, particularly the using of anti-fibrinolytic agents, such as tranexamic acid (TXA).

Tranexamic acid is a synthetic amino acid that functions by competitively inhibiting the activation of plasminogen, thereby inhibiting clot degradation [5], which has been

* Correspondence: 66799073@qq.com
[†]Xiaozhen Han and Guiqing Gong contributed equally to this work.
[3]Department of Intensive Care Unit, Wuhan No.1 Hospital, No.215 Zhongshan Ave, Wuhan 430022, Hubei, China
Full list of author information is available at the end of the article

identified as effectively reducing blood loss and the risk of adverse outcomes following THA and TKA [6–8].

Tranexamic acid can be administered intravenously (IV), topically (intra-articular), and orally. However, the optimal administration of TXA administration remains controversial [9–11]. Recently, several studies have been published to evaluate the effects of the TXA administration routes between oral and IV-TXA, while the efficacy and safety between two groups are still unknown [12, 13].

In this meta-analysis, we aim to explore whether oral TXA has an equivalent effect to intravenously in reducing blood loss in THA and TKA.

Methods

Search strategy

We performed the current meta-analysis based on the electronic databases: Pubmed, Embase, Cochrane library up to September 2018.The process was established to find all articles based on the MeSH terms and free key words: "Total knee replacement or arthroplasty" AND "Total hip replacement or arthroplasty" OR "tranexamic acid" AND "oral TXA" , AND "intravenous TXA". Moreover, we identified full-text papers from reference materials for further evaluation.

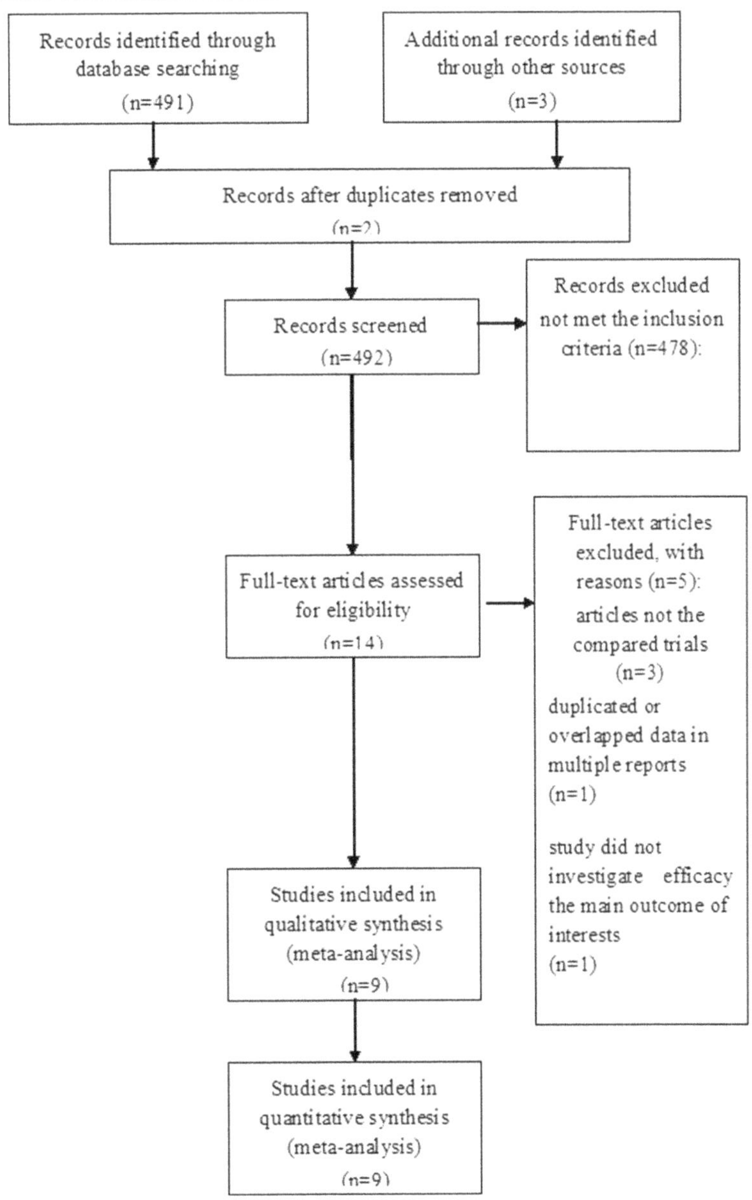

Fig. 1 PRISMA flow chart of selection process to identify studies eligible for pooling

Table 1 the primary characteristics of the eligible studies in more detail

Studies (year)	Study type	Surgery	Treatment regimen (Dosage of TXA)		Treatment regimen (number)		Treatment regimen (Age)	
			oral	intravenous	oral	intravenous	oral	intravenous
Kayupovt, 2017	RCT	THA	1950 mg/kg	1000 mg	40	43	60	55
Yuan, 2017	RCT	TKA	40 mg/kg	20 mg/kg	140	140	63.2	63.7
Fillingham, 2016	RCT	TKA	1950 mg	1000 mg	34	37	62	63
Irwin, 2013	RCS	TKA and THA	25 mg/kg (maximum 2 g)	15 mg/kg (maximum 1.2 g)	302	2698	67.6	68.2
Zohar, 2004	RCT	TKA	4000 mg	10 mg/kg for 12 h	20	20	69	73
Cao, 2018	RCT	THA	2000 mg	20 mg/kg	54	54	55.7	55.7
Gortemoller, 2017	RCS	TKA and THA	1950 mg	1000 mg	165	165	67	68
Luo, 2017	RCS	THA	2000 mg	20 mg/kg	60	60	67.6	66.98
Wang, 2018	RCT	TKA	2000 mg	20 mg/kg	60	60	63.91	66.9

TXA tranexamic acid, *THA* total hip arthroplasty, *TKA* total knee arthroplasty, *RCT* randomized controlled trial, *RCS* retrospective cohort study

Eligibility criteria

Studies were included in the meta-analysis should meet the following criteria: [1] articles that enrolled total knee/hip arthroplasty patients treated with TXA; [2] the studies are designed as comparing TXA administered via intravenous (IV) and oral routes; [3] the outcomes of interest were efficacy (total blood loss, total hemoglobin (Hb) loss, Hb reduction, transfusion rate, length of hospital stay) and toxicity (incidence of deep vein thrombosis (DVT)), and with corresponding 95% CIs were provided; [4] the full-text papers were only included.

Quality assessment

The quality of the search was performed separately by two reviewers. We use the New-castle-Ottawa Quality Assessment Scale recommended by the "Cochrane Intervention Manual Systematic Review".

Data extraction

Two authors independently extracted the relevant data from each trial. Disagreement was resolved by consensus. We extracted the main categories based on the following: first author family name, year of publication, study type, surgery, dosage of TXA patient number, age, and outcomes measures. We extracted the corresponding Std.Mean Difference (SMD) and odds ratios (ORs) with 95% confidence interval (95%CI) to describe the endpoints of interest.

Statistical analysis

The Cochrane Collaborations have offered Review Manager Software (RevMan5.3) for statistical analysis.(Revman; The Cochrane collaboration Oxford, United Kingdom). The chi-square was used to assess the significance of heterogeneity [14]. I^2 value larger than 50% suggested high degree of heterogeneity [15]. When there was high heterogeneity among studies, the randomed-effects model was used. Otherwise, the fixed effects model was used. A P value less than 0.05 was identified as statistically significant difference. Findings of our meta-analysis were shown in forest plots. The Begg test and the Egger test were conducted to evaluate publication bias.

Results

Study selection process

A total of 492 articles were considered possibly eligible. Based on the criteria described in the methods, 14 articles were further eliminated by reading the full articles, but some did not provide enough detail of outcomes of two

Study or Subgroup	Experimental Mean	SD	Total	Control Mean	SD	Total	Weight	Std. Mean Difference IV, Fixed, 95% CI
Fillingham, 2016	3.45	0.93	34	3.31	0.95	37	10.5%	0.15 [-0.32, 0.61]
Kayupovt, 2017	3.67	1.2	40	3.53	1.2	43	12.3%	0.12 [-0.32, 0.55]
Luo, 2017	3.48	1.32	60	3.58	1.07	60	17.8%	-0.08 [-0.44, 0.28]
Wang, 2018	2.91	1.73	60	3.13	0.89	60	17.8%	-0.16 [-0.52, 0.20]
Yuan, 2017	2.9	0.43	140	2.92	0.41	140	41.6%	-0.05 [-0.28, 0.19]
Total (95% CI)			**334**			**340**	**100.0%**	**-0.03 [-0.18, 0.12]**

Heterogeneity: $Chi^2 = 1.59$, df = 4 (P = 0.81); $I^2 = 0\%$
Test for overall effect: Z = 0.43 (P = 0.67)

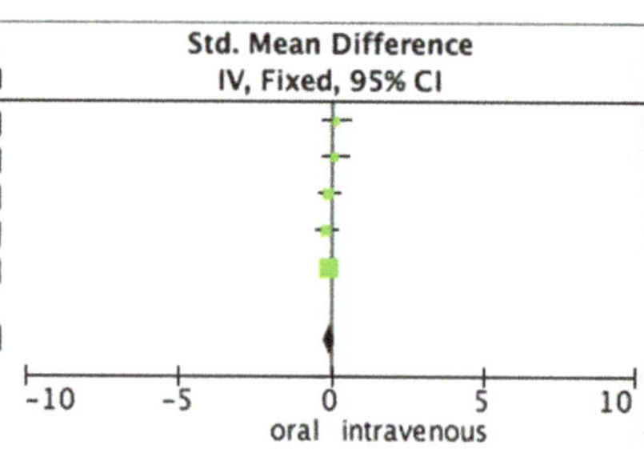

Fig. 2 Pooled analysis of Hb drop between oral administration and intravenous administration

Study or Subgroup	Experimental Mean	Experimental SD	Experimental Total	Control Mean	Control SD	Control Total	Weight	Std. Mean Difference IV, Fixed, 95% CI
Fillingham, 2016	177	50	34	168	56	37	11.8%	0.17 [-0.30, 0.63]
Gortemoller, 2017	2.09	0.9	165	1.97	0.9	165	54.8%	0.13 [-0.08, 0.35]
Kayupovt, 2017	183	57	40	162	63	43	13.6%	0.35 [-0.09, 0.78]
Wang, 2018	2.91	1.13	60	3.13	0.89	60	19.9%	-0.21 [-0.57, 0.14]
Total (95% CI)			**299**			**305**	**100.0%**	**0.10 [-0.06, 0.26]**

Heterogeneity: Chi² = 4.36, df = 3 (P = 0.23); I² = 31%
Test for overall effect: Z = 1.19 (P = 0.24)

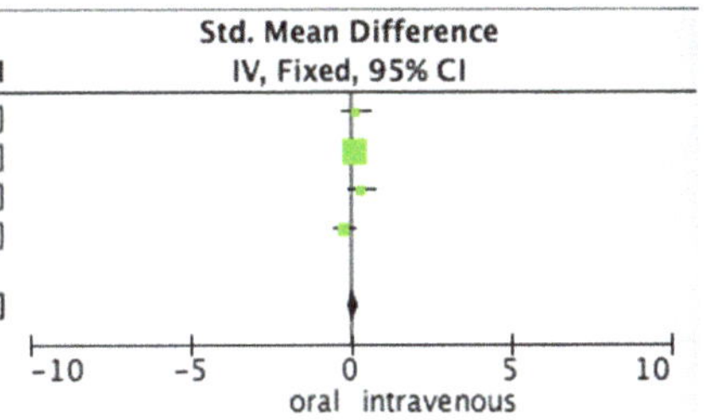

Fig. 3 Pooled analysis of total Hb loss between oral administration and intravenous administration

approaches. Therefore, a final total of 9 studies [11, 16–23] with included (Fig. 1). Table 1 describes a brief description of these eligible studies. All included studies in this study were based on moderate to high quality evidence.

Clinical and methodological heterogeneity

Pooled analysis of Hb drop between oral administration and intravenous administration

Pooled data of the Hb drop from five studies showed that no statistical differences were observed in terms of favoring oral administration compared with the intravenous administration group (SMD = – 0.03,95%CI = – 0.18–0.12, P = 0.67) (Fig. 2).

Pooled analysis of total Hb loss between oral administration and intravenous administration

In terms of total Hb loss, no significant differences compared oral administration and intravenous administration was observed (OR = 0.73; 95% CI = 0.51–1.05; p = 0.09) (Fig. 3).

Pooled analysis of total blood loss between oral administration and intravenous administration

Fixed-effect model was used to pool the total blood loss data, since the heterogeneity across the four studies was insignificant. The pooled data showed that oral administration did not increase total blood loss (SMD = – 0.00,95%CI = – 0.20–0.20, P = 1.00) than intravenous administration therapy (Fig. 4).

Pooled analysis of transfusion rate between oral administration and intravenous administration

The pooling transfusion rate data did not achieve advantage in the oral administration (OR = 0.77,95%CI = 0.54–1.10, P = 0.14). In other words, oral administration compared to intravenous administration did not increase the rate of transfusion (Fig. 5).

Pooled analysis of DVT rate between oral administration and intravenous administration

The pooled data showed that oral administration did not increase the rate of DVT (OR = 0.58,95%CI = 0.19–1.75, P = 0.33) than intravenous administration (Fig. 6).

Pooled analysis of length of hospital stay between oral administration and intravenous administration

The pooling analysis revealed that there was no difference in length of hospital stay between oral administration and intravenous administration (SMD = – 0.05,95%CI = – 0.28–0.17, P = 0.63) (Fig. 7).

Discussion

Tranexamic acid has become a widely used to decrease blood loss and transfusion rates following THA and TKA, mainly administrated in the IV in previous studies [8, 24–26]. Compared with intravenous TXA, oral TXA is convenient to administer, reaches cost-benefit advantage, and increases the safety [11, 19]. However, limited research has been done on the use of oral TXA in total joint arthroplasty, and the optimal regimen for TXA has remained uncertain, which have been extensively explored in recent RCTs [27–29].

Study or Subgroup	Experimental Mean	Experimental SD	Experimental Total	Control Mean	Control SD	Control Total	Weight	Std. Mean Difference IV, Fixed, 95% CI
Fillingham, 2016	1.281	265	34	1.231	353	37	18.0%	0.00 [-0.47, 0.47]
Kayupovt, 2017	1.339	375	40	1.301	424	43	21.1%	0.00 [-0.43, 0.43]
Luo, 2017	1.004	415	60	1.032	350	60	30.5%	-0.00 [-0.36, 0.36]
Wang, 2018	1.004	414	60	1.108	392	60	30.5%	-0.00 [-0.36, 0.36]
Total (95% CI)			**194**			**200**	**100.0%**	**-0.00 [-0.20, 0.20]**

Heterogeneity: Chi² = 0.00, df = 3 (P = 1.00); I² = 0%
Test for overall effect: Z = 0.00 (P = 1.00)

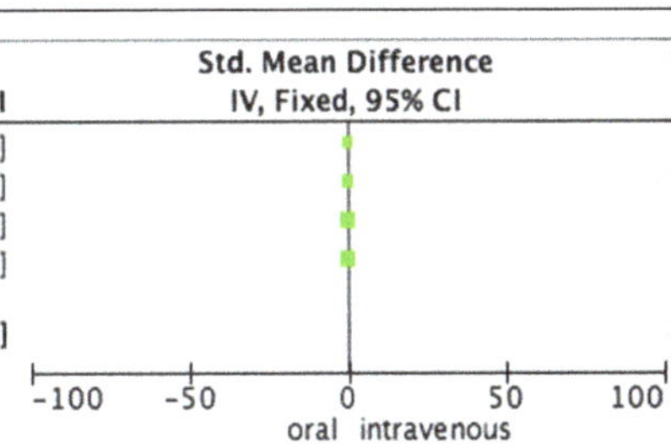

Fig. 4 Pooled analysis of total blood loss between oral administration and intravenous administration

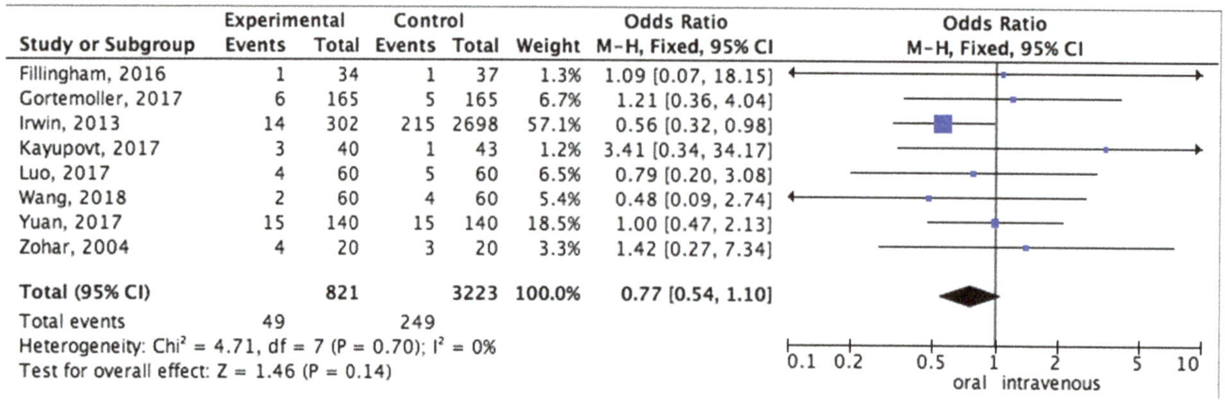

Fig. 5 Pooled analysis of transfusion rate between oral administration and intravenous administration

Our meta-analysis aims to assess the effects of intravenous or topical routes of administration.

The results of this study suggested that no significant differences were found in blood-sparing management between oral and IV TXA. This finding is comparable to the findings of a recent meta-analysis that shown that oral TXA provided equivalent blood-sparing efficacy when compared with intravenous routes [23].

The Hb drop accounted for > 60% of total blood loss in total joint arthroplasty [30, 31]. Due to the blood loss may leading to postoperative hypoxemia, the blood transfusion is required. However, blood transfusion is associated with adverse effects and increases the risk of complications resulting from hypervolemia [32–34]. Hence, rational and effective method for minimizing perioperative blood loss is needed. Previous studies have reported that IV-TXA has beneficial effects on blood-sparing, which has been widely used in patients undergoing both TKA and THA. However, IV administration of TXA has increased the risk of anaphylactic reaction [35]. Moreover, specific equipment is required for IV administration of TXA, which prolong the surgery time.

Recently, some RCTs have demonstrated that oral TXA administration was non-inferior to IV administration in the prevention of perioperative blood loss [11, 18, 19]. Kayupov et al. [18] found that no difference in the reduction of Hb was seen between two groups. Coincidentally, both Yuan et al. [19] and Fillingham et al. [11] have reported the same result. Moreover, these authors further reported that oral TXA meet similar with the IV TXA in terms of the total Hb loss following TKA and THA. Our meta-analysis was consistent with these results.

In terms of the transfusion rate, a RCT carried out by Kayupov et al. [18] found no significant difference between the two routes of administration following THA. Yuan et al. [19] compared the transfusion rate between oral administration and IV administration in patients who received TKA, and this difference was not statistically significantly different. This result was consistent with our findings.

DVT is a common postoperative complication, which may promote the risk of death in TKA and THA [36]. TXA has been reported to be associated with a potential higher risk of thrombotic complication, which might be due to the tendency of DVT, and plays as anti-fibrinolytic agent to promote the risk of clotting. The intravenous administration might be more likely to cause thrombus due to the higher TXA level of blood concentration. Our study found that the two routes of administration of TXA were similar in terms of the risk of DVT.

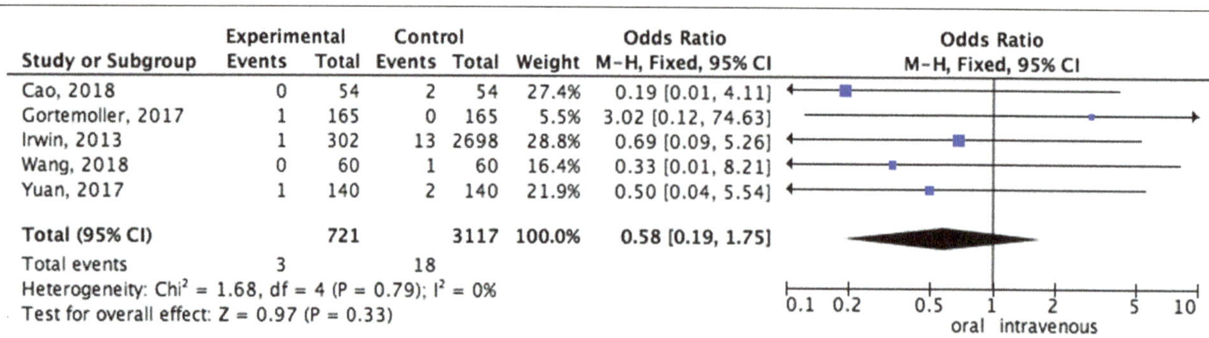

Fig. 6 Pooled analysis of DVT rate between oral administration and intravenous administration

Study or Subgroup	Experimental Mean	SD	Total	Control Mean	SD	Total	Weight	Std. Mean Difference IV, Fixed, 95% CI
Fillingham, 2016	3	1	34	3	1	37	22.8%	0.00 [−0.47, 0.47]
Kayupovt, 2017	2	1	40	2	1	40	25.8%	0.00 [−0.44, 0.44]
Luo, 2017	3.43	0.95	60	3.58	1.17	60	38.5%	−0.14 [−0.50, 0.22]
Zohar, 2004	8	2	20	8	2	20	12.9%	0.00 [−0.62, 0.62]
Total (95% CI)			**154**			**157**	**100.0%**	**−0.05 [−0.28, 0.17]**

Heterogeneity: $Chi^2 = 0.36$, df = 3 ($P = 0.95$); $I^2 = 0\%$
Test for overall effect: $Z = 0.47$ ($P = 0.63$)

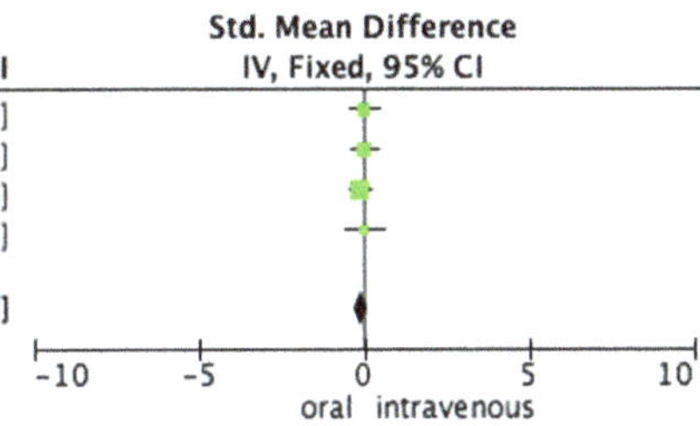

Fig. 7 Pooled analysis of length of hospital stay between oral administration and intravenous administration

Admittedly, there were a few limitations in the current study that should not be ignored. First, the main strength of this article is the use of a well-maintained and updated database. Nevertheless, due to all included studies' retrospective nature, bias still exist, and this may impact the comparison of clinical outcomes. Second, several potential variations, such as hemodilution, dosing strategies and timing of oral TXA, may affect estimated blood loss [20]. However, these variations provided insufficient data. Thus, there was no strong statistical evidence to analyze. Thirdly, the cost is another important evidence to help to inform decision-making when choosing the standard treatment option of TXA. The therapeutic attempts are justifiable if the better efficacy as well as cost savings can be achieved.

Conclusion

Oral TA was non-inferior to IV TA for blood-sparing efficacy without increasing the risk of thromboembolic diseases in THA and TKA. The efficiency, safety, and cost are considered to be crucial parameters during the decision-making of TXA routes, whether oral TXA can stands as an optimal administration of reducing blood loss following the THA and TKA compared with the IV and other forms still remains a matter of debate in future.

Acknowledgements
None.

Funding
This study was supported by Nature Science Foundation of Hubei Province (No. 2018CFB353).

Authors' contributions
XH and ML have made substantial contributions to conception and design of the study; GG, NH and ML searched literature, extracted data from the collected literature and analyzed the data; XH wrote the manuscript; ML revised the manuscript; All authors approved the final version of the manuscript.

Consent for publication
Not applicable.

Competing interests
The authors declare that they have no competing interests.

Author details
[1]Department of Orthopedics, Jinan Zhangqiu District Hospital of Traditional Chinese Medicine, No. 1463 Xiushui Street,Mingshui subdistrict office, Zhangqiu district, Jinan 250200, Shandong, China. [2]Clinical Laboratory, Jinan Zhangqiu District Hospital of Traditional Chinese Medicine, No. 1463 Xiushui Street,Mingshui subdistrict office, Zhangqiu district, Jinan 250200, Shandong, China. [3]Department of Intensive Care Unit, Wuhan No.1 Hospital, No.215 Zhongshan Ave, Wuhan 430022, Hubei, China.

References

1. Singh JA. Epidemiology of knee and hip arthroplasty: a systematic review. Open Orthop J. 2011;5(1):80–5.
2. Kirksey M, Chiu YL, Ma Y, et al. Trends in in-hospital major morbidity and mortality after total joint arthroplasty: United States 1998-2008. Anesth Analg. 2012;115(2):321–7.
3. Ponnusamy KE, Kim TJ, Khanuja HS. Perioperative Blood Transfusions in Orthopaedic Surgery. J Bone Joint Surg Am Vol. 2014;96(21):1836.
4. Carson JL, Duff A, Poses RM, et al. Effect of anaemia and cardiovascular disease on surgical mortality and morbidity. Lancet. 1996;348(9034):1055–60.
5. Okamoto S, Hijikataokunomiya A, Wanaka K, et al. Enzyme-controlling medicines: introduction. Semin Thromb Hemost. 1997;23(06):493–501.
6. Irisson E, Hémon Y, Pauly V, et al. Tranexamic acid reduces blood loss and financial cost in primary total hip and knee replacement surgery. Orthop Traumatol Surg Res Otsr. 2012;98(5):477–83.
7. Diblasi JF, Smith RP, Garavaglia J, et al. Comparing cost, efficacy, and safety of intravenous and topical tranexamic acid in Total hip and knee arthroplasty. Am J Orthop. 2016;45(7):E439–43.
8. Yue C, Kang P, Yang P, et al. Topical application of tranexamic acid in primary total hip arthroplasty: a randomized double-blind controlled trial. J Arthroplasty. 2014;29(12):2452–6.
9. Chen JY, Chin PL, Moo IH, et al. Intravenous versus intra-articular tranexamic acid in total knee arthroplasty: a double-blinded randomised controlled noninferiority trial. Knee. 2016;23(1):152–6.
10. Lin ZX, Woolf SK. Safety, efficacy, and cost-effectiveness of tranexamic acid in orthopedic surgery. Orthopedics. 2016;39(2):119–30.
11. Fillingham YA, Kayupov E, Plummer DR, et al. The James a. Rand young Investigator's award: a randomized controlled trial of Oral and intravenous tranexamic acid in Total knee arthroplasty: the same efficacy at lower cost? J Arthroplasty. 2016;31(9):26–30.
12. Kim JL, Park JH, Han SB, et al. Allogeneic blood transfusion is a significant risk factor for surgical-site infection following Total hip and knee arthroplasty: a meta-analysis. J Arthroplasty. 2017;32(1):320.
13. Chen Y, Chen Z, Cui S, et al. Topical versus systemic tranexamic acid after total knee and hip arthroplasty:a meta-analysis of randomized controlled trials. Medicine. 2016;95(41):e4656.
14. Higgins JPT, Thompson SG. Quantifying heterogeneity in a meta-analysis. Stat Med. 2002;21:1539–58.
15. Higgins JPT, Thompson SG, Deeks JJ, Altman DG. Measuring inconsistency in meta-analyses. BMJ. 2003;327:557.
16. Zohar E, Ellis M, Ifrach N, et al. The postoperative blood-sparing efficacy of oral versus intravenous tranexamic acid after total knee replacement. Anesth Analg. 2004;99(6):1679.
17. Irwin A, Khan SK, Jameson SS, et al. Oral versus intravenous tranexamic acid in enhanced-recovery primary total hip and knee replacement: results of 3000 procedures. Bone Joint J. 2013;95-B(11):1556–61.

18. Kayupov E, Fillingham YA, Okroj K, et al. Oral and intravenous tranexamic acid are equivalent at reducing blood loss following Total hip arthroplasty: a randomized controlled trial. J Bone Joint Surg Am Vol. 2017;99(5):373–8.
19. Yuan X, Li B, Wang Q, et al. Comparison of 3 Routes of Administration of Tranexamic Acid on Primary Unilateral Total Knee Arthroplasty: A Prospective, Randomized, Controlled Study. J Arthroplasty. 2017;32(9):2738–43.
20. Cao G, Huang Z, Xie J, et al. The effect of oral versus intravenous tranexamic acid in reducing blood loss after primary total hip arthroplasty: a randomized clinical trial. Thromb Res. 2018;164:48.
21. Gortemoller MA, Allen B, Forsyth R, et al. Comparison of Oral and intravenous tranexamic acid for prevention of perioperative blood loss in Total knee and Total hip arthroplasty. Ann Pharmacother. 2018;52(3):246–50.
22. Luo ZY, Wang HY, Wang D, et al. Oral vs Intravenous vs Topical Tranexamic Acid in Primary Hip Arthroplasty: A Prospective, Randomized, Double-Blind, Controlled Study. J Arthroplasty. 2017;33(3):786–93.
23. Wang D, Wang HY, Cao C, et al. Tranexamic acid in primary total knee arthroplasty without tourniquet: a randomized, controlled trial of oral versus intravenous versus topical administration. Sci Rep. 2018;8(1):13579.
24. Imai N, Dohmae Y, Suda K, et al. Tranexamic acid for reduction of blood loss during total hip arthroplasty. J Arthroplasty. 2012;27(10):1838–43.
25. Malhotra R, Kumar V, Garg B. The use of tranexamic acid to reduce blood loss in primary cementless total hip arthroplasty. Eur J Orthop Surg Traumatol. 2011;21(2):101–4.
26. Alshryda S, Mason J, Vaghela M, et al. Topical (intra-articular) tranexamic acid reduces blood loss and transfusion rates following total knee replacement: a randomized controlled trial (TRANX-K). J Bone Joint Surg Am Vol. 2013;95(21):1961–8.
27. Wang J, Wang Q, Zhang X, et al. Intra-articular Application is More Effective Than Intravenous Application of Tranexamic Acid in Total Knee Arthroplasty: A Prospective Randomized Controlled Trial. J Arthroplasty. 2017;32(11):3385–9.
28. Sun Q, Yu X, Wu J, et al. Efficacy of a Single Dose and an Additional Dose of Tranexamic Acid in Reduction of Blood Loss in Total Knee Arthroplasty. J Arthroplasty. 2016;32(7):2108–12.
29. Sun Q, Yu X, Nie X, et al. The efficacy comparison of tranexamic acid for reducing blood loss in Total knee arthroplasty at different dosage time. J Arthroplasty. 2016;32(1):33–6.
30. Liu X, Zhang X, Chen Y, et al. Hidden blood loss after total hip arthroplasty. J Arthroplasty. 2011;26(7):1100–1105.e1.
31. Ervens J, Marks C, Hechler M, et al. Effect of induced hypotensive anaesthesia vs isovolaemic haemodilution on blood loss and transfusion requirements in orthognathic surgery: a prospective, single-blinded, randomized, controlled clinical study. Int J Oral Maxillofac Surg. 2010;39(12):1168–74.
32. Lasocki S, Krauspe R, Von HC, et al. PREPARE: the prevalence of perioperative anaemia and need for patient blood management in elective orthopaedic surgery: a multicentre, observational study. Eur J Anaesthesiol. 2015;32(3):160.
33. Spahn DR, Casutt M. Eliminating blood transfusions: new aspects and perspectives. Anesthesiology. 2000;93(1):242–55.
34. Padhi S, Bullock I, Li L, Stroud M, National Institute for H, Care Excellence Guideline Development G. Intravenous fluid therapy for adults in hospital: summary of NICE guidance. BMJ. 2013;347:f7073.
35. Lucaspolomeni MM, Delaval Y, Menestret P, et al. A case of anaphylactic shock with tranexamique acid (Exacyl). Annales Francaises Danesthesie Et De Reanimation. 2004;23(6):607.
36. Wang C, Han Z, Zhang T, et al. The efficacy of a thrombin-based hemostatic agent in primary total knee arthroplasty: a meta-analysis. J Orthop Surg Res. 2014;9(1):90.

20

Growth of epiphysis after epiphyseal-preservation surgery for childhood osteosarcoma around the knee joint

Akihiko Takeuchi*, Norio Yamamoto, Katsuhiro Hayashi, Hidenori Matsubara, Hiroaki Kimura, Shinji Miwa, Takashi Higuchi, Kensaku Abe, Yuta Taniguchi and Hiroyuki Tsuchiya

Abstract

Background: Epiphyseal-preservation surgery for osteosarcoma is an alternative method which has been indicated carefully to selected patients. The tumor-devitalised autograft treated with liquid nitrogen procedure is one of the biological reconstruction method to reconstruct the defect after tumor excision. The limb length discrepancy is usually appeared in children with their growth after limb-sparing surgery. This study was aimed to investigated the growth of residual epiphysis following epiphyseal-preservation surgery for childhood osteosarcoma around the knee joint.

Methods: We retrospectively reviewed 12 patients with osteosarcoma who underwent epiphysis preserving tumor excision (8 in distal femur and 4 in proximal tibia) and reconstructed by using tumor-devitalized autograft treated with liquid nitrogen. The mean patient age was 11 (range, 6 to 14) years. The mean follow-up period were 63 (range, 41 to 90) months. Epiphysis transverse growth rate, epiphysis-width discrepancy (EWD) and collapse of epiphysis were evaluated by using pre- and post-operative whole standing leg radiographs. A retrospective chart review was performed to investigate functional outcome, complications and oncological status.

Results: The mean growth of epiphysis rate was 12.6% (range, 3.3 to 28.0%) of affected side and 12.7% (range, 3.8 to 28.9%) of contralateral side, mean EWD was 0.1 mm (range, − 1.0 to 1.7 mm), mean LLD was + 26.1 mm (range, + 1 to + 48 mm) and two patients with distal femoral reconstruction underwent limb lengthening of tibia. There was no collapse of the residual epiphysis. The mean MSTS score was 27.7 (range, 18 to 30).

Conclusions: Epiphysis transverse growth was not diminished, and there was absence of epiphyseal collapse even after epiphyseal-preservation surgery in this small series of childhood osteosarcoma around the knee. With careful assessment for epiphyseal tumor involvement, epiphyseal-preservation surgery shall be possible, and could be an alternative method worth considering.

Keywords: Pediatric osteosarcoma, Epiphysis growth, Epiphyseal-preservation surgery

Background

The advances in imaging modalities, multi-agent chemotherapy and surgical procedures have made limb-sparing surgery more common in the treatment of osteosarcoma, which is the most common malignant bone tumor [1]. However, osteosarcoma usually occurs in metaphyseal locations and must be excised with the adjacent joint and replaced by an endoprosthesis. Moreover, treatment of skeletally immature children should consider any growth-related complications following tumor surgery. Limb-length discrepancy is a major complication [2], and extendable endoprostheses [3] or distraction osteogenesis [4] have been applied to address this problem.

Recently, the advanced imaging [5], accurate tumor excision [6] and rigid fixation using a locking plate [7] have made it possible to perform the epiphyseal-preservation surgery for selected patients who responded to chemotherapy without tumor

* Correspondence: a_take@med.kanazawa-u.ac.jp
Department of Orthopaedic Surgery, Kanazawa University Graduate School of Medical Sciences, 13-1 Takara-machi, Kanazawa 920-8641, Japan

extension to the epiphysis [8]. This procedure is expected to preserve excellent limb function. To reconstruct the defect after tumor excision, various methods, including allograft [8], distraction osteogenesis [9], tumor-devitalised autograft [10], vascularised fibular graft [11] and custom-made implants [6], have been applied. Tumor-devitalised autograft treated with liquid nitrogen procedure was introduced in 1999 [10] and its usefulness has since been reported [12]. The advantages of frozen autografts include simplicity and the possibility of preserving proteins, including bone morphogenetic protein (BMP) [13]. However, the growth of residual epiphysis in children after epiphyseal-preservation surgery has not been fully studied. The purpose of this study was to investigate the growth of residual epiphysis, limb function, complications and oncological status after epiphyseal-preservation surgery for childhood osteosarcoma around the knee.

Methods

After the approval of our institutional review board, the authors retrospectively reviewed consecutive cases of osteosarcoma in our hospital treated with epiphysis preserving tumor excision and reconstion by using the tumor-devitalised autograft treated with liquid nitrogen procedure at our hospital between 2009 and 2013. All patients received neoadjuvant chemotherapy following our base protocol of five pre-operative courses of intra-arterial or intra-venous cisplatin (120 mg/m^2) and doxorubicin (30 mg/m^2/day × 2 days) [14]. The indications for this procedure were: 1) good radiological responses to neoadjuvant chemotherapy without extend to the physis, described as findings of sclerotic changes or good margination of the tumor observed on plain radiographs, marked shrinkage of tumors extending into soft tissue on MR images, or the disappearance of abnormal accumulation on TI 201 scintigrams [15]; 2) a thickness of their residual epiphysis > 1 cm; 3) a surgical margin of ≥10 mm. When tumor was located within 2 cm of the physis, the osteotomy line was transepiphyseal or passed through the physis, resulted in complete or partial ablation of the physis [16], and 4) either the absence of (Enneking stages IIA and IIB), or a resectable lung metastasis (Enneking stage III) [17]. The inclusion criteria of the present study was patients < 15 years old with open epiphyseal plate, follow-up of > 24 months and who had a tumor located in the distal femur or the proximal tibia. The patients with a diaphyseal osteosarcoma for which the distance of the osteotomy to the epiphyseal plate was < 1 cm were also included. The tumor excision was classified into three types: transmetaphyseal excision (epiphyseal plate preserved), transphyseal excision (epiphyseal plate partially sacrificed) and transepiphyseal excision (epiphyseal plate totally sacrificed) (Fig. 1). Transphyseal and transepiphyseal excision were indicated for tumors that did not extend to the epiphysis [16], as determined by magnetic resonance imaging (MRI) T1-weighted and short tau inversion recovery (STIR) images [5].

Surgical procedure

Two different techniques of tumor-devitalised autograft treated with liquid nitrogen—free freezing [10] and pedicle freezing [18]—were used depending on the location of the tumor.

Free freezing technique

A K-wire was inserted into the osteotomy line under fluoroscopy. The tumor was then excised en bloc using a microsurgical saw along the K-wire. The specimen's soft

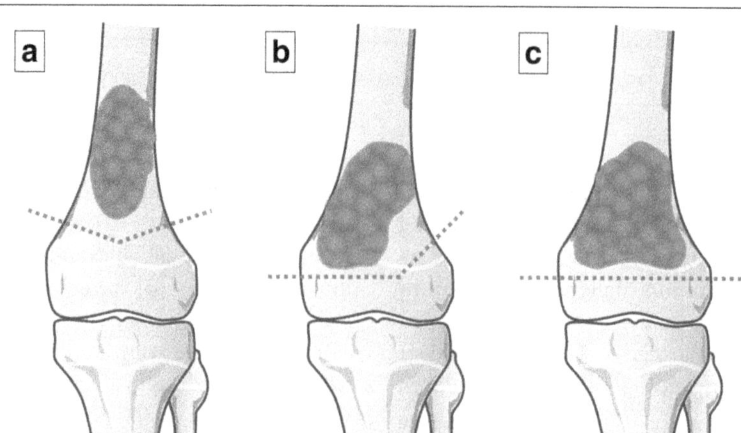

Fig. 1 Diagram showing the classification of tumor excision to preserve the epiphysis. Transmetaphyseal excision (epiphyseal plate preserved) (**a**), transphyseal excision (epiphyseal plate partially sacrificed) (**b**) and transepiphyseal excision (epiphyseal plate totally sacrificed) (**c**). The dotted line indicates the osteotomy line

tissues were removed, and the tumor curetted before freezing. The excised portion was frozen in liquid nitrogen that was stored in sterilized flask right before freezing for 20 min, thawed at room temperature for 15 min, then in distilled water for another 15 min. The frozen autograft was then fixed to the residual limb with double or triple locking plates, and the epiphysis stabilized with two or three screws applied either through the plate or separately (Fig. 2a). For cases of proximal tibial osteosarcoma, the patella tendon was reattached to the frozen autograft by using a screw and spike washer.

Pedicle freezing technique

After the osteotomy of the proximal side of the tumor with adequate surgical margin, the surrounding soft tissues were carefully protected by using surgical sheets and the proximal part of tumor was elevated with isolation by using cotton for cast padding, an Esmarch bandage, and three-layer surgical sheets to prevent tumor contamination and damages to the normal tissue during freezing. The intramedullary canal is subsequently curetted to remove the bone marrow and contents of the tumor in order to prevent a graft-related fracture due to water expansion during freezing. The isolated bony specimen, still in continuity with the distal residual limb, was then carefully rotated and put in a container filled with liquid nitrogen for 20 min. After thawing, reconstruction was performed similarly as for the free freezing technique (Fig. 2b).

The length of resection for free freezing, or of the treated bone for pedicle freezing, was recorded as the length of graft. Additional chemotherapy was administered during the postoperative period. Passive range of motion (ROM) therapy was initiated after the early postoperative period, and active ROM therapy was initiated at 6 weeks postoperatively when the muscle or tendon had to be reattached. The authors encouraged full weight-bearing mobilization after evidence of union. The follow-up protocol consisted of whole standing leg radiographs after 1.5, 3, 6, 9, 12, 16, 20 and 24 months and then every 6 months up to 5 years. Yearly examination was performed up to 10 years thereafter. Graft union was confirmed when the osteotomy line had disappeared in both anteroposterior (AP) and lateral views on

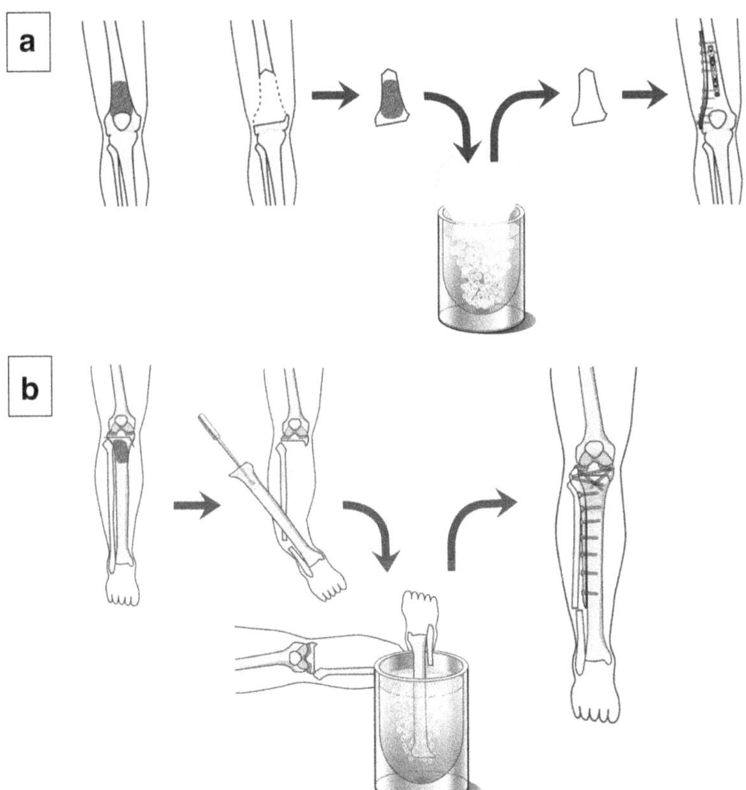

Fig. 2 Schema of surgical procedure of tumor-devitalised autograft treated with liquid nitrogen. Free freezing: Tumor of the distal femur is excised by epiphysis-preserved intercalary osteotomy. After freezing in liquid nitrogen for 20 min, osteosynthesis using plates, screws is performed (**a**). Pedicle freezing: Tumor of the proximal tibia is excised by one- site osteotomy, proximal part of tumor is elevated and the intramedullary canal which contains the tumor, is subsequently curetted. The isolated bony specimen is carefully rotated and put in a liquid nitrogen for 20 min. Osteosynthesis using plate, screws is performed (**b**)

radiography or computed tomography. When it was difficult to evaluate bone union because of the implant shadow, confirmation was achieved by using only one view (either AP or lateral) or computed tomographic scan. Graft union was not evaluated for cases of pedicle freezing for distal femoral tumors because the osteotomy line was only on the proximal side.

The width of the epiphysis of the distal femur was measured with reference to the method of Souryal TO et al. [19]. The distance between the intersection of a line parallel to the joint surface and passing through the medial and lateral cortex at the level of the intercondylar fossa was measured by using whole standing leg radiographs with a 1-mm precision scale. The width of the epiphysis of the proximal tibia was measured from a line perpendicular to the tibial anatomical axis that passed through the medial edge of the medial condyle. At the time of surgery, a locking plate was placed at the lateral side hence the lateral end of the lateral condyle was difficult to detect. So, the distance between the medial end of the medial condyle and the cross point to the mechanical axis was measured on the proximal tibia (Fig. 3). Epiphysis-width discrepancy (EWD) was calculated by comparing the width of the affected side and the width of the unaffected side on radiographs at the latest examination. The epiphysis growth rate was calculated by comparing the width at the latest examination with the width immediately before surgery. To analyse the collapse of the residual epiphysis, the anatomical lateral distal femoral angle (aLDFA) for the distal femoral tumors and medial proximal tibial angle (MPTA) for the proximal tibial tumors at the latest examination were compared with those after surgery (ΔaLDFA/MPTA) [20]. Limb-length discrepancy (LLD) was measured at the latest follow-up. All parameters were measured by using computer software (EV Insite Version 3.1.1.218; PSP Corporation, Tokyo, Japan), which was performed independently by two assessors (AT and TH) blinded to patient information and the assessment was duplicated. Status of the epiphyseal plate at the latest examination, the Musculoskeletal Tumor Society (MSTS) scores [21], complications and oncological statuses were also recorded.

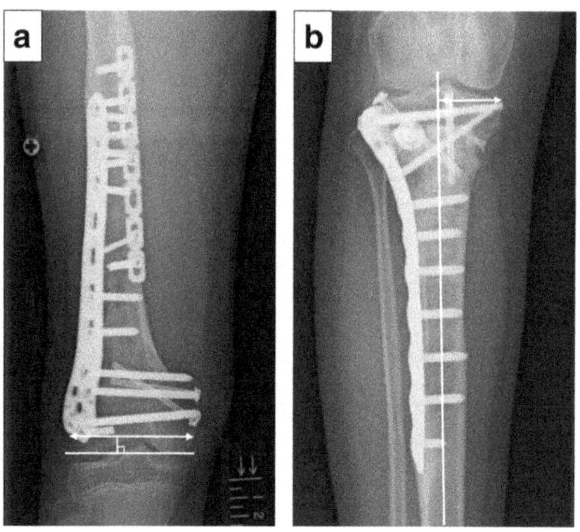

Fig. 3 The width of epiphysis was measured by using whole standing leg radiographs with a 1-mm precision scale. The distance between the intersection of the line that was placed parallel to the joint surface and passed through the medial and lateral cortex at the level of intercondylar fossa in the distal femur before surgery and at the latest examination (a 10-year-old boy with osteosarcoma of the right distal femur, 55 months after surgery) (**a**). The width of the epiphysis of the proximal tibia was measured by a line that was perpendicular to the tibial anatomical axis and passes through the medial edge of the medial condyle. The distance between the ends of the medial and the cross point to the mechanical axis was measured on the proximal tibia before surgery and at the latest examination (an 11-year-old girl with osteosarcoma of the right proximal tibia, 42 months after surgery) (**b**)

Results

Epiphyseal preservation surgery was performed in 18 patients. Six patients were excluded; five were older than 15 years and the other one patient was excluded because the frozen autograft was retrieved at 6 months after surgery due to the deep infection. Twelve patients met our inclusion criteria. The demographics and results are shown in Table 1. The mean patient age was 11 years (range, 6 to 14 years). The mean follow-up period was 61 months (range, 32 to 90 months). Eight tumors were located in the distal femur, and four were in the proximal tibia. Among the 12 patients, 11 (91.7%) were Enneking stage IIB and 1 (8.3%) was Enneking stage III with resectable lung metastases at the time of diagnosis.

Five (41.7%) patients underwent reconstruction using the pedicle-freezing technique, with 2 for distal femoral tumors and 3 for proximal tibial tumors (Fig. 4). A vascularised fibular graft was used in one patient, while two patients underwent cancellous allograft over the osteotomy site. Tumor excision was transmetaphyseal for 3 distal femoral cases, transphyseal for 3 distal femoral cases and 1 proximal tibial cases, and transepiphyseal for 2 distal femoral and 3 proximal tibial cases. The mean length of tumor-devitalised autograft treated with liquid nitrogen was 14.4 cm (range, 8 to 29 cm), and the mean graft union time was 9 months (range, 3 to 35 months). The mean epiphysis growth was 12.6% (range, 3.3 to 28.0%) of affected side and 12.7% (range, 3.8 to 28.9%) of contralateral side, and EWD was 0.1 mm (range, − 1.0 to 1.7 mm). The mean ΔaLDFA/MPTA was 0.6° (range, − 2.4 to 4.0°). These results indicated that the epiphysis transverse growth was preserved without residual epiphyseal collapse, and the preservation or sacrifice of the epiphyseal plate did not influence the epiphysis

Table 1 Dempgrapic data and outcomes

Patient No. /Sex /Age, y	Site	Enneking stage	Type of tumor excision	Freezing method	Graft length, cm	Bone graft	Union time, mo	Epiphysis growth, %		EWD	LLD, mm	Δ aLDFA /MPTA	Epiphyseal plate at laltest examination	MSTS score	Complications /Treatment (mos)	Follow-up, mo	Oncological Outcome
								Affected side	Cotralateral side								
1/F/8	DF	IIB	Trans-metaphyseal	Pedicule	25	VFG	NA	12	13	3	43	4	close	18	Fracture/ORIF (9)	90	CDF
2/F/13	DF	III	Trans-metaphyseal	Pedicule	29	no	NA	3	4	1	18	−2	close	30	Fracture/ ORIF (21)	76	CDF
3/M/11	DF	IIB	Trans-epiphyseal	Free	14	no	35	18	18	−2	38	1	open	30	LLD/ Lenghning (54)	68	CDF
4/M/10	DF	IIB	Trans-physeal	Free	10	no	7	28	29	0	48	−1	open	30	LLD/ Lenghning (53)	64	CDF
5/F/6	DF	IIB	Trans-metaphyseal	Free	17	no	4	22	21	0	42	−1	open	30		48	CDF
6/F/14	DF	IIB	Trans-physeal	Free	8	cancellous allograft	6	7	7	0	1	2	close	27		51	CDF
7/F/9	DF	IIB	Trans-epiphyseal	Free	14	no	3	8	8	1	34	3	open	27	Fracture/ ORIF (35)	48	CDF
8/M/13	DF	IIB	Trans-physeal	Free	14	no	10	4	4	0	24	0	close	27	LR/endoprosthesis replacement (20)	42	NED
9/F/11	PT	IIB	Trans-physeal	Free	8	cancellous allograft	4	13	15	1	17	4	close	30	Infection/ irrigation (44), Fracture/ Cast (68)	90	CDF
10/F/12	PT	IIB	Trans-epiphyseal	Pedicule	11	no	7	9	8	0	6	−1	close	30		90	CDF
11/F/11	PT	IIB	Trans-epiphyseal	Pedicule	8	no	6	6	6	−2	33	−1	open	30		51	CDF
12/F/10	PT	IIB	Trans-epiphyseal	Pedicule	12	no	5	22	20	0	9	0	open	30		41	CDF

Abbreviations: *DF* distal femur, *PT* proximal tibia, *VFG* vascularized fibular graft, *NA* not applicable, *EWD* Epiphysys width discrepancy, *aLDFA* anatomical lateral distal femoral angle, *MPTA* medial proximal Tibial angle, *MSTS* musculoskeletal tumor society, *ORIF* open reduction and internal fixation, *LLD* limb length discrepancy, *LR* local recurrence, *CDF* Continous disease free, *NED* no evidence of disease

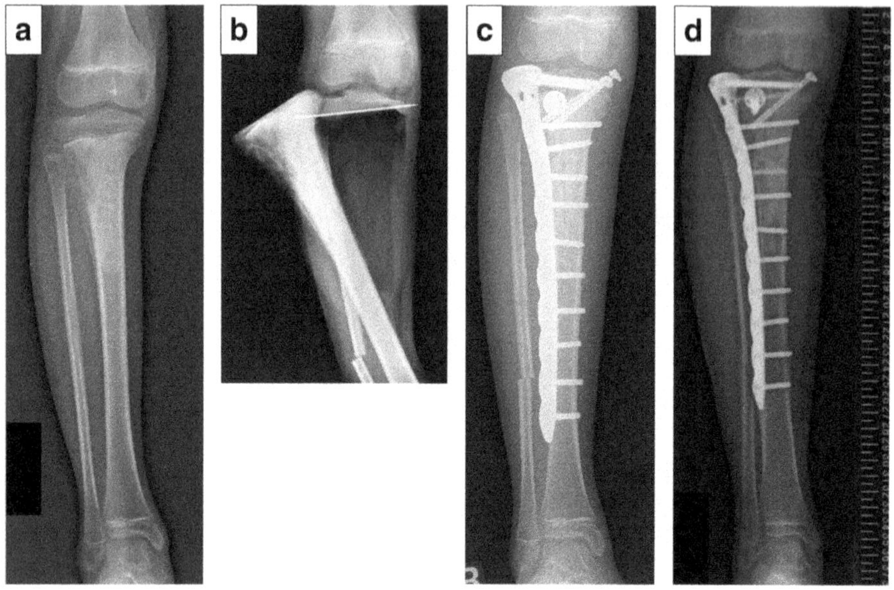

Fig. 4 Patient No. 13. A 10-year old girl with osteosarcoma of the right proximal tibia. Preoperative plain radiograph (epiphysis width: 28.3 mm) (**a**). A radiograph after transepiphyseal excision without osteotomy of the distal tibia for the pedicle freezing. A 1.6-mm Kirschner wire was inserted as a guide, positioned under fluoroscopy. Osteotomy of the distal fibula was performed to expose the proximal part of the tibia (**b**). A radiograph after the reconstruction using a tumor-bearing frozen autograft stabilized with locking plate (aLDFA: 87°) (**c**). Whole-leg radiograph after 37 months (aLDFA: 86°, epiphysis width: 33.9 mm) (**d**)

transverse growth. The mean limb shortening was 26 mm (range, 1 to 48 mm).

Complications that needed additional surgery were observed in 8 (61.5%) patients, that included one deep infection at 6 months after surgery requiring removal of the frozen autograft, and three (25%) fractures. Two of the fracture complications followed pedicle-freezing (Patient No. 1 and 2), and these occurred at the border between the frozen and host bone. One fracture occurred in the frozen bone and was accompanied by plate breakage (Patient No. 7). All three fractures were treated with open reduction and internal fixation combined with allograft or iliac autograft. One local recurrence (8.3%) developed in the surrounding soft tissue in a patient with pathological fracture at the initial presentation, and was treated with re-wide excision including the frozen autograft and reconstruction using an endoprosthesis (Patient No. 8). One superficial infection (8.3%) was managed by irrigation and administration of antibiotics (Patient No. 9). Limb shortening (> 3 cm) was observed in six patients, and two patients (16.7%) (distal femur, 38 mm and 48 mm) underwent limb lengthening of their tibia with three-dimensional external fixation (Taylor Spatial Frame, *Smith and Nephew*, Memphis, USA) (Patient No. 3 and 4). Four cases were managed with shoe lifts. One patient with diaphyseal osteosarcoma underwent initial stabilization of the epiphysis. The screws were removed from the epiphysis after 1.5 years, with subsequent longitudinal growth of epiphysis was observed (Patient No. 5, Fig. 5). The mean MSTS score was 28 (range, 18 to 30). Oncological outcomes were continuous disease free (CDF) in 11 patients and no evidence of disease (NED) in 1 patient at 41 to 90 months follow-up (mean 63 months).

Discussion

In the present study, we found that the transverse growth of the residual epiphysis was observed with almost same rate with contralateral side (12.6% of affected side and 12.7% of contralateral side), and no apparent discrepancy in epiphysis widths was detected even though the epiphyseal plate was totally sacrificed.

Epiphyseal-preservation surgery for metaphyseal osteosarcoma has been reported by several authors, making use of allograft [8], distraction osteogenesis [9], tumor-devitalised autograft [10], vascularised fibular graft [11], and custom-made implants [6] for reconstruction. Muscolo L et al. reported the thirteen cases with a high-grade metaphyseal osteosarcoma of the knee who had been treated with a transepiphyseal resection (partial epiphyseal preservation) and reconstructed with allograft. One patient died of bone and pulmonary metastases with no evidence of local recurrence, while one patient had a soft tissue recurrence with no recurrence in the residual epiphysis [22]. Their group (Aponte-Tinao L et al.) later reported a large series (35 cases) of osteosarcoma of the knee treated with epiphyseal preservation and allograft reconstruction. The mean MSTS score was 26 at final follow up, and no recurrence in residual epiphyses were described. However, a second surgical procedure was performed in 19 patients (54.3%), three to treat oncologic complications (three local recurrences) and 16 to treat orthopaedic complications, including 11 fractures, three diaphyseal nonunions, and two deep infections. The epiphysis was eventually removed in 5 patients (14.3%) because of fracture (3 patients), amputation (1 patient) or infection (1e patient). Their study included 12 paediatric patients (< 15 years old); however, nothing was mentioned about the growth of the residual epiphysis [8]. In another study, Henderson ER et al. reported thirty-eight patients who were performed lower-limb preservation with an expandable endoprosthesis after bone tumor resection including replacement of distal femur in twenty-five and proximal tibia in five patients. Limb length discrepancy was managed by the lengthening of prosthesis (mean, 4.5 cm) and the mean limb-length discrepancy was 0.7 cm at the latest examination. However, sixteen patients (42%) experienced one or more complications: superficial infection without sequelae in five, soft-tissue failures in four, aseptic loosening in four, structural failure in two and failure due to infection in three cases at a mean of twenty-eight months. Ten patients (26%) required prosthesis revision, and two patients required amputation. The mean MSTS score was 26.4 in distal femoral and 26.7 in proximal tibial replacement [23]. Complications in the present study was occurred in eight of thirteen patients (61.5%), however two limb-shortening which needed the additional lengthening was inevitable. Therefore, the authors considered that the incidence of remaining 6 complications (46.2%) including 3 fractures, 1 soft tissue recurrence, 1 superficial infection and 1 deep infection were comparable with those of allograft (54.3%) and expandable prosthesis (42%). Limb reconstruction using tumor-devitalised autograft treated with liquid nitrogen procedure was introduced in 1999 [10], with advantages reported as follows: simplicity, low cost, preservation of osteoinductive [24] and osteoconductive properties, perfect fit between graft and host bone, sufficient biomechanical strength, avoidance of disease transmission, avoidance of immunological rejection, nondependent of bone bank, nondependent of special equipment and strict thermal control, easy attachment of tendons and ligaments to bone, preserving of bone morphogenetic proteins (BMP) [13]. The pedicle freezing technic has the following additional reported advantages as well: shorter operating time, maintaining of joint continuity in selected patients, decreased osteotomy sites, and a lower rate of graft healing complications. The impossibility of histological analysis of the whole specimen (tumor necrosis analysis) and complications similar to those related to allograft implantation are noted disadvantages. Moreover, because a frozen autograft is a tumor-devitalised bone, the strength of the autograft depends on the integrity of the remaining structures following cryogenic sterilization. For this reason, prerequisites for our frozen autograft methods are an osteoblastic lesion and that massive osteolytic destruction has not taken place [18]. Although Yamamoto N, et al. reported that the compression strength of frozen autograft immediately after the treatment was similar to intact bone in animal model [25], the biomechanical strength will be reduced by devitalized tissue with time.

Wong KC et al. reported eight cases of joint-preserving tumor resection in which image-guided computer navigation and reconstruction using a computer-aided design (CAD) prosthesis were performed with excellent limb function (mean MSTS score, 29). They presented a case of continuous growth of the remaining distal femur epiphysis [6]. Puhaindran ME et al. reported nine cases of paediatric osteosarcoma treated by epiphysis preserving tumor excision and reconstructed with fibula grafts supplemented by autoclaved bone grafts infused with bone marrow. They showed one case of latitudinal residual epiphysis growth following distal femur osteosarcoma excision and reconstruction [26]. The epiphysis in a child is composed of articular cartilage, epiphyseal cartilage, a secondary centre of ossification and the physis, all of which are referred to as the articular-epiphyseal cartilage complex [27]. The secondary centre of ossification is supplied by the epiphyseal artery, branches of which end in the proliferating cartilage zone [28]. The groove of Ranvier and the perichondrial ring of LaCroix, both of which support latitudinal growth of the physis, surround the latter. Although the latitudinal growth arrest after damage to the groove of Ranvier and the perichondrial ring of LaCroix caused by physeal injury has been well discussed [29], the latitudinal growth after epiphyseal-preservation surgery has not been fully clarified.

The authors stabilized the residual small epiphysis with a locking plate for preventing loosening or collapse of the epiphysis. Mei J et al. reported their successful treatment of a pediatric distal femoral osteosarcoma with epiphyseal-preservation surgery using a locking plate. They preserved the epiphyseal plate with temporary screw fixation, and removed the screw after 14 weeks. Subsequently, the distal end of the plate had moved superior to the epiphysis accompanied by bone growth [7]. In the present study, one case showed the longitudinal growth of the epiphysis following removal of the screws from the epiphysis (Fig. 5). Despite temporarily stabilization of the epiphysis across the epiphyseal plate after transmetaphyseal excision, longitudinal growth can be expected following removal of the epiphyseal screw. Limb shortening was a major problem, but two cases of distal femoral reconstruction in the present study were successfully salvaged by distraction osteogenesis of the

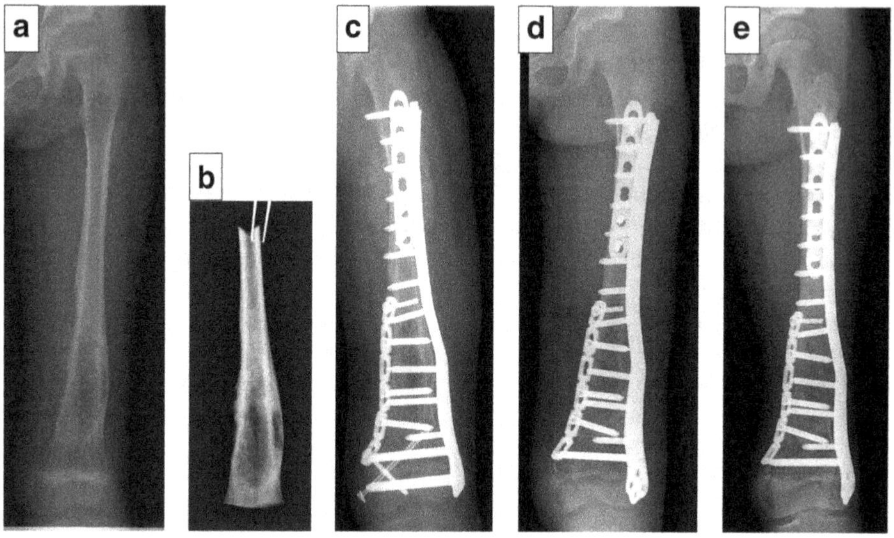

Fig. 5 Patient No. 5. A 6-year-old girl with osteosarcoma of the left distal femur (transmetaphyseal excision). Preoperative plain radiograph (epiphysis width: 53.2 mm) (**a**). A radiograph of resected tumor-bearing segment of femur after transmetaphyseal excision (**b**). A radiograph after the reconstruction using a tumor-bearing frozen autograft stabilized with triple-locking plates and a cancellous allograft (aLDFA: 80°) (**c**). A radiograph after 18 months. Screws in the epiphysis were removed (**d**). A radiograph taken 48 months. Latitudinal and longitudinal growth were observed (aLDFA: 83°, epiphysis width: 63.4 mm) (**e**)

tibia (Patients No. 3 and 4). Four cases were managed with shoe lifts. In lieu of expandable prostheses, excessive limb shortening shall require additional salvage surgery such as distraction osteogenesis. However, we believe our biological reconstruction has several benefits that help preserve excellent limb function as shown by the MSTS score.

The long-term safety of close surgical margin resection including epiphyseal preservation surgery in the treatment of osteosarcoma is yet to be clarified. The most important consideration is to evaluate tumor extension to the epiphysis accurately. Jesus-Garcia R, et al. reported the epiphyseal plate invasion was detected 44% radiologically in their study, whereas histological examination detected 84%. However, the epiphyseal involvement was evaluated by using the routine radiographs [30]. Hoffer FA et al. reported that epiphyseal extension of an osteosarcoma could be detected on MRI as a dark signal on T1 and a bright signal on STIR in MRI. [5] These findings have led to a consensus that epiphyseal-preservation surgery can be performed [11]. Before this consensus, a few studies have reported use of epiphyseal-preservation surgery, including physeal distraction, when removing the tumor [31]. Andreou D et al. reported that the close margins did not lead to increased local recurrence in their 123 of 1355 cases of osteosarcoma treated with close surgical margin resection [32]. In the present study, our method was indicated for those patients who responded to neoadjuvant chemotherapy and with no tumor extension to the epiphysis. All patients were alive within the mean follow-up period of 61 months (range, 32 to 93 months).,However one (8.3%) of 12 patients underwent removal of the residual epiphysis due to soft tissue recurrence at 20 months after the initial surgery. Careful assessment of tumor extension to the epiphysis by using MRI and more long-term analyses are mandatory to evaluate the safety of this method.

This study had some limitations. The number of patients was small; the patient age at the time of surgery, type of excision used for preservation of the epiphysis and the follow-up term varied and the follow-up periods were relatively short. The growth of residual epiphysis was evaluated by measuring the two-dimensional latitudinal growth only by using plain radiography. Moreover, the epiphysis of the proximal tibia was investigated only by examining half of the entire epiphysis width due to the shadow of the plate. Although Computed tomography (CT) scan is more accurate, we did not routinely preform CT scan to reduce radiation exposures. We did not analyse the longitudinal growth of the residual epiphysis because this study contained three types of osteotomy, and it was also difficult to measure the longitudinal growth after achieving bony union with a transepiphyseal excision. Despite its limitations related to its retrospective nature, the present study provides the possibility of continued residual growth of epiphysis after epiphyseal-preservation surgery in childhood osteosarcomas around the knee. Further prospective studies in a larger series of patients with long-term follow-up should be conducted.

Conclusion

Epiphysis transverse growth was not diminished, and there was no collapse following epiphyseal-preservation surgery in this limited series of childhood osteosarcoma around the knee. Although careful assessment is necessary to evaluate the extent of tumor involvement of the epiphysis, epiphyseal-preservation surgery has the advantage of preserving adjacent joint function with excellent limb function. Epiphysis-preservation surgery should be considered in children.

Abbreviations

aLDFA: Anatomical lateral distal femoral angle; EWD: Epiphysis-width discrepancy; LLD: Limb-length discrepancy; MPTA: Medial proximal tibial angle; MRI: Magnetic resonance imaging; MSTS: the Musculoskeletal Tumor Society

Acknowledgements

The authors would like to thank Dr. Mamer Rosario for review and comment on the manuscript prior to submission. The authors also thank Mr. Toshiya Nomura for drawing the figures.

Authors' contributions

AT performed the study design, data collection, analysis of data, paper drafting. TH carried out the analysis of the radiogram. NY, KH, HM, SM, KA and YT analyzed data and edited the manuscript. HT performed the study design and manuscript review. All authors approved the final manuscript.

Competing interests

The authors declare that they have no competing interests.

References

1. Ayerza MA, Farfalli GL, Aponte-Tinao L, Luis Muscolo D. Does increased rate of limb-sparing surgery affect survival in osteosarcoma? Clin Orthop Relat Res. 2010;468:2854–9.
2. Kang S, Lee JS, Park J, Park S-S. Staged lengthening and reconstruction for children with a leg-length discrepancy after excision of an osteosarcoma around the knee. Bone Joint J. 2017;99-B:401–8.
3. Pala E, Henderson ER, Calabrò T, Angelini A, Abati CN, Trovarelli G, et al. Survival of current production tumor endoprostheses: complications, functional results, and a comparative statistical analysis. J Surg Oncol. 2013; 108:403–8.
4. Han C, Chung D, Lee J, Jeong B. Lengthening of intercalary allograft combined with free vascularized fibular graft after reconstruction in pediatric osteosarcoma of femur. J Pediatr Orthop B. 2010:61–5.
5. Hoffer FA, Nikanorov AY, Reddick WE, Bodner SM, Xiong X, Jones-Wallace D, et al. Accuracy of MR imaging for detecting epiphyseal extension of osteosarcoma. Pediatr Radiol. 2000;30:289–98.
6. Wong KC, Kumta SM. Joint-preserving tumor resection and reconstruction using image-guided computer navigation tumor. Clin Orthop Relat Res. 2013;471:762–73.
7. Mei J, Ni M, Jia GY, Chen YX, Zhu XZ. Intermittent internal fixation with a locking plate to preserve epiphyseal growth function during limb-salvage surgery in a child with osteosarcoma of the distal femur. Medicine (Baltimore). 2015;94:1–4.
8. Aponte-tinao L, Ayerza MA, Muscolo DL, Farfalli GL. Survival, recurrence, and function after epiphyseal preservation and allograft reconstruction in osteosarcoma of the knee. Clin Orthop Relat Res. 2015:1789–96.
9. Tsuchiya H, Abdel-Wanis ME, Sakurakichi K, Yamashiro T, Tomita K. Osteosarcoma around the knee. Intraepiphyseal excision and biological reconstruction with distraction osteogenesis. J Bone Joint Surg Br. 2002;84: 1162–6.
10. Tsuchiya H, Wan SL, Sakayama K, Yamamoto N, Nishida H, Tomita K. Reconstruction using an autograft containing tumour treated by liquid nitrogen. J Bone Joint Surg Br. 2005;87:218–25.
11. Kiss S, Terebessy T, Szöke G, Kiss J, Antal I, Szendröi M. Epiphysis preserving resection of malignant proximal tibial tumours. Int Orthop. 2013;37:99–104.
12. Igarashi K, Yamamoto N, Shirai T, Hayashi K, Nishida H, Kimura H, et al. The long-term outcome following the use of frozen autograft treated with liquid nitrogen in the management of bone and soft-tissue sarcomas. Bone Joint J. 2014;96 B:555–61.
13. Takata M, Sugimoto N, Yamamoto N, Shirai T, Hayashi K, Nishida H, et al. Activity of bone morphogenetic protein-7 after treatment at various temperatures: freezing vs. pasteurization vs. allograft. Cryobiology. 2011;63: 235–9.
14. Tsuchiya H, Tomita K, Mori Y, Asada N, Yamamoto N. Marginal excision for osteosarcoma with caffeine assisted chemotherapy. Clin Orthop Relat Res. 1999;358:27–35.
15. Miwa S, Takeuchi A, Shirai T, Taki J, Yamamoto N, Nishida H, et al. Prognostic value of radiological response to chemotherapy in patients with osteosarcoma. PLoS One. 2013;8
16. Kumta SM, Chow TC, Griffith J, Li CK, Kew J, Leung PC. Classifying the location of osteosarcoma with reference to the epiphyseal plate helps determine the optimal skeletal resection in limb salvage procedures. Arch Orthop Trauma Surg. 1999;119:327–31.
17. Enneking WF, Spanier SS, Goodman MA. A system for the surgical staging of musculoskeletal sarcoma. Clin Orthop Relat Res. 1980;(153):106–20.
18. Tsuchiya H, Nishida H, Srisawat P, Shirai T, Hayashi K, Takeuchi A, et al. Pedicle frozen autograft reconstruction in malignant bone tumors. J Orthop Sci. 2010;15:340–9.
19. Souryal TO, Freeman TR. Intercondylar notch size and anterior cruciate ligament injuries in athletes. A prospective study. Am J Sports Med. 1993;21: 535–9.
20. Paley D, Herzenberg JE, Tetsworth K, McKie J, Bhave A. Deformity planning for frontal and sagittal plane corrective osteotomies. Orthop Clin North Am. 1994;25:425–65.
21. Enneking WF, Dunham W, Gebhardt MC, Malawar M, Pritchard DJ. A system for the functional evaluation of reconstructive procedures after surgical treatment of tumors of the musculoskeletal system. Clin Orthop Relat Res. 1993;(286):241–6.
22. Muscolo DL, Ayerza MA, Aponte-Tinao LA, Ranalletta M. Partial epiphyseal preservation and intercalary allograft reconstruction in high-grade metaphyseal osteosarcoma of the knee. J Bone Joint Surg Am. 2005;87 Suppl 1 (Pt 2):226–36.
23. Henderson ER, Pepper AM, Marulanda G, Binitie OT, Cheong D, Letson GD. Outcome of lower-limb preservation with an expandable endoprosthesis after bone tumor resection in children. J Bone Joint Surg Am. 2012;94:537–47.
24. Tanzawa Y, Tsuchiya H, Shirai T, Hayashi K, Yo Z, Tomita K. Histological examination of frozen autograft treated by liquid nitrogen removed after implantation. J Orthop Sci. 2009;14:761–8.
25. Yamamoto N, Tsuchiya H, Tomita K. Effects of liquid nitrogen treatment on the proliferation ofosteosarcoma and the biomechanical properties of normal bone. J Orthop Sci. 2003;8:374–80.
26. Puhaindran ME, Pho RWH. Biological reconstruction for children with osteosarcoma around the knee. Ann Acad Med Singap. 2014;43:499–505.
27. Carlson CS, Hilley HD, Henrikson CK. Ultrastructure of normal epiphyseal cartilage of the articular-epiphyseal cartilage complex in growing swine. Am J Vet Res. 1985;46:306–13.
28. Chung SM. The arterial supply of the developing proximal end of the human femur. J Bone Joint Surg Am. 1976;58:961–70.
29. Peterson HA. Anatomy and Growth. In: Peterson HA, editor. Epiphyseal growth plate fractures. Heidelberg: Springer; 2007. p. 7–17.
30. Jesus-Garcia R, Seixas MT, Costa SR, Petrilli AS, Filho JL. Epiphyseal plate involvement in osteosarcoma. Clin Orthop Relat Res. 2000;373:32–8.
31. Cañadell J, Forriol F, Cara JA. Removal of metaphyseal bone tumours with

preservation of the epiphysis. Physeal distraction before excision. J Bone Joint Surg Br. 1994;76:127–32.

32. Andreou D, Bielack SS, Carrle D, Kevric M, Kotz R, Winkelmann W, et al. The influence of tumor- and treatment-related factors on the development of local recurrence in osteosarcoma after adequate surgery. An analysis of 1355 patients treated on neoadjuvant Cooperative Osteosarcoma Study Group protocols. Ann Oncol. 2011:1228–35.

Consensus on draft OMERACT core domains for clinical trials of Total Joint Replacement outcome by orthopaedic surgeons: a report from the International consensus on outcome measures in TJR trials (I-COMiTT) group

Jasvinder A. Singh[1,2*], Michael Dohm[3] and Peter F. Choong[4,5]

Abstract

Background: There are no core outcome domain or measurement sets for Total Joint Replacement (TJR) clinical trials. Our objective was to achieve an International consensus by orthopaedic surgeons on the OMERACT core domain/area set for TJR clinical trials.

Methods: We conducted surveys of two orthopaedic surgeon cohorts, which included (1) the leadership of international orthopaedic societies and surgeons (IOS; cohort 1), and (2) the members of the American Academy of Orthopaedic Surgeons' Outcome Special Interest Group (AAOS-Outcome SIG), and/or the Outcome Research Interest Group of the Orthopaedic Research Society (ORS; cohort 2). Participants rated OMERACT-endorsed preliminary core area set for TJR clinical trials on a 1 to 9 scale, indicating 1–3 as domain of limited importance, 4–6 being important, but not critical, and 7–9 being critical.

Results: Eighteen survey participants from the IOS group and 69 participants from the AAOS-Outcome SIG/ORS groups completed the survey questionnaire. The median (interquartile range [IQR]) scores were seven or higher for all six proposed preliminary core areas/domains across both groups, IOS and AAOS-Outcome SIG/ORS, respectively: pain, 8 [8, 9] and 8 [7, 9]; function, 8 [8, 8] and 8 [7, 9]; patient satisfaction, 8 [7, 9] and 8 [7, 8]; revision surgery, 7 [6, 9] and 8 [6, 8]; adverse events, 7 [5, 8] and 7 [6, 9]; and death, 7 [7, 9] and 8 [5, 9]. Respective median scores were lower for two additional optional domains: patient participation, 6.5 [5, 7] and 6 [5, 8]; and cost, 6 [5, 7] and 6 [5, 7].

Conclusions: This study showed that two independent surveys dervied from three groups of orthopaedic surgeons with international representation endorsed a preliminary/draft OMERACT core domain/area set for Joint Replacement clinical trials.

Keywords: OMERACT, Core domain, Clinical trails, Total Joint Arthroplasty, TJR

* Correspondence: jasvinder.md@gmail.com
[1]University of Alabama at Birmingham, Birmingham, AL, USA
[2]Birmingham Veterans Affairs Medical Center, Birmingham, AL, USA
Full list of author information is available at the end of the article

Background

Total Joint Replacement (TJR) is one of the most common elective procedures performed in the US and worldwide. The rate of utilization of this highly cost effective and clinically successful procedure has, in part, been attributed to the increasing prevalence of osteoarthritis, obesity, and an aging population [1–3]. Despite the recognition that the measurement of pain and function after TJR is very important and the common practice is to assess these outcomes in clinical practice, there is no consensus as to which domains or outcome measures should be included in every TJR trial. Consistency in measurement is essential for enabling valid comparisons between TJR clinical trials and head-to-head studies, which currently is hampered by the heterogeneity of outcome measures [4], and the inability to pool data for meta-analysis. A TJR outcome Working Group (WG) first met at the OMERACT-9 meeting in 2008 where this critical issue was discussed in detail [5]. Based on the strategy outlined, we have continued the work in this area within our WG for the last 8 years.

The method of development of TJR trial core domain set was a multi-step, data-driven process that required a consensus by key stakeholders, including but not limited to orthopaedic surgeons and patients; step-by-step details are available in a previous publication [6]. Consensus for core domains was defined as the agreement of different stakeholders (and different groups of the same stakeholder type, i.e., two groups of patients or two groups of physicians) for a similar set, if not the same, core domains. In case of a discrepancy in ratings, we would discuss with various stakeholders to agree to a final common domain set, i.e., consensus. We performed two surveys among 1) orthopaedic surgeons and 2) patients, clinicians, orthopaedic surgeons, and methodologists [7] that identified seven potential domains for a draft TJR trial core domain set (including joint-specific quality of life). At the OMERACT-2014 meeting in Budapest, a multi-stakeholder group including orthopaedic surgeons, patients, academic researchers and industry scientists, discussed in detail and by consensus endorsed a preliminary core domain set for TJR clinical trials [6]. The TJR clinical trial preliminary core domain set included six core domains, namely, pain, function, patient satisfaction, revision surgery, adverse events and death [6]. Other domains were considered but not endorsed for inclusion in the core set were patient expectations, joint-specific quality of life and generic quality of life [6]. Joint-specific quality of life was thought to be redundant with functional ability, pain and patient satisfaction and therefore not included in core domain set, details of the discussion are provided elsewhere [6]. We previously determined that the next step in this consensus process was to obtain further input from more independent groups from two important stakeholder communities, the orthopaedic surgeons and the patients.

The objective of the current study was to assess whether a broader orthopaedic community will engage in further development of the draft TJR trial core domain set, endorse or propose modification. We performed two separate surveys with three groups of orthopaedic surgeons to obtain a consensus on the draft TJR trial core domain set. We surveyed: (1) the present/past leadership of international orthopaedic societies (IOS) (survey 1); and (2) the members of the American Academy of Orthopaedic Surgeons' Outcome Special Interest Group (AAOS-Outcome SIG) and the Outcome Research Interest Group of the Orthopaedic Research Society (ORS) at the annual meetings (survey 2), using each groups' email list.

Methods

Setting

We surveyed three groups of orthopaedic surgeons, key stakeholders for this consensus, by performing two separate surveys. These surgeons included not only clinicians, but also orthopaedic clinical trialists and leading total joint registry investigators. We met orthopaedic surgeons face to face at the AAOS meeting and subsequently obtained email lists for three groups of orthopaedic surgeons, categorized as follows for two independent surveys: (1) the present/past IOS leadership (survey 1); and (2) the members of the AAOS-Outcomes SIG and the Outcome Research Interest Group of the ORS (survey 2), who attended the respective meetings at the AAOS-2015.

Survey and analyses

We pre-tested a survey questionnaire that queried the importance of six core domains/areas (pain, function, patient satisfaction, revision surgery, adverse event and death) and two optional areas (patient participation in life/social activities, cost) for reporting in joint replacement clinical trials. Ratings were on a 1–9 scale, 1–3 indicating domain of limited importance, 4–6 being important domain, and 7–9 being critically important domain. If both groups of orthopaedic surgeons were to rate each core domain "7–9", i.e., critical, it would indicate complete consensus, and the TJR core domain set would be considered endorsed by orthopaedic surgeons at this stage. If a majority of the six core domains, but not all, were rated as critical by both orthopaedic surgeon groups, it would indicate incomplete consensus and would lead to discussion with surgeons regarding whether we needed modification of the draft TJR trial core domain set. In case of lack of consensus, modification of core domain set would be done. A similar approach was planned for the future, in case of lack of complete consensus between surgeon and patient surveys for the draft TJR trial core domain set, leading either to its endorsement or modification (separate surveys of the same core domain set in patients) (Singh JA, et al. Patient Endorsement of the Outcome Measures in Rheumatology

(OMERACT) Total Joint Replacement (TJR) Clinical Trial Draft Core Domain Set, submitted).

Summary statistics are calculated for the two cohorts of survey participants. We calculated the median (interquartile range) ratings for each of the preliminary core domain/area within each group, the orthopaedic surgeon/registry leadership group and the AAOS-Outcome SIG/ORS orthopaedic surgeon groups.

Results

There were 18 survey participants from the IOS group and 69 participants from the AAOS-Outcomes SIG/ORS outcome groups who completed the questionnaire. Of the survey respondents, respectively, 100 and 78% were male, >90% in both were arthroplasty researcher/surgeons, and 67 and 64% were 55 years and older (Table 1).

The pattern of endorsement and ratings of both core domains and optional domains for measurement in arthroplasty RCTs were similar across the two diverse groups of orthopaedic surgeons (Table 2). All six proposed preliminary core domains of pain, function, patient satisfaction, revision surgery, adverse event and death achieved a median score of 7 or 8 on a 0–9 scale in both groups, i.e., were rated as critically important. The median score for two additional optional domains, patient participation and cost, achieved a median score of 6–6.5 in both groups (Table 2).

Several important comments were provided by survey respondents, which shed further insight into this issue (Table 3). Additional core domains brought up for consideration by 1 respondent each were: caregiver impact; venous thromboembolism occurrence; return to work; quality of life; and range of motion. Some participants commented that the domains of revision (at some specified time/s after TJR) and patient participation (social vs. work) need to be defined clearly.

Table 1 Participant characteristics

# survey participants	Orthopaedic surgeon leadership group N = 18	Orthopaedic surgeons (AAOS outcomes SIG/ORS group) N = 69
% male[a]	100%	78%
Age category[a]		
18–24	0%	0%
25–34	0%	1%
35–44	0%	17%
45–54	33%	17%
55–64	67%	41%
65–74	0%	19%
≥75	0%	4%
Background[b]		
Arthroplasty surgeon, private practice	56%	18%
Arthroplasty surgeon, academic practice	39%	43%
Arthroplasty researcher	11%	49%
Orthopaedic surgeon, not focused on arthroplasty, private practice	11%	8%
Orthopaedic surgeon, not focused on arthroplasty, academic practice	17%	7%
Patient	0%	7%
Policy maker	0%	3%
Time spent planning/conducting arthroplasty trials		
0–10%	67%	57%
11–20%	28%	16%
21–30%	0%	16%
31–50%	0%	4%
>50%	6%	6%
Years practicing/doing research in arthroplasty		
< 5	6%	4%
5–<10	0%	13%
10–20	18%	23%
>20	77%	59%

[a]Missing values for AAOS-Outcome SIG and OMERACT cohorts: sex: 5 vs. none; age, 4 vs. none; [b]Background, people could choose more than one option

Discussion

TJR clinical trials often report outcomes that are heterogeneous and difficult to combine and compare across trials in a systematic review or comparative analysis [4, 5]. This heterogeneity is not only a major barrier to accurate comparison between trials but also an impediment to the development of consensus, which is critical for the collective analysis of the important findings that TJR trials may bring. The various international joint replacement registries have recognized the importance of harmonizing outcome collection and reporting based on expert consensus and have initiated a collaborative approach to establishing a framework [8]. To date, such an effort has not been completed for a core measurement set in TJR clinical trials.

The OMERACT TJR Working Group, an International group with patient partnership, is pursuing this goal through International collaboration with groups such as the AAOS-Outcome SIG, the ORS, the International Society of Arthroplasty Registries (ISAR), and Functional Outcomes in Total Joint Replacement (FORCE-TJR). In the last few meetings, the OMERACT TJR WG has made significant progress in assembling a multi-stakeholder group and completed the literature reviews examining the frequency of reporting of various domains (pain, function, revision etc.) in TJR clinical trials (Richards B, et al. Outcome measures

Table 2 Preliminary core areas/domains for TJR clinical trials

	Orthopaedic surgeon leadership group Median [IQR]	Orthopaedic surgeons (AAOS, ORS group) Median [IQR]
Main Domains to be reported in every TJR clinical trial		
Joint Pain	8 [8, 9]	8 [7, 9]
Function or functional ability (ability to function in society, work; work productivity, employability; disability; work disability)	8 [8, 8]	8 [7, 9]
Patient Satisfaction (satisfaction with the outcome, satisfaction with the procedure)	8 [7, 9]	8 [7, 8]
Revision surgery	7 [6, 9]	8 [6, 8]
Adverse events	7 [5, 8]	7 [6, 9]
Death	7 [7, 9]	8 [5, 9]
Additional domains for consideration for reporting in TJR clinical trials		
Patient Participation	6.5 [5, 7]	6 [5, 8]
Cost	6 [5, 7]	6 [5, 7]

used in arthroplasty trials: Systematic review of the 2008 and 2013 literature, submitted; Wall P, et al. Do outcomes reported in randomised controlled trials of joint replacement surgery fulfil the OMERACT 2.0 Filter? A review of the 2008 and 2013 literature, submitted).

At OMERACT 2014 TJR WG, a preliminary core domain set for TJR clinical trials was developed based on systematic literature reviews, the OMERACT filter 2.0, and two separate surveys at orthopaedic surgery meetings and the OMERACT pre-meeting [6]. This proposed draft TJR core domain set (pain, function, patient satisfaction, revision, adverse events, death, joint-specific quality of life) was discussed with a multi-stakeholder group at OMERACT-2014 TJR WG that included patients who had undergone arthroplasty, orthopaedic surgeons (in an academic setting or community-based practice), psychometricians, physical/occupational therapists, other clinicians and arthroplasty researchers, and finally endorsed with six core domains [6]. This multi-stakeholder OMERACT group helped develop the draft TJR clinical trial core domain set including experts in the development of clinical trial core domain sets and following a well-described methodology based on a solid framework of the OMERACT filer 2.0 [9–11].

In the current study, both groups of orthopaedic surgeons achieved consensus on the six TJR clinical trial core domains (scores of 7 or above) and did not propose any new core domains. These are very important findings, since these Delphi involved two groups of orthopaedic surgeons independent of those who had participated in the development of the preliminary TJR clinical trial core domain set. This is not surprising since this TJR core domain set was developed over several years after multiple systematic reviews and with multi-stakeholder input consisting of orthopaedic surgeons, patients who had undergone arthroplasty and methodologists who have an extensive experience with developing and validating core domain and measurement sets. The OMERACT's philosophy of a multi-stakeholder involvement from the beginning of the process, and a data driven approach, are key to successfully achieving a broad stakeholder consensus on this draft TJR clinical trial core domain set. This evidence indicates that preliminary TJR core domain set initially developed with multi-stakeholder input and endorsed at OMERACT 2014 meeting was endorsed independently by orthopaedic surgeons.

Core domain sets are those domains that should be reported in every clinical trial for the condition, regardless of the intervention, as they are critical to the conceptualization of the condition/disease. One must not confuse a core domain with the primary outcome for each clinical trial, which is always specific to each research question. In some studies, core domain measures will be primary outcome, since they are the focus of the research question; in other studies, they may be secondary study outcomes. Our work indicates that this draft TJR core domain set is now ready for the next phase, namely, the identification and validation of measures that accurately reflect each core domain, and further dissemination of this TJR core domain set to key stakeholders.

We received qualitative feedback from the surveys, which has helped us with further specification of two core domains. One suggestion was to consider any reoperation, not just revision, due to its relevance to patients- this indicates that the core domain would be revision/reoperation. Another suggestion was to specify whether death was procedure-related vs. not procedure-related. With further refinement of the core domains, these two proposals will be the subject of future WG discussions. It is interesting and reassuring that several of domains brought up one participant each (caregiver impact; venous thromboembolism occurrence; return to work; quality of life; and range of motion) were considered previously. Based on Delphi and detailed discussions with surgeons, patients and other stakeholders,

Table 3 Additional Comments from Delphi Process

Main core domains	Additional domains
AAOS-Outcomes SIG/ORS Orthopaedic surgeon group	
Change in function, change in pain duration of improvement	Cost is a very nebulous area, particularly since cost varies by how you measure it and what part of the country the research is performed in
Patient satisfaction is nebulous unless everyone is using the same instrument to measure it.	I am not sure what patient participation means, so I stayed neutral. I suspect this refers to charges and in that case, there needs to be a cost to charge ratio applied
I believe that limping is important and has a tendency to drown in the available scores used	Limping for total hip and stiffness (joint fibrosis) for TKA
Patient-reported outcomes using validated instruments should have a very high priority and would cover the upper (first) two items.	Unclear what is meant by patient participation so unable to score
PROM function and patient satisfaction are important but both are often affected by factors not directly related to the outcome of surgery. Thus it depends on the type of clinical trial if they are essential or not. Revision surgery indicates that both the patient and the physician agreed on that the initial procedure had been unsuccessful, Death and adverse events are very important but uncommon. For a new technique or approach such information is essential but maybe not for every clinical trial.	Participation in rehabilitation is important to functional outcome, but the trial focus may or may not require collection of these data. If patients are randomized to a drug trial, for example, then participation levels should be random and the focus is on the endpoints/outcomes (pain, function, AE) not on the level of participation.
Family function; Caregiver impact	Medical and surgical complications should be reported separately
Venous thromboembolism occurrence–What is the Best VTE prophylaxis?	Need more definition around how cost will be measured and reported Cost is variable from state to state and center to center within a state or city
Revision should probably be re-designated as "reoperation for any reason" as patients often care more if they had to have repeat surgery for what ever the reason, and not as much whether implant parts (if any) are swapped out or exchanged	Patient participation is very unreliable on higher levels of participation
Implant revision is impractical unless the trial involves many years of follow-up. However, surgical AEs (manipulation, etc.) are important. Death is important, but very rare	
Of importance for the patient: To which degree are expectations fulfilled	
Return to work or avoidance of environment modification for the older patient	
Quality of life, 8 Work disability and employability are very culture- and society-dependent issues and therefore suit poorly as core domains. Function should be assessed in more general and patient-specific terms	
Range of motion	
Patient Satisfaction should not be a core domain and should not be reported by all arthroplasty trials should be optional	
Longevity of arthroplasty–similar to revision surgery	
For the first two listed (joint pain and function), I think it would be very important to measure those outcomes not only at 6–12 months after surgery, but also at an earlier time interval after surgery (ex. 6 weeks) for patients interested in the extent to which they can expect rapid recovery.	
My rating is in part weighted by how accessible the information is. For example, revision surgery or death may take place years or decades after the initial surgery, and hence may not be related or the index procedure may not be available to the researcher. Secondly, there is little consensus of what is a "revision surgery". A German colleague demonstrated that an I & D was considered a revision surgery in France, but not in other countries. Similar for	

Table 3 Additional Comments from Delphi Process *(Continued)*

"adverse events". Would this include a post-op infection resulting in an infection? Obviously you have a lot of work here—what periods are being suggested? I know that the spine surgeons may consider 2 years as acceptable follow-up. Not sure what this group is considering. 1 year? 2 years? 5 years? At what point is the patient's status no longer relevant to the surgery? Good luck Mike. These are my perspectives and may not be representative of the physicians involved. Stan	
Orthopaedic leadership group	
The importance of death is social situation dependent. For two identical patients but for one having dependent family and the other not, the impact of death would be different, and might affect the decision to have surgery	Cost should be cost-effectiveness. These two terms are not necessarily interchangeable and there is an important difference in arthroplasty. A cheaper cemented stem and cup in a young person is not cost effective
Death as long as related to surgery. Patient satisfaction probably one question item. Link revision to joint registries if they exist in the country–a better question may be any other surgery related to joint where revision surgery not an option (i.e. ankle arthroplasty)	Cost is such a veritable worldwide. It will be difficult to quantify it accurately based on the various deals and accountancy practices in different hospitals. I'm not sure as part of a clinical review of the performance
I believe patient satisfaction and function of secondary only to the relief of osteoarthritic pain.. Adverse events I think a slightly less important as they reflect on the anesthetic care and this is going ability rather than the prosthetic	
Function domain needs to be relative to the involved joint and attempt to capture non joint limiting disabilities	

they were recommended not for inclusion in the core domain set, since they were not considered to represent an independent core domain, above and beyond the six domains already included.

We noted that both groups independently rated the additional non-core domains (patient participation, cost) as important but not critical; the median scores were 6 to 6.5, appropriately lower than the core domains, since these are not core domains. Non-core domains are those domains that may be additionally reported in a TJR clinical trial, depending on the clinical question being asked.

Our study findings must be interpreted with caution, since they may not be generalizable to other groups. Our orthopaedic surgeon samples were 78 and 100% male, which may limit the generalizability of the findings to all surgeons. The gender distribution among orthopaedic surgeons is not balanced in general. We developed this draft TJR core domain set for clinical trials; it is possible that with validation and future work, this set or a similar set may be endorsed for observational studies as well.

Our study has several strengths, including use of the same survey in two groups of stakeholders, inclusion of both leaders of orthopaedic societies as well as the group of orthopaedic surgeons and researchers from community and academic practices.

Conclusions

In conclusion, the current study shows further independent endorsement of the draft TJR core domain set for reporting of TJR clinical trials. The next steps in this process, are a wider endorsement of these by OMERACT and/or orthopaedic organizations that we have been collaborating with. This will be followed by the development of a valid, data- and consensus-driven TJR clinical trial core outcome measurement set. Our group will aim to complete this step over the next 2 years. The process will be completed with multi-stakeholder input with a particular emphasis of involvement of patients and TJR surgeons.

Abbreviations

AAOS: American Academy of Orthopaedic Surgeons' Outcome Special Interest Group; NRS: Numeric Rating Scale; OA: Osteoarthritis; OMERACT: Outcome measures in rheumatology; ORS: Outcome Research Interest Group of the Orthopaedic Research Society; SIG: Special Interest Group; TJR: Total Joint Replacement; TKA: Total knee arthroplasty; WG: Working group; WOMAC: Western Ontario and McMaster Universities Osteoarthritis Index

Acknowledgements

We thank the orthopaedic surgeons for their time and participation in this survey study.

Funding

There is no direct funding for this study. This study was supported by the resources and use of facilities at Birmingham VA Medical Center at Birmingham, Alabama, USA.

Authors' contributions

All authors have read and approved the manuscript. JS: development of study question and protocol. JS, MD: modification and finalization of study protocol. JS, MD, PC: Data collection. JS: Data programming, data analysis. JS, MD, PC: Interpretation of data analysis. JS: First Draft of manuscript. JS, MD, PC: Critical revisions and approval of the final version of the manuscript.

Authors' information

JAS is the co-chair of the OMERACT TJR Working group assessing the outcome measures in arthroplasty and has served as expert/lead on task forces for the specialty societies and the US FDA. Other authors have no other relevant information.

Each author certifies that his or her institution has approved the human protocol for this investigation and that all investigations were conducted in conformity with ethical principles of research.

"The views expressed in this article are those of the authors and do not necessarily reflect the position or policy of the Department of Veterans Affairs or the United States government."

Names, Degrees and Academic title:

JA Singh, MBBS, MPH Professor of Medicine and Epidemiology.

M Dohm, MD, FAAOS, ABOS Assistant Professor of Orthopaedic Surgery, Assistant Professor of Medicine.

P F Choong, MBBS, MD, FRACS, FAOrthA Professor of Surgery.

Competing interests

JAS has received research grants from Takeda and Savient and consultant fees from Savient, Takeda, Regeneron, Merz, Bioiberica, Crealta and Allergan pharmaceuticals, WebMD, UBM LLC and the American College of Rheumatology. JAS serves as the principal investigator for an investigator-initiated study funded by Horizon pharmaceuticals through a grant to DINORA, Inc., a 501 (c)(3) entity. JAS is a member of the executive of OMERACT, an organization that develops outcome measures in rheumatology and receives arms-length funding from 36 companies; a member of the American College of Rheumatology's (ACR) Annual Meeting Planning Committee (AMPC); Chair of the ACR Meet-the-Professor, Workshop and Study Group Subcommittee; and a member of the Veterans Affairs Rheumatology Field Advisory Committee. MD receives no direct funding and has no financial conflicts. He is a member of the American Joint Replacement Registry (AJRR) and Chairman of the Data Elements Committee as well as an associate member of the International Society of Arthroplasty Registers (ISAR), is a member of the evidence based practice committee for AAHKS and Chairman of the AAOS Outcome Special Interest Group. PC has received consultancy fees from DePuy, Zimmer and Stryker as part of surgeon design or research teams. PC's institution has received research grant funding from Allergan, DePuy and Medacta. None of the authors have any non-financial disclosures. JAS is a Section Editor for BMC Musculoskeletal Disorders.

Consent for publication

Not applicable.

Author details

[1]University of Alabama at Birmingham, Birmingham, AL, USA. [2]Birmingham Veterans Affairs Medical Center, Birmingham, AL, USA. [3]Department of Orthopaedic Surgery, University of Arizona, Tucson, AZ, USA. [4]Department of Surgery, University of Melbourne, Melbourne, Australia. [5]Department of Surgery, St. Vincent's Hospital, Melbourne, Australia.

References

1. Kurtz S, Ong K, Lau E, Mowat F, Halpern M. Projections of primary and revision hip and knee arthroplasty in the United States from 2005 to 2030. J Bone Joint Surg Am. 2007;89:780–5.
2. Healthcare Cost and Utilization Project (HCUP). HCUP Facts and Figures 2009- Section 3: Inpatient Hospital Stays by Procedure. Exhibit 3.1 Most Frequent All-listed Procedures. Rockville: Agency for Healthcare Research and Quality; 2012. Updated February 2012. http://hcup-us.ahrq.gov/reports/factsandfigures/2009/pdfs/FF_2009_section3.pdf. 10 Feb 2014.
3. Ethgen O, Bruyere O, Richy F, Dardennes C, Reginster JY. Health-related quality of life in total hip and total knee arthroplasty. A qualitative and systematic review of the literature. J Bone Joint Surg Am. 2004;86-A:963–74.

4. Riddle DL, Stratford PW, Bowman DH. Findings of extensive variation in the types of outcome measures used in hip and knee replacement clinical trials: a systematic review. Arthritis Rheum. 2008;59:876–83.
5. Riddle DL, Stratford PW, Singh JA, Strand CV. Variation in outcome measures in hip and knee arthroplasty clinical trials: a proposed approach to achieving consensus. J Rheumatol. 2009;36:2050–6.
6. Singh JA, Dohm M, Sprowson AP, Wall PD, Richards BL, Gossec L, et al. Outcome Domains and Measures in Total Joint Replacement Clinical Trials: Can We Harmonize Them? An OMERACT Collaborative Initiative. J Rheumatol. 2015;42(12):2496–502.
7. Singh JA, Dohm M. Towards Consensus on the Reporting of Core Outcome Domains in Total Joint Replacement Clinical Trials: The Derivation of the Preliminary Core Outcome Domain Set. J Arthritis. 2016;5:6.
8. Rolfson O, Wissig S, van Maasakkers L, Stowell C, Ackerman I, Ayers D, et al. Defining an International Standard Set of Outcome Measures for Patients with Hip or Knee Osteoarthritis: Consensus of the International Consortium for Health Outcomes Measurement Hip and Knee Osteoarthritis Working Group. Arthritis Care Res (Hoboken). 2016;68:1631–9.
9. Boers M, Kirwan JR, Wells G, Beaton D, Gossec L, d'Agostino MA, et al. Developing core outcome measurement sets for clinical trials: OMERACT filter 2.0. J Clin Epidemiol. 2014;67:745–53.
10. Boers M, Kirwan JR, Gossec L, Conaghan PG, D'Agostino MA, Bingham 3rd CO, et al. How to choose core outcome measurement sets for clinical trials: OMERACT 11 approves filter 2.0. J Rheumatol. 2014;41:1025–30.
11. Singh JA, Taylor WJ, Simon LS, Khanna PP, Stamp LK, McQueen FM, et al. Patient-reported outcomes in chronic gout: a report from OMERACT 10. J Rheumatol. 2011;38:1452–7.

A qualitative study of patient education needs for hip and knee replacement

Deborah Kennedy[1,2,3*], Amy Wainwright[1,3], Lucy Pereira[1], Susan Robarts[1], Patricia Dickson[1,4], Jennifer Christian[5] and Fiona Webster[6]

Abstract

Background: Quality health information is key to patient engagement, self-management and an enhanced healthcare experience. There is strong evidence to support involving patients and their families in the development and evaluation of health-related educational material. These factors were the impetus for our high volume joint replacement centre to undertake a qualitative study to elicit patient experiences to inform the development of effective strategies and education along the care continuum for hip and knee replacement.

Methods: Purposively selected patients from postoperative follow-up clinics were recruited to participate in a focus group or telephone interview. We developed a semi-structured interview guide that addressed four specific aspects of the patient's experience with educational material: pre-surgery, hospital stay, recovery period and future recommendations. The focus groups and interviews continued to the point of saturation and were audio-recorded and transcribed verbatim. Interview transcripts were coded and then inductively organized into larger categories using thematic analysis.

Results: Six focus groups and seven telephone interviews were conducted, totalling 32 participants. One of the key themes that emerged was a need for more education concerning pain management post-operatively; specifically, patients wanted more information on expected levels of pain, pain medication usage, management of side effects and guidelines for weaning off the medication. There was surprising variability in patients' descriptions of their pre-surgery, surgery and recovery experiences. These corresponded to an equally diverse range of preferences for educational content, delivery and timing. Many patients reported using the web while others preferred traditional formats for information delivery. There was some interest in receiving education using mobile technology.

Conclusions: Our findings validate the importance of multi-modal patient education tailored to individual preferences and experiences, which may differ according to such characteristics as gender and age. The gap in pain management information is a critical finding for healthcare providers working with patients undergoing joint replacement. Developing pain management education in different formats that addresses frequently asked questions will enhance patient engagement and, their overall experience and recovery.

Keywords: Patient engagement, Hip and knee replacement, Education, Pain management, Person-centred care

* Correspondence: Deborah.kennedy@sunnybrook.ca
[1]Sunnybrook Holland Orthopaedic and Arthritic Centre, 43 Wellesley Street East, Toronto, ON M4Y 1H1, Canada
[2]School of Rehabilitation Science, McMaster University, 1400 Main St. W, Hamilton, ON L8S 1C7, Canada
Full list of author information is available at the end of the article

Background

In our increasingly complex healthcare environment, patients require high quality information to successfully manage their health. Although access to information on the web and other sources has increased, it has not necessarily translated to increased understanding. Often patient health information has been created from the lens of the providers without patient consultation.

In 2015, the World Health Organization released a global strategy on people-centred and integrated health services calling for a fundamental shift in the way health services are managed and delivered [1]. The current focus for healthcare organizations is a person-centred care approach, where the patient's values, knowledge, preferences and needs are central to their care. There is strong evidence to support the importance of involving patients and their families in the development and evaluation of educational material for health purposes [2, 3].

Currently, there is limited literature exploring the education needs of patients and their families in many patient populations including that of hip and knee replacement. This information would be extremely useful in the design of effective strategies that support and educate patients both prior to, in hospital and after discharge. Given the growing prevalence of this surgery, along with shortening lengths of stay, patients need this type of information for shared decision-making.

These factors were the impetus for our team to undertake a qualitative study at our high volume joint replacement centre and seek the voice of our patients about their educational needs and preferences. Our study question was, "What are the informational needs and delivery preferences for education of families and patients undergoing hip or knee replacement?"

Methods

Design and setting

The study was conducted in a large Canadian orthopaedic centre specialized in joint replacement surgery. Using descriptive qualitative methods [4], purposefully selected patients were recruited from outpatient clinics at their 6 week to one-year follow-up visits post joint replacement.

Sampling

Using purposeful sampling, a small percentage of patients were invited to participate in the study to explore their experiences and preferences for education following hip or knee replacement surgery [5]. Maximum variation sampling was used to ensure we had participants who differed by age, gender, affected joint, and marital status. This helped to ensure that the patients we interviewed were similar to those regularly seen at our facility. We did not collect information about socio-economic status. We conducted focus groups as well as telephone interviews to accommodate those who did not reside within the urban setting of the hospital. One spouse attended a focus group at the participant's request as she did not feel sufficiently comfortable with English but wanted to share her story. One focus group was composed entirely of men. Six focus groups and seven telephone interviews were conducted totalling 32 participants, at which point our team decided we had generated sufficient data to reach saturation while maintaining a manageable final dataset within this project's timeframe. The mean age of the 32 participants was 67.9 (standard deviation ±7.82; min 46, max 78) years. There was equal distribution of men and women (n = 16 each) and similarly, hip and knee replacements. Regarding time point of participation, 44% of the patients were up to 3 months postoperatively, another 44% between 3 months to 9 months and 12% greater than 9 months up to 1 year.

Ethics

Local Research Ethics Board approval was obtained for this study. Patients were approached for consent during their follow-up visits. The clinic secretary asked the patient if they would be willing to receive a consent form, and have someone from research speak to them about participating in a focus group or interview.

Focus groups

We developed a focus group guide to address four specific aspects of the patient's experience with educational material [6]. The guide (see Additional file 1) began with open, broader questions about the patient's educational needs and experiences leading up to surgery and then questions were asked about each stage of the hospital and recovery process. Finally, a series of questions were asked in relation to the patient's preferences for future educational materials, including videos and internet resources. All questions were meant to be exploratory and relied on probes to allow differences between patients in perceptions and experiences to emerge during the course of the interview. The focus group guide was pilot tested with one patient identified by our research team. The objective of pilot testing was to confirm the length of each interview and to ensure that the questions were clear and comprehensible. FW, who is a trained qualitative interviewer, performed the pilot interview with one patient and facilitated several of the focus groups and telephone interviews; other focus groups were conducted by an experienced Research Associate, JC. Members of the healthcare team did not solicit or conduct interviews. All interviews and focus groups were audio-taped and professionally transcribed verbatim.

Data analysis

Data collection and analysis were conducted concurrently. Three members of the research team (DK, FW and JC) read transcriptions of the pilot interview independently to identify codes. The researchers then met to compare their independent analyses and develop a coding framework for use in the subsequent analysis. JC then coded the remaining interviews, keeping memo notes of any potential changes to the coding framework that she identified. After all interviews had been coded, the larger research team held several meetings in which they interpreted the data to identify similarities and differences across the interviews. We combined our codes into themes and identified predominant ones. The relationships between the themes were also summarized in these team meetings.

Our team performed several steps to ensure rigour [6]. To ensure *reliability*, more than one investigator performed each key step. Our analysis was *reflexive* as our team was multidisciplinary, consisting of clinicians, educators and researchers, which allowed us to consider our personal biases during data analysis throughout the memoing and data summarizing steps [6].

Results

Although some people preferred to be interviewed one-on-one rather than in a focus group, we did not find any significant differences in their accounts. For the purposes of this study, using both data collection approaches allowed us to achieve both depth and breadth, increasing the number of participants we could speak with over a relatively short period of time [7]. While qualitative interviews and focus groups are not inter-changeable we did not find significant differences in the data we obtained across using the two approaches. We organized our findings into four main themes: 1) education gaps relating to pain management 2) participant's validation of existing organizational education materials; 3) informal sources of information; and 4) interest in new delivery modes for education, such as mobile health applications.

Theme 1: Educational gaps around pain management

An important finding that emerged from our interviews and focus groups was an identified need to have more education around pain management post-operatively. In particular, participants expressed an interest in education related to expected levels of post-operative pain, the purpose of the prescribed medications, information on how to take the medications, their side effects and how to "wean off" pain medications. In the following account, the patient describes how she needed more information to manage her pain,

> *"Well, if there was possibility to deal with the pain part more effectively ... that might have been of help. I think [the surgeon] did say if I had any questions ... I could phone them, I just don't think I did because I thought there wasn't really much they could do about, you know, the pain stuff ..."* (Participant #1, Interview #4, Female)

Another participant describes his perception of other people's negative experiences of medication side effects. In the following excerpt, he is suggesting that patients are both afraid to ask about medication and are without recourse regarding pain medication once they leave the hospital. He says,

> *"I mean, I got off those white little pills as fast as I possibly could. I took Tylenol Extra Strength for whatever, and now maybe once a week or so I'll take a couple Tylenol Extra Strength. But two things, one is a lot of the people that go to rehab, they get sick from them, they get sick from those white little pills, whatever they are, OxyContin or oxy-something, they get sick, but the doctor told them to take them and they continue to take them ... but there's no recourse back, and they're afraid to ask, they're definitely afraid to ask about the pills ... So again it's education about medication."*
> (Participant #1, Focus Group #1, Male)

Participants suggested that nobody provided them with information about how to "wean" themselves off their pain medication once they were back at home.

> *"...The first time around I expected someone to say to me, "Once you get your pain medication here's a method of getting off of it. Here's a way of weaning yourself off of that," but nobody did this. ..., it was maybe at six weeks I was still taking Oxy. The first time [the pharmacist] go, "You gotta stop doing this," I go, "What do you mean?" No one had told me [that]. ... even this time when I had my hip nobody would give me a method of weaning myself off of it, I had to go back to the pain specialist."* (Participant #3, Focus Group #1, Male)

While participants did acknowledge they received information that they would need to reduce their pain medication, they frequently felt that these instructions lacked crucial information about how they would accomplish this in terms of practical steps. As one participant shared,

> *"I think I started to wean off on my own without realizing it. It was every four hours, I think, if I remember. And then I realized afterwards I had*

forgotten one time, and I thought, "Oh, okay, I've been an hour without it," so I took it then because I felt pain. So the next day I really tested it out ... Now, I was fortunate ... But it was a nurse here, before I left, when I got the prescription, who said to me, "You'll want to wean yourself off," but not how." (Participant #6, Focus Group #1, Female)

Theme 2: Participants' validation of existing materials

Despite identifying a gap in pain management education, patients did validate the usefulness of the existing patient education tools (www.sunnybrook.ca/holland) offered in different mediums both pre and post-operatively. These included a comprehensive guide (organized into preoperative, hospital stay and post discharge sections), a preoperative education class, as well as, a short animated educational YouTube video developed by our organization in partnership with Dr. Mike Evans. Of note, not all participants attended the workshop or recalled seeing the video.

2a) guide for patients having hip or knee replacement

The following participant highlights that the Guide is useful across various stages of the pre to post surgery process and was something she referred to throughout her recovery.

> *"I like having the book because you don't remember everything you read the first time, and you don't remember everything a month later, so I could go back to the book, especially about preparing and getting ready. So it was nice to have the printed material that I could look at."*
> (Participant #1, Interview #2, Female)

2b) the preoperative education class

Participants commented on the benefits of attending the Preoperative Education class. They commented on how appropriate preparation *"built their confidence"* (Participant #1, Focus Group #1, Male). This confidence building was important given how many people were initially fearful of having surgery. In the following account, the participant stresses the importance of hearing from another patient and described how valuable it was to have the expertise of the rehabilitation staff.

> *"I was terrified like I think most people are, and there was a person who'd gone through the surgery who was able to answer any questions that most people had. The physiotherapist and the OT were, you know, incredibly gracious and able to sit down and really, you know, relax most of the patients there."* (Participant #1, Pilot Interview, Female)

2c) Dr. Mike Evans' 'preparing you for your hip or knee replacement surgery' (www.sunnybrook.ca/holland/hipknee)

Participants who had viewed the Dr. Mike Evans' video expressed that they had found it helpful, especially as it emphasized and was consistent with the information they had received in the Guide.

> *"...I think it repeated a lot of what was in the pamphlet, but you could see it. You know, it's concrete, tangible, you see it, very step-by-step, and so it helped me..."* (Participant #2, Focus Group #4, Female)

Theme 3: Favoured sources of patient information

Patients identified several sources of information that they drew on most frequently. Not surprisingly, and consistent with other studies, these included family and friends; information they found on the internet (referred to by several participants as "Dr. Google") as well as surgeons.

3a) family and friends

Patients frequently identified friends and families as an important source of information. Hearing stories from other people that their surgeries had been successful seemed to go a long way toward reassuring participants, as the following account exemplifies,

> *"I think my bigger source was other people that had the same operation...what you do is you gather information, which is all part of the decision-making process, but you gather information from multiple sources and you start to get confident in the things that are consistently heard from everybody, so that's where I got my information."*
> (Participant #1, Focus Group #2, Female)

At the same time, they voiced their concern that experiential accounts were not necessarily medically valid. Related to this, many voiced a desire to access a bank of patient "testimonials" that the hospital could curate, hence increasing its reliability from a patient perspective. Several noted that they wanted to hear both "good and indifferent" experiences from others:

> *"What I think is going to be helpful for me is testimonials, good and indifferent ... so testimonials from past patients who have had whatever type of surgery, whether it's hip or knee ..."*
> (Participant #3, Focus group #2, Male)

3b) "Dr. Google"

The majority of participants had searched Google for information on the surgery or recovery process. Many did not question the validity or accuracy of this information.

For some participants, mostly men, they wanted to actually watch the surgery *"to see what goes on in the operating room"*.

Women were more likely to indicate that they specifically did not want to view the surgery online, as the following quote exemplifies:

> *"I just kind of Googled "total knee replacement surgery" or, "required devices required after total knee replacements." "... I didn't look up what the procedure looked like because I thought I might chicken out then." "No, I don't want to see that!""*
> (Participant#1, Interview #4, Female)

Not all people thought that accessing information on the internet was useful and in some instances it reinforced the fear they already felt about the upcoming surgery.

3c) surgeons as a source of education

Some participants identified the surgeon as their main source of information. While patients felt that surgeons were an important source of knowledgeable information, they often described mixed experiences of how much time they felt surgeons could or did provide.

Theme 4: Interest in new delivery modes for education, such as social media

Several participants were interested in accessing information from newer technologies including mobile health applications and social media. A small number of people said that they would in the future use an app. As one participant noted,

> *"[It would be] easy access to information to compare notes with other patients who've gone through it ... either from apps or ... Twitter ..."*
> (Participant #4, Focus group #2, Male)

Other participants, however, were uncertain as to how social media would be useful for them. Some noted that they were comfortable with the computer but did not own smartphones or other technology that would enable them to use newer forms of social media/mobile apps. The following quotes were typical of what we heard during the focus groups.

> *"I use a computer extensively and I look up a lot of stuff on the Internet, so a website that I can go to is fine, I just don't do the social media, I don't want to get involved, and I don't have a smartphone, don't want one. So for me, you know, that's just my level and my choice. But it might benefit somebody else. We're not dealing too often with younger people who are more into those things."* (Participant #3, Focus Group #3, Female)*"I'm not sure. I'm still learning all these apps. Right now it's information overload."* (Participant #6, Focus Group #1, Female)

Discussion

Our experiences and findings with this study have validated the importance of engaging our patients to fully understand their educational needs and delivery preferences. The largest gap that patients identified related to pain medication education, especially for the time-period after they had left the hospital and were at home recovering. This finding was very interesting to the team as historically, we had been very intentional to include information about pain management in our comprehensive guide and preoperative education classes. However, upon reviewing our materials, we realized that although we covered some core concepts, we did not provide enough details around specific medications or weaning steps.

Chan et al. [8] found that more than half of patients after knee replacement reported the first 2 weeks at home as being the most painful time-period after surgery. Poorly managed pain decreases patient satisfaction, the ability to progress functionally [8, 9] and has been found to increase the likelihood of persistent pain following joint replacement [10]. Chan et al's study of over one hundred patients following knee replacement, after hospital discharge found there was suboptimal use of pain medication and non-pharmacological strategies, misconceptions of pain medication usage, disturbing side effects and inadequate information provided to manage pain at home [8]. Similarly, our patients voiced a need for more information on pain medication usage, side effects and how to wean off at the appropriate time. Given the shortening lengths of stay, these topics are becoming even more important as patients are managing acute pain while at home.

The importance of multiple modalities (pamphlets, classes, videos, Apps) available to patients in plain, clear language has been demonstrated in other populations [11]. Our findings also supported the importance of providing multi-modal education to patients that can be tailored to their individual learning preferences and experiences. Prior research investigating the information needs of patients undergoing arthroplasty found that although a core set of questions could be defined; the information needs across patients was quite variable [12, 13]. While this idea is not novel, we still have to broaden our understanding of the social and cultural differences between patients and how to address these in education.

Participants valued the organization's educational materials, including the comprehensive guide, the YouTube video and the pre-operative education classes. The guide enabled patients to review materials at different stages of recovery. All participants described using this guide repeatedly along the continuum of care. The preoperative education session was highly regarded and reduced fears by enabling patients to ask questions, clarify issues and interact with others undergoing similar surgeries. Several studies have shown the importance of preoperative education in reducing anxiety and improving satisfaction, however study findings are variable as demonstrated in a recent meta-analysis [14–16].

Other sources of information patients accessed included; families and friends, the internet and their surgeons. They strongly favoured learning from the experiences of other patients; often these were friends. For this reason, many suggested that having access to a curated set of patient vignettes or "stories" available on a hospital website would be useful. This would allow them to learn from peer experiences while having the added benefit of providing legitimacy to these accounts, an issue many struggled with in relation to the medical validity of the lay accounts they heard from others or by browsing the web. There was interest in using technology to deliver education such as mobile health apps. Although, not all patients have access to smartphones or tablets, the use of mobile technology is increasing annually. The latest Government of Canada statistics indicated that in 2014, 66% of Canadians owned a smartphone and 49% owned a tablet [17].

The study findings have been the impetus for a number of quality improvement projects. We have strengthened the role of patient and family advisors to improve the care experience. To address the gap in our pain management education, patient advisors and team members co-designed new materials in multimodal formats. We introduced a new brochure and video addressing the top 10 questions about pain medication after joint replacement, the information of which is also available online (www.sunnybrook.ca/hipkneepain). Concurrently, we provided widespread staff education about the new resources.

These experiences have reinforced the importance of including the patient voice, as the healthcare team's focus was not always reflective of patients' preferences. We have also launched a mobile app (with a web-based version to follow shortly) that includes a daily health check with recommendations based on responses and a library of resources on key patient identified topics to empower patients to better manage their recovery. The new pain management information is located in the education library of the mobile app.

Our study had several limitations. Due to resource implications, we recruited only English speaking patients (except in one instance in which an English-speaking spouse participated); future studies might focus on non-English speaking patients. We did not specifically target younger patients for whom the use of mobile technology and social media might be more relevant. Finally, we did not collect data about individual participant's demographic details such as home support, occupation, marital status and level of education and therefore did not stratify our analysis across these differences. We did however obtain rich, in-depth information about the experiences of our patients, with the goal of providing insight into their experiences, rather than on obtaining statistical generalizability. For this reason, the core concepts from our research should be transferable to other centres wanting to develop more patient-centred education materials.

Conclusion

Patients undergoing hip and knee replacement have a wide range of preferences for educational content, modes of delivery and timing to successfully engage and manage their recovery. The findings of our study underscore the importance of multi-modal patient education that can be tailored to individual preferences and experiences. It is important to offer traditional formats for information delivery as well as alternatives using web and mobile technology.

Patients emphasized the need for more comprehensive education concerning pain management following discharge from hospital. Management of acute postoperative pain remains a significant challenge, particularly for those undergoing knee replacements. Given the trend of shortening lengths of stay, patients are coping with acute pain at home; therefore, they require more information on pain medication usage, side effects and guidelines for weaning off the medications. Since completing this study, our site has introduced a new pain management brochure and video, which are also available online and through our new mobile App.

Acknowledgements

Funding for this study was provided by the Canadian Orthopaedic Foundation whose mission is to achieve excellence in bone and joint health, mobility, and function for all Canadians through the advancement of research, education, and care.

We are grateful to the interprofessional team members for all of their contributions to developing patient-centred educational materials. Of course, without our patients this study would not have been possible, and we thank them for all their support and willingness to participate.

Funding

Funding for this study was provided by the Canadian Orthopaedic Foundation. The Canadian Orthopaedic Foundation was not involved in the design, conduct, data interpretation or publication.

Authors' contributions

DK conceived the idea, designed the study, supervised data collection, assisted with data analysis, and prepared and wrote the manuscript with AW. AW was also involved in qualitative data analysis. LP, SR, PD were involved in study conception and design as well as manuscript review. JC conducted the focus groups and interviews and assisted in the qualitative data analysis and manuscript preparation. FW was involved in study conception, design, conducted and/or supervised focus groups and interviews, led the qualitative data analysis and contributed to writing the manuscript. All authors read and approved the final manuscript.

Consent for publication

Consent for publication was contained in the original consent form to participate in the study.

Competing interests

The authors declare that they have no competing interests.

Author details

[1]Sunnybrook Holland Orthopaedic and Arthritic Centre, 43 Wellesley Street East, Toronto, ON M4Y 1H1, Canada. [2]School of Rehabilitation Science, McMaster University, 1400 Main St. W, Hamilton, ON L8S 1C7, Canada. [3]Department of Physical Therapy, University of Toronto, 500 University Avenue, Toronto, ON M5G 1V7, Canada. [4]Department of Occupational Science and Occupational Therapy, University of Toronto, 500 University Avenue, Toronto, ON M5G 1V7, Canada. [5]Centre for Addiction and Mental Health, 33 Russell Street, Toronto, ON M5S 2S1, Canada. [6]Institute of Health Policy Management and Evaluation, Dalla Lana School of Public Health, University of Toronto, 155 College Street, Toronto, ON M5T 3M7, Canada.

References

1. World Health Organization global strategy on integrated people-centred health services 2016–2026 [http://www.who.int/servicedeliverysafety/areas/people-centred-care/global-strategy/en/]. Accessed 29 June 2016.
2. Making the Case for Information: The evidence for investing in high quality health information for patients and the public [http://www.pifonline.org.uk/the-case-for-information-investment-in-patient-information-improves-outcomes-and-reduces-costs/]. Accessed 23 Sept 2015.
3. Macdonnell M, Darzi A. A key to slower health spending growth worldwide will be unlocking innovation to reduce the labor-intensity of care. Health Aff (Millwood). 2013;32(4):653–60.
4. Sandelowski M. Whatever happened to qualitative description? Res Nurs Health. 2000;23(4):334–40.
5. Coyne IT. Sampling in qualitative research. Purposeful and theoretical sampling; merging or clear boundaries? J Adv Nurs. 1997;26(3):623–30.
6. Guba EG. Criteria for assessing the trustworthiness of naturalistic inquiries. Educ Commun Technol. 1981;29:75–91.
7. Morgan DL. Focus groups. Ann Rev Sociol. 1996;22:129–52.
8. Chan EY, Blyth FM, Cheow SL, Fransen M. Postoperative pain following hospital discharge after knee replacement surgery: a patient survey. Pain Manag. 2013;3(3):177–88.
9. Chan EY, Blyth FM, Nairn L, Fransen M. Acute postoperative pain following hospital discharge after total knee arthroplasty. Osteoarthr Cartil. 2013;21(9):1257–63.
10. Clarke H, Woodhouse LJ, Kennedy D, Stratford P, Katz J. Strategies aimed at preventing chronic post-surgical pain: comprehensive Perioperative pain management after Total joint replacement surgery. Physiother Can. 2011;63(3):289–304.
11. Gaglio B, Glasgow RE, Bull SS. Do patient preferences for health information vary by health literacy or numeracy? A qualitative assessment. J Health Commun. 2012;17(Suppl 3):109–21.
12. Macario A, Schilling P, Rubio R, Bhalla A, Goodman S. What questions do patients undergoing lower extremity joint replacement surgery have? BMC Health Serv Res. 2003;3(1):11.
13. Soever LJ, Mackay C, Saryeddine T, Davis AM, Flannery JF, Jaglal SB, Levy C, Mahomed N. Educational needs of patients undergoing total joint arthroplasty. Physiother Can. 2010;62(3):206–14.
14. McDonald S, Page MJ, Beringer K, Wasiak J, Sprowson A. Preoperative education for hip or knee replacement. Cochrane Database Syst Rev. 2014;5:CD003526.
15. McGregor AH, Rylands H, Owen A, Dore CJ, Hughes SP. Does preoperative hip rehabilitation advice improve recovery and patient satisfaction? J Arthroplast. 2004;19(4):464–8.
16. Spalding NJ. Reducing anxiety by pre-operative education: make the future familiar. Occup Ther Int. 2003;10(4):278–93.
17. Go C. Smartphone and tablet ownership on the rise. Ottawa, Canada: Government of Canada; 2015.

23

Application of postoperative autotransfusion in total joint arthroplasty reduces allogeneic blood requirements

Weiping Ji[1], Xianfeng Lin[2], Ruoxia Zhang[2], Pan Tang[2], Jian Mo[2], Xinyi Teng[2], Qiuping Fan[1], Bo Wang[1], Shunwu Fan[2], Jianfeng Zhang[2], Shuai Chen[2*] and Kangmao Huang[2*]

Abstract

Background: Total joint arthroplasty is associated with significant blood loss and often requires blood transfusion. However, allogeneic blood transfusion (ABT) may lead to severe problems, such as immunoreaction and infection. Postoperative autotransfusion, an alternative to ABT, is controversial. We conducted a meta-analysis to evaluate the ability of postoperative autotransfusion to reduce the need for ABT following total knee arthroplasty (TKA) and total hip arthroplasty (THA).

Methods: Systematic literature searches for randomized controlled trials were performed using PubMed, Embase, and the Cochrane Library until February 2016. Relative risks (RRs) and weighted mean differences with 95% confidence intervals (CIs) were calculated using fixed-effect or random-effect models; we also evaluated publication bias and heterogeneity.

Results: Seventeen trials with a total of 2314 patients were included in the meta-analysis. The pooled RRs of ABT rate between autotransfusion and the regular drainage/no drainage groups for TKA and THA were 0.446 (95% CI = 0.287, 0.693; $p < 0.001$) and 0.757 (95% CI = 0.599, 0.958; $p = 0.020$), respectively. In the subgroup analysis performed in TKA patients according to control interventions, the pooled RRs were 0.377 (95% CI = 0.224, 0.634; $p < 0.001$) (compared with regular drainage) and 0.804 (95% CI = 0.453, 1.426, $p = 0.456$) (compared with no drainage). In the subgroup analysis performed for THA, the pooled RRs were 0.536 (95% CI = 0.379, 0.757, $p < 0.001$) (compared with regular drainage) and 1.020 (95% CI = 0.740, 1.405, $p = 0.904$) (compared with no drainage).

Conclusions: Compared to regular drainage, autotransfusion reduces the need for ABT following TKA and THA. This reduction is not present when comparing autotransfusion to no drainage. However, the reliability of the meta-analytic results concerning TKA was limited by significant heterogeneity in methods among the included studies.

Keywords: Postoperative autotransfusion, Total knee arthroplasty, Total hip arthroplasty

* Correspondence: cs30518310@163.com; huangkangmao@zju.edu.cn
[2]Department of Orthopaedic Surgery, Sir Run Run Shaw Hospital, Medical College of Zhejiang University, Hangzhou, China
Full list of author information is available at the end of the article

Background

Total knee arthroplasty (TKA) and total hip arthroplasty (THA) are major orthopedic surgeries. Both procedures are associated with significant blood loss, generally from bone osteotomies, severed muscles, periosteal bleeding, and some patient-related factors such as bleeding disorders and comorbidities [1, 2]. It is estimated that perioperative blood loss is between 1000 mL and 1500 mL in TKA and that 18–95% of patients require donor transfusions [3]. Following primary THA, the rate of allogeneic blood transfusion (ABT) can be as high as 30–40% [4, 5]. However, ABT can lead to infection with human immunodeficiency virus and hepatitis C [6], allergic reactions, anaphylaxis, hemolytic reactions, lung injury, or graft-versus-host disease [7]. Not only may these conditions undermine the success of the surgery, but can also result in death. Moreover, allogeneic blood resources are limited and expensive.

To establish stable postoperative hemoglobin (Hb) levels and to reduce the need for ABT, various alternatives to donor transfusion have been proposed. For example, there has been support for preoperative blood donation [8, 9], acute normovolemic hemodilution [10], erythropoietin injections [11], autologous transfusion systems [12–18], correction of preoperative anemia [19], and pharmacologic agents such as tranexamic acid [20]. The optimal combination of techniques for particular patients and cost-effectiveness remains a matter of debate.

Recently, the concept of reinfusing blood collected from drains following TKA and THA has gained the interest of orthopedists. Drains are used to prevent hematoma accumulation and decrease the possibility of prolonged wound healing and infection [21]. Recent studies have reported that the transfusion of autologous blood has no effect in the majority of cases, but some studies support the method [22–24]. Furthermore, the usefulness of autotransfusion is uncertain due to methodological difficulties, such as no formal power analysis for study size and significance level, different transfusion triggers, and different autotransfusion devices [23]. In order to clarify the issue, we performed a meta-analysis that evaluated ABT rate, postoperative Hb, and adverse effects after total joint arthroplasty when using autotransfusion drainage, and the use of regular drainage or no drainage.

Methods

Database search

A systematic review was performed in accordance with guidelines [25]. All holdings of PubMed, the Cochrane Library, and Embase were searched for relevant trials published until February 2016 using the following terms: (1) "autotransfusion," "autologous blood transfusion," "blood transfusion," or "autologous transfusion"; (2) "total knee arthroplasty," "total knee replacement," "TKA," "total hip arthroplasty," "total hip replacement," or "THA"; and (3) "postoperative," or "post-operation." Only English studies with full texts were included in the final analysis. We chose the most recent study if several publications reported on the same set of patients. The search strategy is provided in Additional file 1.

Inclusion and exclusion criteria

Eligible literature was carefully identified and selected according to the flow chart in Fig. 1. Studies were included on the basis of the following criteria: (1) a randomized controlled trial (RCT) was designed; (2) the comparison was between a postoperative autotransfusion system and no drainage/regular drainage (i.e., suction drainage, vacuum drainage, hemovac drainage); (3) the results included key data such as transfusion rate; and (4) patients underwent total joint replacement. The exclusion criteria were as follows: (1) an anticoagulant was added to the autotransfusion system; (2) patients underwent bilateral surgery or revision surgery; and (3) patients underwent TKA without a tourniquet because its use would have affected blood loss [26].

Study selection and data extraction

Two authors (Weiping Ji and Xianfeng Lin) reviewed all titles and abstracts independently to determine which articles met the inclusion criteria. All variables and

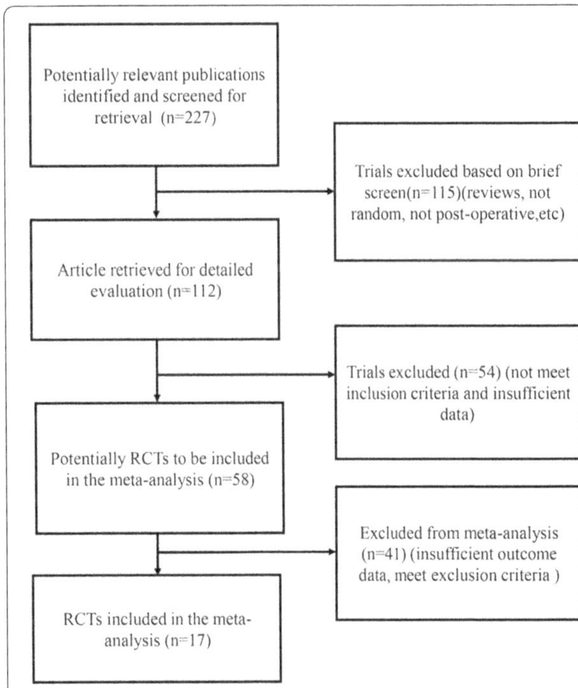

Fig. 1 Flowchart for selecting studies

outcomes of interest were extracted independently. The authors solved disagreements by in-person discussion.

The study group referred to the autotransfusion group and the control group encompassed the regular drainage group and no drainage group. We extracted the following characteristics for all studies: year, country of study, type of surgery, population information (age, sample size and gender), autotransfusion systems, and funding sources. The outcomes included the numbers of patients needing allogeneic transfusion, postoperative Hb levels on day 1, day 2, day 3, and day 5, and adverse effects. In this meta-analysis, the transfusion rate was the primary outcome and defined as the rate of patients receiving allogeneic transfusion in both the study group and regular drainage/no drainage group postoperatively during hospitalization. The adverse events included complications such as wound infection and febrile reactions recorded in-hospital. Data relating to Hb levels and adverse effects were extracted to assess recovery after total joint arthroplasty. Blood loss volume, amount of blood transfusion per patient, length of hospital stay, and adverse reactions such as deep vein thrombosis (DVT) and swelling were extracted (data not shown), but the data were insufficient to be included in the meta-analysis.

Validity assessment

The Cochrane Collaboration's tool was used to assess the bias of all eligible RCTs [27]. The assessment criteria were as follows: (1) the method of randomization was adequate; (2) the treatment allocation was concealed; (3) the groups were similar in the most important prognostic indicators at baseline; (4) the patients were blinded to the intervention; (5) the caregivers were blinded to the intervention; (6) the outcome assessors were blinded to the intervention; (7) co-interventions were controlled; (8) compliance was acceptable in all groups; (9) the dropout rate was described and acceptable; (10) the timing of assessment in all groups was the same; and (11) intention-to-treat analysis was performed. We awarded a score of 1 for each item if it was completely met; scores of 0.5, 0, and N/A were awarded for partly met, not met, and unclear, respectively. The total score of each study was then calculated and the validity scores of >6 were considered to represent a low degree of bias.

Statistical analysis

Statistical analyses were performed with STATA Version 12.0 (StataCorp LP, College Station, TX, USA). Relative risks (RRs) and corresponding 95% confidence intervals (CIs) were estimated by fixed-effect or random-effect meta-analyses. Weighted mean difference was used to perform meta-analysis for continuous outcomes. The significance of the pooled RRs was evaluated by a Z-test and $p < 0.05$. The I^2 statistic was used to evaluate heterogeneity. A random-effect model was used when significant heterogeneity was detected among studies ($p < 0.1$, $I^2 > 50\%$). Otherwise, a fixed-effect model was adopted ($I^2 < 50\%$, $p > 0.1$). The fixed-effect model was adopted if a small number of studies (< 5) were included in the meta-analysis. Considering the source of heterogeneity, the studies were classified by control intervention. To explain some of the clinical heterogeneity observed in the included trials, a subgroup analysis by type of control intervention was performed for the primary outcome. Two sensitivity analyses were performed to assess the stability of pooled effects for TKA and THA. The RRs calculated after excluding a single study were compared with initial effects (before excluding). The results could be considered stable if the RRs did not change significantly (not beyond the initial CI). Egger's test and Begg's test were used to test for publication bias by assessing the association between intervention effects and a measure of study size. Egger's test used actual standardized effect size while Begg's test used ranks of effect sizes and variances. Funnel plots were used to depict asymmetry on visual inspection. A value of >0.05 for Pr > |z| (continuity correct) suggested no publication bias [28]. All p-values were two-sided.

Results

Study characteristics

Seventeen RCTs [2, 7, 12–18, 22–24, 29–33] were assessed and 2314 patients were included in the meta-analysis (Table 1). Sample sizes ranged from 36 to 231. Three studies included two control groups [13, 18, 33]. Another three studies included two types of surgery: TKA and THA [2, 17, 23]. The criteria for transfusion thresholds were varied and based on authors' experiences, anesthetists' protocols, or hospital policies (data not shown). The data of tranexamic acid use were rarely provided in the included studies. All of the included studies were published in 1992 or later. Validity scores are shown in Table 2 and two studies with validity scores of <6 were considered as having a high degree of bias [16, 33].

Meta-analysis findings for TKA

The autotransfusion group had a significantly lower requirement for postoperative ABT ($p < 0.001$; RR = 0.446 [95% CI = 0.287, 0.693]; $I^2 > 50\%$) than the regular drainage/no drainage group (Fig. 2). Although the autotransfusion group did not show superior reductions in ABT requirements when compared with the no-drainage group ($p = 0.456$; RR = 0.804 [95% CI = 0.453, 1.426]; $I^2 < 30\%$), a significant reduction in ABT requirements was noted when compared with the regular drainage group ($p < 0.001$; RR = 0.377 [95% CI = 0.224, 0.634];

Table 1 Characteristics of the studies included in the meta-analysis

Study	Year	Country	Type of surgery	Sample size	Age	Men%	transfusion threshold (Hb)	Study group		Control group	
								Patients number (n)	Autotransfusion system	Patients number (n)	Treatment
Heddle [12]	1992	Canada	TKA	79	70.16	35.4	<9 g/dl	39	Solcotrans	40	Regular drain
Adalberth [13]	1998	Sweden	TKA	73	72	45.6	<9 g/dl	24	Solcotrans	25 24	Regular drain No drain
Thomas [14]	2001	UK	TKA	231	69.63	42.9	<9 g/dl	115	Cell Saver 5 Haemonetics	116	Regular drain
Cheng [15]	2005	Hong Kong	TKA	60	70.53	30	<9 g/dl	26	DONOR	34	Regular drain
Dramis [29]	2006	UK	TKA	49	70.04	30.61	<9 g/dl	32	CellTrans	17	Regular drain
Abuzakuk [30]	2007	UK	TKA	104	68.5	41.34	<9 g/dl	52	Bellovac	52	Regular drain
Moonen [17]	2007	UK	TKA THA	77 83	69.25	14.38	ASA classification	45 35	Bellovac, AstraTech AB Bellovac, AstraTech AB	32 48	Regular drain Regular drain
Smith [16]	2007	UK	THA	158	74.54	48.1	<8 g/dl	76	ABTrans	82	Regular drain
Amin [31]	2008	UK	TKA	178	70.35	46.07	<8 g/dl	92	Bellovac	86	Regular drain
Atay [2]	2010	Turkey	THA TKA	36 41	59.33 66.76	33.33 21.95	<8 g/dl	17 20	Transolog Transolog	19 21	Regular drain Regular drain
Cheung [18]	2010	UK	THA	153	68.12	45.1	Made by the ward doctors	53	Bellovac	52 48	Regular drain No drain
Horstmann [32]	2012	Netherland	THA	100	68.8	27	ASA classification	50	Bellovac	50	No drain
Kleinert [33]	2012	Switzerland	THA	120	65.33	49.17	<8 g/dl	40	Bellovac	40 40	Regular drain No drain
Sarkanovic [7]	2013	Serbia	TKA	112	66.5	23.21	<8.5 g/dl	55	Cell Saver	57	Regular drain
Horstmann [24]	2014	Netherland	TKA	115	68.48	29.57	ASA classification	59	Bellovac	56	No drain
Thomassen [23]	2014	Netherland	TKA THA	165 219	68.9	25.58	<8 g/dl	78 116	Bellovac Bellovac	87 103	No drain No drain
Teetzmann [22]	2014	Norway	THA	161	73	37.94	clinical judgement	74	Sangvia	87	No drain

TKA total knee arthroplasty, *THA* total hip arthroplasty

$I^2 > 50\%$). The sensitivity analyses revealed stable results (Additional file 2: Figure S1), namely that the excluded studies did not influence the pooled RRs. The pooled results of post-operation Hb level (four studies included) suggested that the autotransfusion group had higher post-operative Hb levels than the regular drainage/no drainage group (Additional file 3: Figure S2). Six studies reported wound infections (three studies included) and febrile reactions (three studies included). We found no significant differences between the autotransfusion group and the regular drainage/no drainage group (Additional file 4: Figure S3). The reliability of these results was limited by the small number of studies included (< 5).

Meta-analysis findings for THA

The autotransfusion group had a significantly reduced need for postoperative ABT ($p = 0.020$; RR = 0.757 [95% CI = 0.599, 0.958]; $I^2 < 30\%$) than the regular drainage/no drainage group (Fig. 3). Similar results were found when the autotransfusion group was compared with the regular drainage group and no-drainage groups. Specifically, ABT requirements significantly decreased when the autotransfusion group was compared with the regular drainage group ($p < 0.001$; RR = 0.536 [95% CI = 0.379, 0.757]; $I^2 < 30\%$). However, the autotransfusion group did not demonstrate a significant reduction in ABT requirements compared with the no-drainage group ($p = 0.904$; RR = 1.020 [95% CI = 0.740, 1.405]; $I^2 < 30\%$). Sensitivity analyses proved the results to be stable (Additional file 5: Figure S4). The autotransfusion group also had higher Hb levels (two studies included) compared with the regular drainage/no drainage group (Additional file 6: Figure S5). The pooled results for adverse effects (four studies reporting wound infections and two studies reporting febrile reactions) showed no significant differences between the groups (Additional file 7: Figure S6). The small number of included studies (< 5) limited the reliability of these results.

Publication bias

Egger's and Begg's tests suggested a lack of publication bias with respect to ABT rate (Additional file 8: Table S1). According to this analysis, the included studies were relatively comprehensive and yielded statistically reliable results. The funnel plots did not reveal obvious asymmetry of the included studies (Additional file 9: Figure S7 and Additional file 10: Figure S8).

Table 2 Risk of bias in included studies

Study	Year	A	B	C	D	E	F	G	H	I	J	K	Total score
Heddle [12]	1992	1	1	1	0	0	N/A	1	1	N/A	1	1	7
Adalberth [13]	1998	1	1	0.5	1	1	N/A	1	1	N/A	1	1	8.5
Thomas [14]	2001	1	1	0	0.5	1	N/A	1	1	N/A	1	1	7.5
Cheng [15]	2005	1	1	0.5	1	0	N/A	0.5	1	N/A	1	1	7
Dramis [29]	2006	1	N/A	0.5	N/A	N/A	N/A	1	1	0.5	1	1	6
Abuzakuk [30]	2007	1	1	0.5	0.5	0.5	N/A	1	N/A	N/A	1	1	6.5
Moonen [17]	2007	1	1	1	N/A	N/A	N/A	1	1	0.5	1	1	7.5
Smith [16]	2007	1	1	0.5	N/A	N/A	N/A	1	N/A	N/A	1	1	5.5
Amin [31]	2008	1	1	0.5	1	1	N/A	1	N/A	N/A	1	1	7.5
Atay [2]	2010	1	1	0.5	N/A	N/A	N/A	1	1	N/A	1	1	6.5
Cheung [18]	2010	1	1	0.5	N/A	0	N/A	1	1	N/A	1	1	6.5
Horstmann [32]	2012	1	1	0.5	1	0.5	N/A	1	N/A	N/A	1	1	7
Kleinert [33]	2012	1	N/A	0.5	N/A	N/A	N/A	1	N/A	N/A	1	1	4.5
Sarkanovic [7]	2013	1	1	1	N/A	N/A	N/A	1	N/A	N/A	1	1	6
Horstmann [24]	2014	1	1	0	0.5	1	N/A	1	1	N/A	1	1	7.5
Thomassen [22]	2014	1	1	0.5	N/A	N/A	1	1	1	N/A	1	1	7.5
Teetzmann [23]	2014	1	N/A	0.5	N/A	N/A	N/A	1	1	1	1	1	6.5

RCT randomized controlled trial, *N/A* not clear

Eleven Cochrane Back Review Group criteria: (A) the method of randomization was adequate; (B) the treatment allocation was concealed; (C) the groups were similar in the most important prognostic indicators at the baseline; (D) the patients were blinded to the intervention; (E) the caregivers were blinded to the intervention; (F) the outcome assessors were blinded to the intervention; (G) co-interventions were controlled; (H) compliance was acceptable in all groups; (I) the dropout rate was described and acceptable; (J) the timing of assessment in all groups was the same; and (K) intention-to-treat analysis was performed

Discussion

We conducted a meta-analysis to determine the effectiveness and safety of postoperative autotransfusion for TKA and THA. The findings revealed that postoperative autotransfusion could significantly reduce the number of patients who require postoperative ABT for TKA and THA compared with patients who receive regular drainage. However, the effect was not sustained when comparing autotransfusion with no drainage. The autotransfusion group had higher Hb levels than the regular

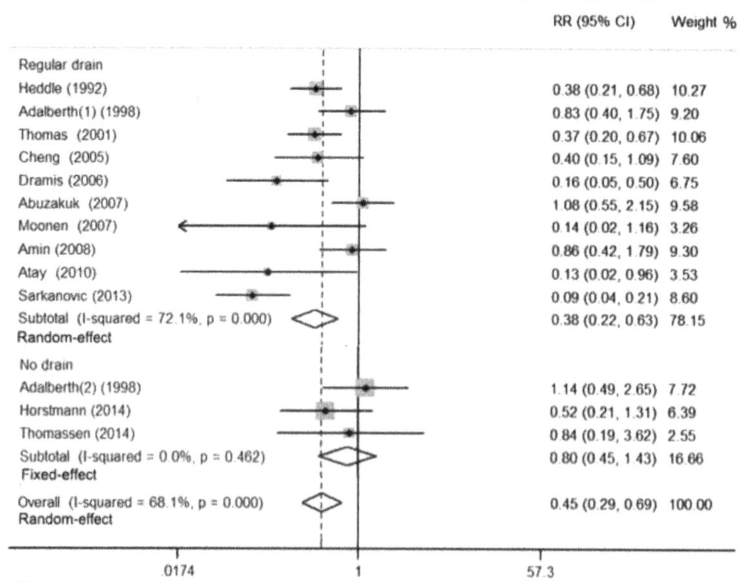

Fig. 2 Relative risk (RR) of postoperative ABT requirements in TKA. ABT, allogeneic blood transfusion; TKA, total knee arthroplasty

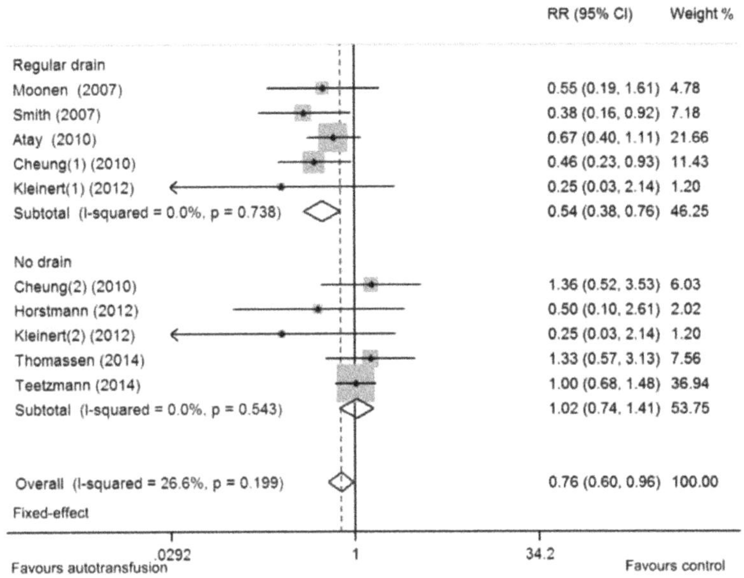

Fig. 3 Relative risk (RR) of postoperative ABT requirements in THA. ABT, allogeneic blood transfusion; THA, total hip arthroplasty

drainage/no drainage group, and no significant difference in adverse reactions was observed between the two groups.

Although our results were positive for autotransfusion, the heterogeneity of the RRs for ABT rate in TKA was a limitation of the meta-analysis. Thus, the reliability of our meta-analytic estimates concerning TKA is questionable due to significant heterogeneity in methodologies. To reduce this heterogeneity in future trials, factors such as the type of system used, Hb triggers, comparison groups, and anesthesia methods should be taken into account. With this in mind, we performed subgroup and sensitivity analyses of the transfusion rates in TKA and THA. We believe that the variability in autotransfusion systems was an important consideration as at least seven autotransfusion systems were used in the 17 RCTs. Moreover, the skill of the operator performing blood re-infusion varied, which could have caused the differences in the volumes of re-infused blood among the studies. Insufficient data from existing RCTs limited our ability to analyze the effects of the different systems.

A previous meta-analysis drew different and incomplete conclusions regarding the benefits of autotransfusion. Zhao et al. and Markar et al. showed that autotransfusion drainage effectively reduced the demand for ABT after total joint arthroplasty when compared with regular drainage [34, 35]. However, Li et al. found no statistically significant differences in ABT rate between autotransfusion drainage and no/regular drainage in THA [36], which could be explained by the fact that only one study was included in the comparison [33].

Our meta-analysis revealed some distinct differences from the findings of previous studies. First, in this study, strict inclusion and exclusion criteria were observed in order to omit studies that implemented anticoagulants in the autotransfusion system [37, 38] or were performed without a tourniquet. Anticoagulants and tourniquets would affect blood loss during total joint arthroplasty. Second, two new RCTs were published [22, 23], neither of which showed a significant effect of the autotransfusion system compared with no drainage. In addition, few systematic reviews have considered the differences between autotransfusion drainage and no drainage for both TKA and THA. Finally, our research synthetically analyzed all related studies and gathered comprehensive results regarding the effects of autotransfusion in patients who underwent total joint arthroplasty.

The most important finding of this meta-analysis was that there was no significant difference in ABT rate between autotransfusion drainage and no-drainage. Recently, Thomassen et al. examined 575 patients who underwent primary hip and knee replacement with autotransfusion or no drainage [23]. The authors did not identify any significant difference in the need for ABT between the groups, which is in accordance with our results and those of many other studies (e.g., [13, 18, 22, 24, 32, 33]. Although the autotransfusion group had a significant reduction of ABT rate compared with the regular drainage/no drainage group in our meta-analysis, it is clear that autotransfusion drainage and no drainage have similar effects on ABT reduction.

To date, it remains controversial whether autotransfusion is superior to regular drainage. Atay et al. and

Moonen et al. reported that the need for ABT was decreased by autotransfusion in both TKA and THA [2, 17]. Heddle et al. and others reported the same results for TKA alone [12, 14]. In contrast, some studies have shown that the use of an autotransfusion system fails to reduce the need for ABT after TKA [30, 31] or THA [18, 33]. This meta-analysis identified a statistically significant reduction in ABT requirements in patients who underwent autotransfusion drainage when compared with those who received regular drainage following TKA or THA. The previous meta-analyses performed by Markar et al. and Zhao et al. reported the same results for TKA alone [34, 35]. Other meta-analyses also compared regular drainage and no drainage for TKA [39] and THA [40], but there was no support for regular drainage in these reports. In conclusion, autotransfusion drainage and no drainage were superior to regular drainage. The mechanisms underlying these results should be explored in the future.

Adverse reactions including wound infection and febrile reactions were similar in the two groups, which mirrors the findings of previous meta-analyses [35, 36]. However, significant differences were noted by Zhao et al. between autotransfusion drainage and suction drainage in TKA with regard to febrile reactions [34]. This echoes Soosman's report [41], which suggested a higher rate of febrile reactions than previous reports. Considering the low incidence of febrile reactions and wound infections in our results, we can only infer that autotransfusion drainage had a similar degree of safety when compared with regular drainage/no drainage. Notably, the number of included studies was small, limiting the reliability of these results. Further studies with sufficient data are required to evaluate the safety of autotransfusion systems.

We did not pool the data regarding blood loss volume, amount of blood transfusion per patient, length of hospital stay, and adverse reactions such as DVT and swelling because of insufficient data. Most RCTs stated the protocol for transfusion triggers, but whether strict transfusion rules were followed remains unknown. In addition, the transfusion triggers were not identical among the different RCTs. Thus, a subgroup analysis of transfusion triggers was not appropriate.

This meta-analysis has some limitations. First, the reliability of pooled results concerning TKA is limited by significant heterogeneity in methodological approaches. Second, the number of studies including data related to secondary outcomes was small. Thus, further meta-analyses including more studies and more information on safety outcomes are required in the future. Third, the results were based on many unadjusted factors. A more precise analysis should be conducted that allows for the time of randomization, drain insertion time, timing of drain opening and closing, and financial factors. Finally, the protocol for the systematic review was not prospectively registered. Thus, the transparency of our approach cannot be ascertained.

Conclusion

Autotransfusion systems reduce the need for ABT compared with regular drainage, but this reduction is not maintained in comparison to procedures that employ no drainage. The use of autotransfusion is characterized by a reduced need for ABT, higher Hb levels, and similar adverse reactions when compared with control groups (regular drainage and no drainage). However, the reliability of our assessment of secondary outcomes was limited by the inclusion of a small number of studies including these data. Transfusion triggers and the operation procedure should be explored in future study.

Additional files

Additional file 1: Search strategy. (DOCX 14 kb)

Additional file 2: Figure S1. Sensitivity analysis of postoperative ABT requirements in TKA. ABT, allogeneic blood transfusion; TKA, total knee arthroplasty. (TIFF 106 kb)

Additional file 3: Figure S2. Weighted mean differences (WMDs) of postoperative hemoglobin (Hb) level in TKA. TKA, total knee arthroplasty. (TIFF 190 kb)

Additional file 4: Figure S3. Relative risk (RR) of postoperative adverse reactions in TKA. TKA, total knee arthroplasty. (TIFF 82 kb)

Additional file 5: Figure S4. Sensitivity analysis of postoperative ABT requirements in THA. ABT, allogeneic blood transfusion; THA, total hip arthroplasty. (TIFF 84 kb)

Additional file 6: Figure S5. Weighted mean differences (WMDs) of postoperative hemoglobin (Hb) level in THA. THA, total hip arthroplasty. (TIFF 124 kb)

Additional file 7: Figure S6. Relative risk (RR) of postoperative adverse reactions in THA. THA, total hip arthroplasty. (TIFF 78 kb)

Additional file 8: Table S1. Publication bias determined using the Egger and Begg's tests. (DOCX 18 kb)

Additional file 9: Figure S7. Funnel plot of included studies for TKA. TKA, total knee arthroplasty. (TIFF 40 kb)

Additional file 10: Figure S8. Funnel plot of included studies for THA. THA, total hip arthroplasty. (TIFF 39 kb)

Additional file 11: Dataset. The dataset supporting the conclusions of this article. (XLSX 14 kb)

Additional file 12: Table S2. The transfusion thresholds and funding source of included studies. (DOCX 87 kb)

Abbreviations

ABT: Allogeneic blood transfusion; CIs: Confidence intervals; DVT: Deep vein thrombosis; Hb: Hemoglobin; PRISMA: Preferred Reporting Items for Systematic Reviews and Meta-Analyses; RR: Relative risk; THA: Total hip arthroplasty; TKA: Total knee arthroplasty

Acknowledgements

Not applicable.

Funding

Zhejiang Province education department subject (Y201017108).

Authors' contributions
Conceived and designed the analysis: WPJ XFL RXZ. Performed the analysis: WPJ XFL RXZ. Revised the paper/Analysis tools: PT JM XYT QPF BW SWF JFZ SC KMH. Wrote the paper: WPJ XFL RXZ. All authors read and approved the final manuscript.

Consent for publication
Not applicable.

Competing interests
The authors declare that they have no competing interests.

Author details
[1]Department of Orthopaedic Surgery, Lishui City People's Hospital, the Sixth Affiliated Hospital of Wenzhou Medical University, Lishui, China. [2]Department of Orthopaedic Surgery, Sir Run Run Shaw Hospital, Medical College of Zhejiang University, Hangzhou, China.

References

1. Lotke PA, Faralli VJ, Orenstein EM, Ecker ML. Blood loss after total knee replacement. Effects of tourniquet release and continuous passive motion. J Bone Joint Surg Am. 1991;73(7):1037–40.
2. Atay EF, Guven M, Altintas F, Kadioglu B, Ceviz E, Ipek S. Allogeneic blood transfusion decreases with postoperative autotransfusion in hip and knee arthroplasty. Acta Orthop Traumatol Turc. 2010;44(4):306–12.
3. Aksoy Y, Altinel L, Kose KC. The comparison of the effects of intraoperative bleeding control and postoperative drain clamping methods on the postoperative blood loss and the need for transfusion following total knee arthroplasty. Acta Orthop Traumatol Turc. 2011;45(3):190–4.
4. Sehat KR, Evans RL, Newman JH. Hidden blood loss following hip and knee arthroplasty. Correct management of blood loss should take hidden loss into account. J Bone Joint Surg Br. 2004;86(4):561–5.
5. Rosencher N, Kerkkamp HE, Macheras G, Munuera LM, Menichella G, Barton DM, Cremers S, Abraham IL. Orthopedic surgery transfusion hemoglobin European overview (OSTHEO) study: blood management in elective knee and hip arthroplasty in Europe. Transfusion. 2003;43(4):459–69.
6. Dodd RY. Current estimates of transfusion safety worldwide. Dev Biol (Basel). 2005;120:3–10.
7. Sarkanovic ML, Gvozdenovic L, Savic D, Ilic MP, Jovanovic G. Autologous blood transfusion in total knee replacement surgery. Vojnosanit Pregl. 2013;70(3):274–8.
8. Toy PT, Kaplan EB, McVay PA, Lee SJ, Strauss RG, Stehling LC. Blood loss and replacement in total hip arthroplasty: a multicenter study. The preoperative autologous blood donation study group. Transfusion. 1992;32(1):63–7.
9. Woolson ST, Pottorff G. Use of preoperatively deposited autologous blood for total knee replacement. Orthopedics. 1993;16(2):137–41. discussion 141-132
10. Oishi CS, D'Lima DD, Morris BA, Hardwick ME, Berkowitz SD, Colwell CW Jr. Hemodilution with other blood reinfusion techniques in total hip arthroplasty. Clin Orthop Relat Res. 1997;339
11. Sparling EA, Nelson CL, Lavender R, Smith J. The use of erythropoietin in the management of Jehovah's witnesses who have revision total hip arthroplasty. J Bone Joint Surg Am. 1996;78(10):1548–52.
12. Heddle NM, Brox WT, Klama LN, Dickson LL, Levine MN. A randomized trial on the efficacy of an autologous blood drainage and transfusion device in patients undergoing elective knee arthroplasty. Transfusion. 1992;32(8):742–6.
13. Adalberth G, Bystrom S, Kolstad K, Mallmin H, Milbrink J. Postoperative drainage of knee arthroplasty is not necessary: a randomized study of 90 patients. Acta Orthop Scand. 1998;69(5):475–8.
14. Thomas D, Wareham K, Cohen D, Hutchings H. Autologous blood transfusion in total knee replacement surgery. Br J Anaesth. 2001;86(5):669–73.
15. Cheng SC, Hung TS, Tse PY. Investigation of the use of drained blood reinfusion after total knee arthroplasty: a prospective randomised controlled study. J Orthop Surg (Hong Kong). 2005;13(2):120–4.
16. Smith LK, Williams DH, Langkamer VG. Post-operative blood salvage with autologous retransfusion in primary total hip replacement. J Bone Joint Surg Br. 2007;89(8):1092–7.
17. Moonen AF, Knoors NT, van Os JJ, Verburg AD, Pilot P. Retransfusion of filtered shed blood in primary total hip and knee arthroplasty: a prospective randomized clinical trial. Transfusion. 2007;47(3):379–84.
18. Cheung G, Carmont MR, Bing AJ, Kuiper JH, Alcock RJ, Graham NM. No drain, autologous transfusion drain or suction drain? A randomised prospective study in total hip replacement surgery of 168 patients. Acta Orthop Belg. 2010;76(5):619–27.
19. Strumper D, Weber EW, Gielen-Wijffels S, Van Drumpt R, Bulstra S, Slappendel R, Durieux ME, Marcus MA. Clinical efficacy of postoperative autologous transfusion of filtered shed blood in hip and knee arthroplasty. Transfusion. 2004;44(11):1567–71.
20. Ralley FE, Berta D, Binns V, Howard J, Naudie DD. One intraoperative dose of tranexamic acid for patients having primary hip or knee arthroplasty. Clin Orthop Relat Res. 2010;468(7):1905–11.
21. Beer KJ, Lombardi AV Jr, Mallory TH, Vaughn BK. The efficacy of suction drains after routine total joint arthroplasty. J Bone Joint Surg Am. 1991;73(4):584–7.
22. Teetzmann R, Sorensen B, Liseth K, Opheim E, Hervig T. Effects of the Sangvia blood collection system on patients undergoing elective hip surgery. Transfus Apher Sci. 2014;51(2):91–6.
23. Thomassen BJ, den Hollander PH, Kaptijn HH, Nelissen RG, Pilot P. Autologous wound drains have no effect on allogeneic blood transfusions in primary total hip and knee replacement: a three-arm randomised trial. Bone Joint J. 2014;96-B(6):765–71.
24. Horstmann W, Kuipers B, Ohanis D, Slappendel R, Kollen B, Verheyen C. Autologous re-transfusion drain compared with no drain in total knee arthroplasty: a randomised controlled trial. Blood Transfus. 2014;12(Suppl 1):s176–81.
25. Moher D, Liberati A, Tetzlaff J, Altman DG. Preferred reporting items for systematic reviews and meta-analyses: the PRISMA statement. Int J Surg. 2010;8(5):336–41.
26. Smith TO, Hing CB: A meta-analysis of tourniquet assisted arthroscopic knee surgery. Knee 2009, 16(5):317–321.
27. van Tulder M, Furlan A, Bombardier C, Bouter L. Updated method guidelines for systematic reviews in the cochrane collaboration back review group. Spine (Phila Pa 1976). 2003;28(12):1290–9.
28. Higgins JPT GSe: Cochrane Handbook for Systematic Reviews of Interventions Version 5.1.0 [updated March 2011]. The Cochrane Collaboration 2011, Available from http://www.handbook.cochrane.org/.
29. Dramis A, Plewes J. Autologous blood transfusion after primary unilateral total knee replacement surgery. Acta Orthop Belg. 2006;72(1):15–7.
30. Abuzakuk T, Senthil KV, Shenava Y, Bulstrode C, Skinner JA, Cannon SR, Briggs TW. Autotransfusion drains in total knee replacement. Are they alternatives to homologous transfusion? Int Orthop. 2007;31(2):235–9.
31. Amin A, Watson A, Mangwani J, Nawabi DH, Ahluwalia R, Loeffler M. A prospective randomised controlled trial of autologous retransfusion in total knee replacement. J Bone Joint Surg Br. 2008;90(4):451–4.
32. Horstmann WG, Kuipers BM, Slappendel R, Castelein RM, Kollen BJ, Verheyen CC. Postoperative autologous blood transfusion drain or no drain in primary total hip arthroplasty? A randomised controlled trial. Int Orthop. 2012;36(10):2033–9.
33. Kleinert K, Werner C, Mamisch-Saupe N, Kalberer F, Dora C. Closed suction drainage with or without re-transfusion of filtered shed blood does not offer advantages in primary non-cemented total hip replacement using a direct anterior approach. Arch Orthop Trauma Surg. 2012;132(1):131–6.
34. Haien Z, Yong J, Baoan M, Mingjun G, Qingyu F. Post-operative auto-transfusion in total hip or knee arthroplasty: a meta-analysis of randomized controlled trials. PLoS One. 2013;8(1):e55073.
35. Markar SR, Jones GG, Karthikesalingam A, Segaren N, Patel RV. Transfusion drains versus suction drains in total knee replacement: meta-analysis. Knee Surg Sports Traumatol Arthrosc. 2012;20(9):1766–72.
36. Li N, Li P, Liu M, Wang D, Xia L. Comparison between autologous blood transfusion drainage and no drainage/closed-suction drainage in primary total hip arthroplasty: a meta-analysis. Arch Orthop Trauma Surg. 2014;134(11):1623–31.

37. Rs M, Ic C, Jh N. Postoperative collection and reinfusion of autologous blood in total knee arthroplasty. Ann R Coll Surg Engl. 1991;6
38. Newman JH, Bowers M, Murphy J, Newman JH, Bowers M, Murphy J. The clinical advantages of autologous transfusion. Acoustics Speech & Signal Processing Newsletter IEEE. 1997;79(4):630–2.
39. Quinn M, Bowe A, Galvin R, Dawson P, O'Byrne J. The use of postoperative suction drainage in total knee arthroplasty: a systematic review. Int Orthop. 2015;39(4):653–8.
40. Kelly EG, Cashman JP, Imran FH, Conroy R, O'Byrne J. Systematic review and meta-analysis of closed suction drainage versus non-drainage in primary hip arthroplasty. Surg Technol Int. 2014;24:295–301.
41. So-Osman C, Nelissen RG, Eikenboom HC, Brand A. Efficacy, safety and user-friendliness of two devices for postoperative autologous shed red blood cell re-infusion in elective orthopaedic surgery patients: a randomized pilot study. Transfus Med. 2006;16(5):321–8.

24

More complications in uncemented compared to cemented hemiarthroplasty for displaced femoral neck fractures: a randomized controlled trial of 201 patients, with one year follow-up

Sophie Moerman[1*], Nina M. C. Mathijssen[1], Dieu D. Niesten[1], Roeland Riedijk[2], Willard J. Rijnberg[3], Sander Koëter[4], Keetie Kremers van de Hei[4], Wim E. Tuinebreijer[5], Tim L. Molenaar[1], Rob G. H. H. Nelissen[6] and Anne J. H. Vochteloo[7]

Abstract

Background: It is unclear whether cemented or uncemented hemiarthroplasty is the best treatment option in elderly patients with displaced femoral neck fractures. Previous randomized trials comparing cemented and uncemented hemiarthroplasty have conflicting results. We conducted a randomized controlled trial to compare cemented and uncemented hemiarthroplasty.

Methods: This multicenter parallel-randomized controlled trial included patients of 70 years and older with a displaced femoral neck fracture (Garden type III or IV). Inclusion was between August 2008 and June 2012. Patients were randomized between a cemented hemiarthroplasty, type Müller Straight Stem or an uncemented hemiarthroplasty, type DB-10. Primary outcomes were complications, operation time, functional outcome (measured by Timed-Up-and-Go (TUG) and Groningen Activity Restriction Scale (GARS)) and mid-thigh pain. Health Related Quality of Life (HRQoL, expressed with the SF-12) was measured as an secondary outcome. Follow up was 1 year.

Results: In total 201 patients were included in the study (91 uncemented, 110 cemented hemiarthroplasties) The uncemented group showed more major local complications (intra- and postoperative fractures and dislocations) odds ratio (95% confidence interval) 3.36 (1.40 to 8.11). There was no difference in mean operation time (57.3 vs 55. 4 min). There were no differences in functional outcomes (TUG 12.8 (9.4) vs. 13.9 (9.0), GARS 43.2 (19.7) vs. 39.2 (16.5)) and mid-thigh pain (18.6 vs 21.6%). Physical component SF-12 HRQoLwas lower in the uncemented group (30.3 vs. 35.3 $p < 0.05$ after six weeks, 33.8 vs 38.5 $p < 0.05$ after 12 weeks).

Conclusion: A cemented hemiarthroplasty in elderly patients with a displaced femoral neck fracture results in less complications compared to an uncemented hemiarthroplasty.

Keywords: Hip fracture, Arthroplasty, Bone cement, Complication

* Correspondence: sophie.moerman@rdgg.nl
[1]Department of Orthopaedics, Reinier de Graaf Group, Reinier de Graafweg 5, 2625 AD Delft, The Netherlands
Full list of author information is available at the end of the article

Background

Hip fractures are a rising problem in our aging society. An increase in the incidence of hip fractures in Europe from 615.000 in 2010 to 815.000 in 2025 (+32%) due to demographic changes is expected [1]. Elderly patients with a dislocated femoral neck can be treated effectively with hemiarthroplasty [2]. However, there is a persistent controversy regarding the use of cement [3].

In cemented hemiarthroplasties, polymethylmethacrylate bone cement is used during surgery to create a solid bone-implant interface. A potential advantage of cement is less post-operative mid-thigh pain, as the hemiarthroplasty is more firmly fixed within the femur [4]. A potential negative effect of using cement is the Bone Cement Implantation Syndrome (BCIS), characterized by hypoxia and/or hypotension in combination with an unexpected loss of consciousness which occasionally occurs following cement insertion [5]. This complication may be fatal.

Uncemented hemiarthroplasties are placed press-fit in the femur. In the weeks after the surgery the bond between femur and the stem is dependent on osseous integration [6]. However, bone quality is generally poor in elderly hip fracture patients, which may lead to periprosthetic fractures during press-fit placement or inadequate bony in-growth post-operatively [7].

Both NICE and AAOS guidelines advise to use cemented implants [2, 8]. However, despite these guidelines, database studies show that 22 to 34% of the hemiarthroplasties are used without cement [9, 10].

The Cochrane review of 2011 included six trials comparing cemented and uncemented hemiarthroplasty and demonstrated a reduction of the amount of postoperative pain, an improvement in postoperative function and less implant-related complications when cement was used, but a longer operation time. There was no difference in adverse events or mortality [3]. After this review three more randomized trials were published. One found no difference in functional outcome, complications and mortality [11]. Another found more complications (subsidence, intraoperative fracture and postoperative fracture) in the uncemented group, with no differences in pain or mortality [12]. The third trial found better functional outcomes and less intraoperative fractures in the cemented group [13]. Thus the controversy whether to use an cemented or uncemented hemi arthroplasty in the older patients with a displaced femoral neck fracture persists.

Therefore, we compared uncemented and cemented hemiartroplasties in a parallel randomized controlled trial. We hypothesized that an uncemented hemiarthroplasty for a displaced femoral neck fracture in elderly patients would have at least comparable radiological and functional outcomes and complication rate as a cemented hemiarthroplasty and that non-cementing of hemiarthroplasty would result in a shorter operation time [14].

Methods

This multicenter parallel randomized controlled trial included patients with a displaced femoral neck fracture. The study was approved by the Regional Ethics Committee (NL19200.098.07, METC07 –118). The trial was registered in the Netherlands Trial Registry NTR 1508 (http://www.trialregister.nl). The protocol was published before start of the study [14].

All patients were admitted to one of the participating hospitals (Reinier de Graaf hospital, Delft; Rijnstate hospital, Arnhem and Canisius Wilhelmina hospital, Nijmegen), large district hospitals in the Netherlands. Inclusion was between August 2008 and June 2012. Included were patients aged 70 years or older, with a displaced femoral neck fracture (Garden type III or IV) suitable for hemiarthroplasty. Excluded were patients with a pathological fracture, a fracture older than seven days or ASA-IV or V classification. Orthopedic residents, trained for this study, performed inclusion.

All patients gave informed consent. In case of (mental) incompetence of the patient, his or her legal representative was consulted to obtain informed consent. Patients were randomized following a simple randomization procedure in the operation theatre by the orthopedic surgeon through opaque sealed envelopes. These were prepared by A.J.V. and kept at the operation theatre of each of the three hospitals. 200 opaque sealed envelopes were prepared. However, 16 patients could not be included in our trial due to variable reasons (Fig. 1), which forced us to prepare another 16 envelopes.

The patients were blinded for the type hemiarthroplasty they received, although we acknowledge the possibility that they might be able to tell after seeing their radiographs during the outpatient clinic visits. Surgeons and outcome assessors were aware of the allocated arm.

Patients received a cemented hemiarthroplasty, type Müller Straight Stem (Zimmer - Biomet, 1800 West Center St. Warsaw, Indiana, USA) or an uncemented hemiarthroplasty, type DB-10 (Zimmer- Biomet, 1800 West Center St. Warsaw, Indiana, USA). The cemented hemiarthroplasty, the Muller straight stem has a small proximal collar and two longitudinal grooves to enable good cement adhesion. The non-cemented DB-10 is a straight collared stem with metaphyseal anchoring and on the surface full hydroxyapatite coating on macro-structured titanium and grooves. If complications occurred during the procedure, the surgeon could change the procedure to ensure best medical practice. Operating technique was according to the manufacturer instruction. In the participating hospitals there was experience

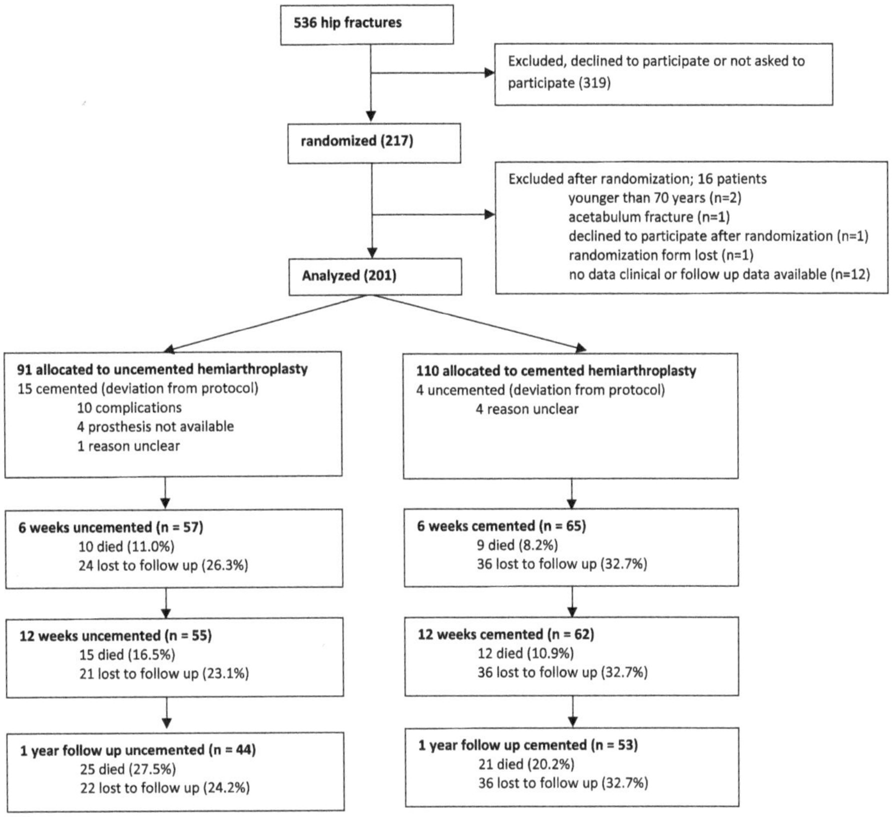

Fig. 1 Flowchart of the recruitment and flow of patients with femoral neck fractures during the study

with both cemented and uncemented hip arthroplasty. Either an orthopedic surgeon or registrar performed the operation. Cementing technique involved vacuum mixing, cement plug, saline pulsed lavage and retrograde introduction of cement with a cement gun. The approach was up to the surgeon's preference, as Parker's Cochrane analysis has shown that insufficient evidence is available for superiority of either approach [3].

Each patient received physiotherapy therapy, analgesia and trombo-embolic prophylaxis according to the protocol of the hospital in which they were treated.

Preoperatively, social demographic data (age, sex, place of residence), ASA— (American Society of Anesthesiologists) classification [15], Body Mass Index (BMI), Minimal Mental State Examination (MMSE) [16] were obtained. Patients were asked to score their pre-fracture mobility and Health Related Quality of Life (HRQoL) using the New Mobility Score (NMS) [17], Groningen Activity Restriction Scale (GARS) [18] and the SF-12 [19]. Patients were asked if they mobilized with an aid indoors and outdoors with or without aid and whether they received homecare. The baseline hemoglobin level was measured. The surgical approach, the type of surgeon (consultant or registrar) and kind of anesthesia were registered.

Outcomes measured during operation were operation time (defined as skin-to-skin surgical time, measured in minutes) and blood loss (in centiliter, estimated by the surgeon).

Length of stay, decrease in hemoglobin level and transfusion rate were measured postoperatively.

All patients were invited for follow up at six, 12 and 52 weeks postoperatively. When the patient was not able to visit the outpatient clinic, the questionnaires were mailed to the patient or its relatives. During follow-up functional outcome was measured using Timed-Up and-Go (TUG) score [20], GARS [18] and NMS [17]. HRQoL, expressed in the SF-12 [19], was measured. The SF-12 was divided in a Physical Component summary Score (PCS) and a Mental Component summary Score (MCS). Mid-thigh pain (defined as pain explicitly in the front and mid part of the femur) pain and place of residence were registered. Complications during surgery, hospital stay and the year thereafter were recorded. The complications were defined and ranked in the modified Elixhauser mode, as described by Parvizi [21]. Mortality was scored meticulously by repeated consultation of the population registers of the counties in the region of the hospital as well as the hospital's patient registration systems for the full length of follow-up.

A radiograph was obtained on the first postoperative day and after six weeks, 12 weeks and 1 year. Adequate positioning of the stem was defined as within 10° varus or valgus position with respect to the femoral axis. Fissures, fractures, subsidence and loosening were noted.

Analysis

Primary outcomes were complications, operation time, functional outcome and post-operative mid-thigh pain. A Bonferroni correction was applied for the eight primary outcome measures (4 types of complications, operation time, GARS, TUG and mid-thigh pain at 1 year) making $p < 0.006$ significant. Secondary outcomes were return to place of residence as percentage of pre-fracture situation, HRQoL and adequate radiological positioning of the hemiarthroplasty [14].

Determination of sample size

The complete power calculation is published in our protocol [14] We expected (based on the literature in 2008) that midthigh pain in uncemented prosthesis would be 30% and in cemented prosthesis 7.5%.

$$\pi 1 = 30\%, \pi 2 = 7.5\%, \pi = (30\% + 7.5\%)/2 = 18.75\%$$

$$n1 = n2 \geq 21 * \left(0,1875 * (1-0,1875)\right)/(0,225)2 = 63.2.$$

While we expected 25% 1-year mortality and 10% lost-to follow-up we raised this number by 35%. Thus a total of 86 patients a group were needed. The calculations for the other three primary outcome measures (duration of surgery, functional outcome and complications) produced lower patients numbers [14]. From a practical point of view we choose a total of 100 patient per group.

Statistical analysis

All analyses were performed using SPSS software (SPSS Inc., Chicago, IL, USA). The differences in outcome measures were analyzed using an independent sample student *T*-test (for continuous data) and Chi-Square Test (for categorical data), setting the level of significance at $p < 0.05$ for secondary outcomes. All outcomes analyses were done twice: both for as treated analysis and for intention to treat. The numbers given in the results section represent the intention to treat analysis. We will report explicitly if differences exist between as treated analysis and intention to treat analysis.

Results

In total 201 patients were analyzed (Fig. 1) 91. Were randomized to an uncemented, 110 to a cemented hemiarthroplasty. In 15 of the 91 (16%) patients randomized to an uncemented hemiarthroplasty a cemented hemiarthroplasty was used instead. In ten patients this was due to intraoperative complications (i.e. fracture of the femur). In four patients the necessary instruments or prosthesis were not present and in one patient the reason was unknown. Four of the 110 (4%) patients randomized to a cemented hemiarthroplasty received an uncemented hemiarthroplasty. In none of these cases the reason for this breach of the protocol was clear.

Table 1 shows baseline characteristics of both groups.

Primary outcomes

Complications

The 1-year complication rate per category as categorized by Parvizi is shown in Table 2 [21]. Major local complications were more frequent in the uncemented hemiarthroplasty group; (odds ratio; 95% CI) (3.36; 1.40 to

Table 1 Baseline characteristics

	Uncemented (91)	Cemented (110)
Age (mean (SD))	84.0 in 91 (6.7)	83.0 in 110 (6.2)
Sex female (number, %)	61 out of 91 (67%)	82 out of 110 (75%)
ASA classification (number, %)		
I	7 out of 91 (8%)	6 out of 110 (6%)
II	51 out of 91 (56%)	71 out of 110 (65%)
III	33 out of 91 (37%)	33 out of 110 (30%)
BMI (mean (SD))	24.3 in 60 (3.5)	24.1 in 73 (3.4)
MMSE < 24 (number, %)	15 out of 44 (34%)	23 out of 56 (41%)
Mobile without aid indoors (number, %)	32 out of 73 (44%)	41 out of 81 (51%)
Mobile without aid outdoors (number, %)	21 out of 73 (29%)	32 out of 81 (40%)
NMS (mean (SD))	5.2 in 71 (2.7)	5.5 in 77 (3.0)
GARS (mean (SD))	41.1 in 71 (16.8)	41.7 in 78 (18.6)
SF-12, Physical Component (mean (SD))	37.1 in 65 (11.2)	37.9 in 65 (12.3)
SF-12, Mental Component (mean (SD))	46.8 in 65 (10.9)	48.3 in 65 (12.1)
Living at home (number, %)	52 out of 73 (71%)	58 out of 84 (69%)
No domestic or homecare (number, %)	37 out of 64 (58%)	39 out of 75 (52%)
Hemoglobin level (g/dL) (mean (SD))	12.8 in 91 (1.5)	12.7 in 110 (1.8)
Surgical approach (number, %)		
Straight lateral	41 out of 90 (46%)	49 out of 110 (45%)
Postero lateral	45 out of 90 (50%)	61 out of 110 (56%)
Anterior	4 out of 90 (5%)	4 out of 110 (4%)
Consultant (vs. registrar) (number, %)	24 out of 91 (26%)	43 out of 110 (39%)
Spinal anesthesia (vs. general) (number, %)	68 out of 90 (76%)	80 out of 107 (75%)

Table 2 One-year complication rate per category as categorized by Parvizi

		Uncemented (91)	Cemented (110)	*P*
Major systemic	Death	25	21	(0.18)
	Tachyarrhythmia	1	4	
	Myocardial infarction	4	2	
	Pulmonary embolus	1	6	
	Acute renal failure	3	2	
	Stroke and/or TIA	3	3	
	Bowel obstruction	0	1	
	Total number of patients with >/=1 major systemic complication [a]	29 out of 91 (31.9%)	29 out of 110 (26.4%)	0.41
Minor systemic	Anemia	30	39	
	Urinary tract infection	14	22	
	Mental status change	23	21	
	Gastric hypomotility	0	2	
	Deep venous thrombosis	0	1	
	Pneumonia	14	12	
	Social complication	2	9	
	Others	2	2	
	Total number of patients with >/=1 minor systemic [a]	73 out of 91 (80.2%)	89 out of 110 (80.9%)	0.92
Major local	Peripheral nerve injury	0	1	
	Infection leading to revision	0	1	
	Periprosthetic fracture	14	3	
	intraoperatively	*12*	*0*	
	postoperatively	*2*	*3*	
	Dislocation	5	3	
	Total number of patients with >/= 1 major local complication [a]	19 out of 91 (20.9%)	8 out of 110 (7.3%)	0.005
Minor local	Hematoma	1	6	
	Persistent wound drainage	3	4	
	Superficial wound infection	3	6	
	Skin blisters	1	1	
	Other	6	2	
	Total number of patients with >/= 1 minor local complication [a]	12 out of 91 (13.2%)	19 out of 110 (10.9%)	0.42

[a]The number of patients with a complication in a category is not equal to the sum of complications in a category, while some patients had more than 1 complication

8.11). In the uncemented group there were 14 periprostetic fractures. 12 were noticed perioperative, in ten of these patients the procedure was converted to a cemented procedure, in two patients a cerclage wire was used. In two patients of the uncemented group and 3 of the cemented group a fracture was noted postoperative, these patients were treated with protected weight baring. Analysis according the as treated analysis approach (instead of intention to treat) showed no differences between cemented and uncemented hemiarthroplasty regarding major local complications. Minor local complications (0.73; 0.33 to 1.59), major systemic (1.31; 0.71 to 2.41) and minor systemic complications (0.96; 0.47 to 1.93) were comparable between groups. The 1-year mortality rate was higher in the uncemented group (25 (27.4%)) compared to the cemented group (21 (19.0%)) but did not reach significance ($p = 0.18$). One major systemic complication was a patient who died just after injecting the cement into the femoral canal, potentially caused by BCIS, however autopsy was not performed.

Operation time

The mean (95% CI) operation time was comparable between uncemented and cemented hemiarthroplasty: 57.3 min (52.8–61.9) and 55.4 min (52.0–58.9) respectively.

Functional outcome

At no point of follow-up a difference was found in functional outcome, expressed in the TUG and GARS score (Table 3). The pre-defined clinically relevant worsening from 30 to 42 of the TUG was not met in a single patient in one of the groups. TUG was poorly registered (53% at six weeks, 51% at 12 weeks, 48% at 1 year, corrected for mortality).

* $P<0.05$ The NMS was at all moments of follow-up comparable (Table 3).

Post-operative mid-thigh pain

There was no difference in post-operative mid-thigh pain between both groups at any time during follow up. It was present in 43 patients (36%) after six weeks, which decreased to 31% after 12 weeks and 20% after 1 year (Table 3).

Secondary outcomes;

There was no difference in the number of patients who returned to their baseline place of residence after 1 year (28 patients (72%) vs. 37 patients (80%) $p = 0.88$).

The SF-12 MCS did not differ between the cemented and the uncemented group. (Table 3) However, the SF-12 PCS was lower at six and 12 weeks postoperatively in the uncemented hemiarthroplasty group. This difference resolved after 1 year (Table 3 and Fig. 2). Analyzing the results according the as treated analysis showed a lower PCS for uncemented hemiarthroplasty at six weeks (30.3 vs. 34.8 $p = 0.01$), and a difference at 12 weeks (34.0 vs. 37.9) which nearly did reach significance ($p = 0.056$). There was no difference at 1 year after surgery (36.6 vs.37.6 $p = 0.65$).

Radiographs were taken direct post-operative and after 6 and 12 weeks and 1 year. Five patients deceased before the post-operative radiograph was obtained. Eight varus or valgus deviations in the uncemented group and seven in the cemented group ($p = 0.76$) were found on the post-operative radiograph. Loosening or subsidence was observed in 13 (20%) of the uncemented and five (6%) of the cemented hemiarthroplasties ($p = 0.007$) any time during follow up. Four (2%) revision operations were performed: three due to loosening (all in the uncemented group) and one for infection (in the cemented group) ($p = 0.162$).

There were no differences in length of stay between both groups (mean 11 (SD 7.7) days uncemented vs. 11 days (SD 8.3) cemented $p = 0.83$), loss in hemoglobin

Table 3 Functional outcome measures at six, 12 weeks and 1 year and radiological outcome post-operative and any time during follow up

		Uncemented			Cemented			
		Mean (SD)	97.5% CI	Number	Mean (SD)	97.5% CI	Number	P
Timed up and go	6 weeks	18.7 (13.8)	13.9–23.5	45	18.7 (12.9)	14.6–22.9	51	0.99
	12 weeks	16.2 (12.4)	11.5–20.9	38	15.5 (8.5)	12.7–18.2	50	0.74
	1 year	12.8 (9.4)	8.9–16.7	33	13.9 (9.0)	10.1–16.7	41	0.79
GARS* (iADL)	6 weeks	53.1 (14.9)	48.5–57.8	54	50.0 (15.3)	45.7–54.4	65	0.27
	12 weeks	45.7 (17.0)	40.3–51.2	52	45.3 (16.6)	40.4–50.1	62	0.88
	1 year	43.2 (19.7)	36.2–50.2	43	39.2 (16.5)	34.0–44.4	53	0.28
NMS	6 weeks	3.7 (2.5)	2.9–4.4	53	3.5 (2.4)	2.8–4.1	64	0.65
	12 weeks	4.5 (2.8)	3.6–5.4	51	4.8 (3.1)	3.8–5.7	59	0.68
	1 year	4.7 (3.2)	3.6–5.8	44	5.7 (2.9)	4.8–6.7	50	0.12
SF-12 Physical component	**6 weeks**	**30.3 (6.9)***	**27.9–32.6***	**47**	**35.3 (9.3)***	**32.4–38.2***	**54**	**0.003**
	12 weeks	**33.8 (9.8)***	**30.6–37.1***	**48**	**38.5 (9.9)***	**35.4–41.6***	**54**	**0.018**
	1 year	36.8 (10.7)	32.9–40.8	40	37.5 (9.4)	34.3–40.7	50	0.76
SF-12 Mental component	6 weeks	45.0 (13.0)	40.7–49.5	47	47.4 (11.0)	44.0–50.8	54	0.33
	12 weeks	47.7 (11.2)	43.9–51.4	48	49.5 (11.0)	46.0–52.9	54	0.41
	1 year	49.3 (11.2)	45.2–53.4	40	51.4 (10.1)	47.9–54.9	50	0.36
		Number (%)			Number (%)			
Mid-thigh pain	6 weeks	23 out of 55 (42%)			20 out of 63 (32%)			0.26
	12 weeks	19 out of 55 (35%)			17 out of 61 (27%)			0.83
	1 year	8 out of 43 (19%)			11 out of 51 (22%)			0.72
Varus or valgus deviation	Post operative	8 out of 89 (9%)			7 out of 107 (7%)			0.76

*$p < 0.05$

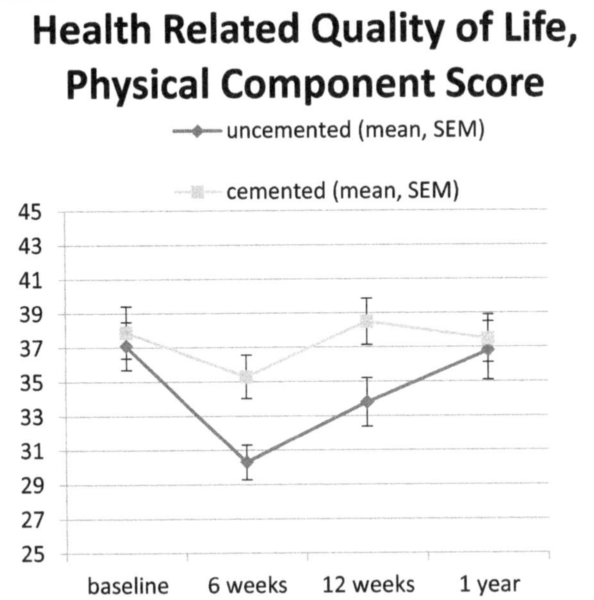

Fig. 2 Health related quality of life, physical component score

level (g/dl) after surgery (uncemented mean 2.2 (SD 1.4) vs. cemented mean 2.0 (SD 1.5) $p = 0.31$) and transfusion rate (uncemented 17 (24%) vs. cemented 22 (26%) $p = 0.74$). Surgeon estimated blood loss was larger in the uncemented group (mean 288 mL (sd 213) vs. mean 220 mL (sd 143) $p = 0.03$) (Additional file 1: Table S1).

Discussion

The most important finding of our study was that major local complications were more frequent (odds ratio; 95% CI) (3.36; 1.40 to 8.11) in the uncemented hemiarthroplasty group compared to the cemented group. In elderly patients with a displaced femoral neck fracture hemiarthroplasty is a widely accepted treatment of choice [2]. Previous randomized trials comparing cemented and uncemented hemiarthroplasty give conflicting results on this [4, 11–13, 22].

A periprosthetic fracture was the most common major local complication in the uncemented group (15%). Previous papers comparing fracture rate are heterogenic. Some studies found a higher fracture rate in the uncemented group, ranging from 5.5 to 12% [3, 12, 13, 23] whereas others demonstrated no difference in fracture rate [4, 11, 22]. The fracture rate in the current study is higher than previous papers demonstrate. The teaching of registrars might have attributed to this. This can be due to the design of the DB-10 stem (proximal fitting) compared to the stems used in the other papers. Furthermore, teaching of registrars might have attributed to this as well: the level of experience of the operation surgeon is not always mentioned, but for example in the studies of Inngul, DeAngelis and Parker the operations were always performed by consultant orthopaedic surgeons [4, 11, 13]. However this high complication rate might better reflect the everyday practice with registrars often performing this type of operations.

One-year mortality rate was higher in the uncemented group (25 (27.4%) compared to the cemented group 21 (19.0%) but did not reach significance ($p = 0.16$). This is in contrast to other randomized controlled trials [4]. The register studies show higher mortality in the first operative days in cemented hemi arthroplasty [24–26]. However the Australian and British register shows lower mortality in cemented hemiarthroplasty the year thereafter [10, 27]. Power analysis in our study was not performed on finding differences in mortality. In our trial one patient died intraoperatively, probably due to Bone Cement Implantation Syndrome (BCIS). BCIS is a major side effect of cement implantation, it has no agreed definition but is characterized by a number of clinical features with amongst others hypoxia, hypotension, cardiac arrhythmias, increased pulmonary vascular resistance and cardio-respiratory collapse [5]. Guidelines to minimize the risk for BCIS by both surgeon and anesthetist are recently published [28].

In contrast to our hypothesis and literature, we did not find a difference in operation time between groups [3, 22]. Intraoperative complications in the uncemented group might have affected this, however equality in the mean operation time persisted when we analyzed our data in an As Treated analysis. Teaching residents during might have affected the operation time in such way that the difference disappeared.

Functional outcome (GARS score and TUG test) was not different between both groups. However TUG was measured only in 53% of all patients at 6 weeks, 51% at 12 weeks and 48% at 1 year. Probably TUG is not a very useful outcome measure in this frail population as mobility was too poor to measure well. Mobility expressed as the NMS was comparable between the two groups. In literature different outcome measures for functional outcome have been used (Oxford or Harris Hip Score [12, 13, 22] Older Americans Resources and Services Instrument [11] Barthel Index [22]) A meta-analysis pooled results of five trials (491 patients) and found that patients with an cemented hemiarthroplasty had a better hip function after 1 year [7].

Mid-thigh pain is known to be more prevalent in uncemented prostheses, however the reported incidence differs tremendously [4, 7, 29]. In our study presence of mid-thigh pain was comparable between groups. Several factors can be of influence on postoperative mid-thigh pain such as sizing, design and stiffness of a prosthesis [29].

Radiological follow up showed loosening or subsidence in 13 uncemented hemiarthroplasty, which led to a revision in three cases. Subsidence in uncemented (hemi) arthroplasty is a common finding; one trial found a larger subsidence in the uncemented hemiarthroplasty [12]. In The Norwegian Hip Fracture Register patients treated with an uncemented hemiartroplasty had a 2.1 times increased risk of revision compared with patients treated cemented prostheses. This increased risk of re-operation was due to peri-prosthetic fracture HRR 17 and aseptic loosening HHR 17 [30]. A combined analysis of the Norwegian and Swedish registers (33.205 hip fractures in patients older than 60 years treated with hemiarthroplasty) also found more reoperations in uncemented stems (HR2.2) [9].

PCS of HRQoL was lower in patients treated with an uncemented hemiarthroplasty at six weeks and three months after surgery. PCS HRQoL is known to decrease in the first three months and recover thereafter [31]. The larger complication rate might have led to this lower PCS HRQoL, although we would have expected to find a difference in functional and mobility scores as well. One previous trial found higher HRQoL (expressed in EQ5days) in the cemented group [13] at 4 and 12 months, another trial did not [22]. The latter did not find a difference in complications either [22]. HRQoL was an secondary outcome in this trial, thus no power calculations were made and dropout at follow-up was quite high: therefore the difference we found might be due to coincidence and has to be verified in further trials.

The large number of patients, the randomized design and outcome measures on both functional and radiological outcomes make the current study worthwhile. Furthermore, we did not exclude patients with cognitive disorders. The latter makes our study generalizable to all elderly hip fracture patients treated with hemiarthroplasty.

However, our study does have limitations. First, many (293) patients (or their caretakers) declined to participate in our study or were not asked to participate, thus selection bias might be present. Second, poor registration has led to incompleteness of some of the baseline data. This led to the exclusion of 12 patients after randomization because of missing baseline data, 5 patients were excluded after randomiz ation due to other reasons (Fig. 1). Deviation from the protocol occurred in 19 patients (9% of analyzed cases). Therefore both as treated analysis and intention to treat were performed. More deviations from protocol were present in the uncemented group (15 vs. 4) which might have caused a bias.

Furthermore, we had a substantial percentage (24%) of patients who were lost to follow-up. This might be due to the inclusion of patients with cognitive disorders (38% had an MMSE less than 24) and high age of the participators, resulting in their caretakers to refrain from extra stress by those patients by filling in follow-up forms.

This trial adds value to the discussion whether to use a cemented or an uncemented hemiartroplasty in femoral neck fractures. Conflicting evidence on this matter is published the last few years [4, 11–13, 22]. Trial design, prosthesis design, inclusion criteria and whether the trail was performed in a teaching hospital or not might all have been of influence of these published results.

Conclusions

Elderly patients with a displaced femoral neck fracture treated with an uncemented hemiarthroplasty had more periprosthetic fractures, loosening, reoperations and lower quality of life compared to patients with a cemented stem. Operation time, functional outcome and mid-thigh pain were comparable between groups. Based on these findings, and earlier work [3, 12, 13] we conclude that in elderly patients with a displaced femoral neck fracture a cemented hemiarthroplasty is favorable compared to an uncemented stem.

Abbreviations

ASA -classification: American Society of Anesthesiologists -classification; BCIS: Bone cement implantation syndrome; BMI: Body mass index; GARS: Groningen activity restriction scale; HRQoL: Health related quality of life; MCS: Mental component summary score; MMSE: Minimal mental state examination; PCS: Physical component summary score; TUG: Timed-up-and-go

Acknowledgements

Not applicable

Funding

For the reported research no funding was used.

Authors' contributions

AV designed the study, and lead the study. DN, RR, WR, SK, KK were responsible for data collection on of the three participating hospitals. SM and TM collected all data. SM and WT did the statistical analysis. SM, NM, RN and AV wrote the manuscript. All authors read and approved the final manuscript.

Competing interests

The department of Orthopaedic Surgery and the Orthopaedic Research Foundation in Reinier de Graaf Hospital receive grants from Zimmer Biomet. (SM, NM, DD, TM) For the remaining authors and institutions none were declared.

Consent for publication

Not applicable

Author details

[1]Department of Orthopaedics, Reinier de Graaf Group, Reinier de Graafweg 5, 2625 AD Delft, The Netherlands. [2]Tergooi hospital, Hilversum, The

Netherlands. [3]Rijnstate Hospital, Arnhem, The Netherlands. [4]Canisius Wilhelmina Hospital, Nijmegen, The Netherlands. [5]Department of Surgery/ Traumatology, Erasmus MC, Rotterdam, The Netherlands. [6]Leiden University Medical Center, Leiden, The Netherlands. [7]Centre for Orthopedic Surgery OCON, Hengelo, The Netherlands.

References

1. Hernlund E, Svedbom A, Ivergård M, Compston J, Cooper C, Stenmark J, et al. Osteoporosis in the european union: medical management, epidemiology and economic burden: a report prepared in collaboration with the international osteoporosis foundation (IOF) and the european federation of pharmaceutical industry associations (EFPIA). Arch Osteoporos. 2013;8:136.
2. AAOS. Management of Hip Fractures in the Elderly Evidence- based clinical practice guidelines. AAOS. 2014. http://www.aaos.org/cc_files/aaosorg/research/guidelines/hipfxguideline.pdf. Accessed 11 Apr 2015.
3. Parker MJ, Gurusamy KS, Azegami S. Arthroplasties (with and without bone cement) for proximal femoral fractures in adults. Cochrane Database Syst. Rev. 2010;6:CD001706.
4. Parker MI, Pryor G, Gurusamy K. Cemented versus uncemented hemiarthroplasty for intracapsular hip fractures: a randomised controlled trial in 400 patients. J Bone Joint Surg Br. 2010;92:116–22.
5. Donaldson AJ, Tomson HE, Harper NJ, Kenny NW. Bone cement implantation syndrome (BCIS). Br J Anaesth Bone. 2009;102:12–22.
6. Sporer SM, Paprosky WG. Biologic fixation and bone ingrowth. Orthop Clin North Am. 2005;36:105–11.
7. Li T, Zhuang Q, Weng X, Zhou L, Bian Y. Cemented versus uncemented hemiarthroplasty for femoral neck fractures in elderly patients: a meta-analysis. PLoS One. 2013;8:1–13.
8. National Institute for Health and Care Excellence. Hip fracture: the management of hip fracture in adults. 2011. NICE clinical guideline 124.
9. Gjertsen J-E, Fenstad AM, Leonardsson O, Engesæter LB, Kärrholm J, Furnes O, et al. Hemiarthroplasties after hip fractures in Norway and Sweden: a collaboration between the Norwegian and Swedish national registries. Hip Int. 2014;24:223–30.
10. White SM, Moppett IK, Griffiths R. Outcome by mode of anaesthesia for hip fracture surgery. An observational audit of 65 535 patients in a national dataset. Anaesthesia. 2014;69:224–30.
11. DeAngelis JP, Ademi A, Staff I, Lewis CG. Cemented versus uncemented hemiarthroplasty for displaced femoral neck fractures. J Orthop Trauma. 2012;26:135–40.
12. Taylor F, Wright M, Zhu M. Hemiarthroplasty of the Hip with and without cement: a randomized clinical trial. J Bone Jt Surg. 2012;94:577.
13. Inngul C, Blomfeldt R, Ponzer S, Enocson A. Cemented versus uncemented arthroplasty in patients with a displaced fracture of the femoral neck: a randomised controlled trial. Bone Joint J. 2015;97-B:1475–80.
14. Vochteloo AJH, Niesten D, Riedijk R, Rijnberg WJ, Bolder SBT, Koëter S, et al. Cemented versus non-cemented hemiarthroplasty of the hip as a treatment for a displaced femoral neck fracture: design of a randomised controlled trial. BMC Musculoskelet Disord. 2009;10:56.
15. Owens WD, Felts JA, Spitznagel EL. ASA physical status classifications: a study of consistency of ratings. Anesthesiology. 1978;49:239–43.
16. Folstein MF, Folstein SE, McHugh PR. "Mini-mental state". A practical method for grading the cognitive state of patients for the clinician. J Psychiatr Res. 1975;12:189–98.
17. Parker MJ, Palmer CR. A new mobility score for predicting mortality after hip fracture. J Bone Joint Surg Br. 1993;75:797–8.
18. Suurmeijer TPBM, Doeglas DM, Moum T, Briancon S, Krol B, Sanderman R, et al. The groningen activity restriction scale for measuring disability: its utility in international comparisons. Am J Public Health. 1994;84:1270–3.
19. Mols F, Pelle AJ, Kupper N. Normative data of the SF-12 health survey with validation using postmyocardial infarction patients in the Dutch population. Qual Life Res. 2009;18:403–14.
20. Nygard H, Matre K, Fevang JM. Evaluation of timed Up and Go test as a tool to measure postoperative function and prediction of one year walking ability for patients with hip fracture. Clin Rehabil. 2016;30:472–80.
21. Parvizi J, Mui A, Purtill JJ, Sharkey PF, Hozack WJ, Rothman RH. Total joint arthroplasty: when do fatal or near-fatal complications occur? J Bone Joint Surg Am. 2007;89:27–32.
22. Figved W, Opland V, Frihagen F, Jervidalo T, Madsen JE, Nordsletten L. Cemented versus uncemented hemiarthroplasty for displaced femoral neck fractures. Clin Orthop Relat Res. 2009;467:2426–35.
23. Yli-Kyyny T, Ojanpera J, Venesmaa P, Kettunen J, Miettinen H, Salo J, et al. Perioperative complications after cemented or uncemented hemiarthroplasty in hip fracture patients. Scand J Surg. 2013;102:124–8.
24. Talsnes O, Vinje T, Gjertsen JE, Dahl OE, Engesæter LB, Baste V, et al. Perioperative mortality in hip fracture patients treated with cemented and uncemented hemiprosthesis: a register study of 11,210 patients. Int Orthop. 2013;37:1135–40.
25. Yli-Kyyny T, Sund R, Heinänen M, Venesmaa P, Kröger H. Cemented or uncemented hemiarthroplasty for the treatment of femoral neck fractures? Acta Orthop. 2014;85:49–53.
26. Costa ML, Griffin XL, Pendleton N, Pearson M, Parsons NR. Does cementing the femoral component increase the risk of peri-operative mortality for patients having replacement surgery for a fracture of the neck of femur? : data from the national Hip fracture database. J Bone Jt Surg. 2011;93:1405–10.
27. Costain DJ, Whitehouse SL, Pratt NL, Graves SE, Ryan P, Crawford RW. Perioperative mortality after hemiarthroplasty related to fixation method. Acta Orthop. 2011;82:275–81.
28. Griffiths R, White SM, Moppett IK, Parker MJ, Chesser TJS, Costa ML, et al. Safety guideline: reducing the risk from cemented hemiarthroplasty for hip fracture 2015. Anaesthesia. 2015;70:623–6.
29. Brown T, Larson B, Shen F, Moskal J. Thigh pain after cementless total hip arthroplasty: evaluation and management. J Am Acad Orthop Surg. 2002;10: 385–92.
30. Gjertsen J-E, Lie SA, Vinje T, Engesæter LB, Hallan G, Matre K, et al. More re-operations after uncemented than cemented hemiarthroplasty used in the treatment of displaced fractures of the femoral neck: an observational study of 11,116 hemiarthroplasties from a national register. J Bone Joint Surg Br. 2012;94:1113–9.
31. Peasgood T, Herrmann K, Kanis JA, Brazier JE. An updated systematic review of health state utility values for osteoporosis related conditions. Osteoporos Int. 2009;20:853–68.

25

Frailty as a predictor of hospital length of stay after elective total joint replacements in elderly patients

Han Ting Wang[1*], Josée Fafard[1], Stéphane Ahern[1], Pascal-André Vendittoli[2] and Paul Hebert[3]

Abstract

Background: Total joint replacement procedures are increasing in number because of population aging and osteoarthritis development. Defined as a lack of physiological reserves and the inability to adequately respond to external stressors, frailty may be more common than expected in older patients with degenerative arthritis awaiting total joint replacements.

The aim of the present study was to assess associations between frailty and adverse outcomes, frailty prevalence among elderly patients awaiting elective TJR, and agreement between 2 frailty screening instruments.

Methods: We undertook a prospective, observational, pilot study in our institution. We enrolled patients 65 years or older who were awaiting elective knee or hip replacement surgery and evaluated them in our preoperative clinic with planned postoperative hospital length of stay greater than 24 h. Patients were asked to grade their perceived well-being on the Clinical Frailty Scale and to answer questions on the FRAIL Scale.

Results: The Clinical Frailty Scale classified 40 patients (45.9%) as robust, 43 patients (49.4%) as prefrail and 4 patients (4.5%) as frail, while the FRAIL Scale categorized 12 patients (13.7%) as robust, 54 patients (62.0%) as prefrail, and 20 patients (22.9%) as frail. Robustness, ascertained on the Clinical Frailty Scale was, while the FRAIL Scale was not, significantly associated with shorter hospital length of stay and fewer discharges to the rehabilitation center. Both scales showed moderate mutual agreement.

Conclusion: Screening for frailty identified between 5% and 10% of patients at risk of adverse outcomes. The Clinical Frailty Scale was, while the FRAIL scale was not, significantly associated with hospital length of stay and discharge to rehabilitation center in our cohort of total joint replacement patients.

Keywords: Frailty, Elderly, Total joint replacement, Outcome, Knee arthroplasty, Hip arthroplasty

Background

Total joint replacement (TJR) procedures are increasing in number with population aging and osteoarthritis development. In its 2014 annual report, the Canadian Joint Replacement Registry recorded a 16.5% surge of hip replacements and a 21.5% proliferation of knee replacements in the last 5 years [1] paralleled by increased frailty with advancing age in the general population [2]. Frailty embodies insufficient physiological reserves and the inability to adequately respond to external stressors. Its etiology is complex but is related to aging, faster senescence and acquired illnesses [3, 4]. Its pervasiveness in community-dwelling elders is estimated to be approximately 10%, depending on the study cited [5], and is associated with increased 1-year mortality and institutionalization.

Frailty prevalence is generally considered to be even greater in surgical pre-operative settings, varying from 10% to 46%, depending on the screening instrument selected, the surgical subspecialty/setting, and patient characteristics [6–8]. The choice of "frailty scale" may not be obvious owing to the variety of available instruments with different conceptual underpinnings [9, 10]. Nonetheless, in most studies, frailty is a better predictor

* Correspondence: ht.wang85@gmail.com
[1]Department of Internal medicine and Critical Care Medicine, Centre Integre Universitaire de Sante et Services Sociaux (CIUSSS) de l'est de l'île de Montréal, Hopital Maisonneuve-Rosemont, 5415 boul. l'Assomption, H1T 2M4, Montreal, Quebec, Canada
Full list of author information is available at the end of the article

of post-operative outcomes than co-morbidity scores and even some validated risk model scores specific to certain procedures [6–8].

In orthopedic surgery, especially in patients awaiting TJR, few teams have looked at the association between frailty and post-operative outcomes, such as hospital length of stay (LOS) and disposition at discharge. Frailty may help in selecting vulnerable patients when combined with known predictors in TJR procedures (i.e., pre-operative hemoglobin (Hb) level, American Society of Anesthesiologists score, nutritional status, etc.) [11–13]. The lack of consensus on the different available models of frailty makes it challenging to choose appropriate screening instruments.

Therefore, we undertook a study, with 2 frailty-screening instruments, to assess associations between frailty, hospital LOS and transfer to rehabilitation centre or not among elderly patients awaiting elective, primary TJR. We hypothesized that frail patients are less likely to be discharged home and will have longer LOS. As secondary objectives, we compared the prevalence of frailty with 2 instruments and evaluated their agreement.

Methods

Setting

We conducted a prospective, observational study in our tertiary academic hospital with a pre-operative clinic that sees over 3000 patients per year, and approximatively 20% of them are orthopedics-related.

Study participants

From November 2015 to May 2016, we identified orthopedic participants through routine daily screening of our pre-operative clinic schedule ($N = 419$). A research nurse was trained for screening purposes and performed all frailty assessments. Patients 65 years or older and awaiting primary TJR were enrolled and evaluated in our pre-operative clinic with planned post-operative hospital stay greater than 24 h. For feasibility reasons, we excluded all urgent procedures, patients deemed unfit for surgery by their surgeon or medical consultant, and those unable to understand or provide consent. If they fulfilled eligibility criteria, patients were contacted by phone or in person, and informed consent was obtained. Those who gave consent were subsequently interviewed for frailty assessment. Figure 1 shows the number of patients meeting inclusion and exclusion criteria. In summary, a total of 87 patients accepted to participate and completed the study. Full approval by our local Research Ethics Committee was granted before the study was started.

Frailty assessment

We chose to define frailty as an age-associated, multidimensional syndrome of insufficient reserves giving rise

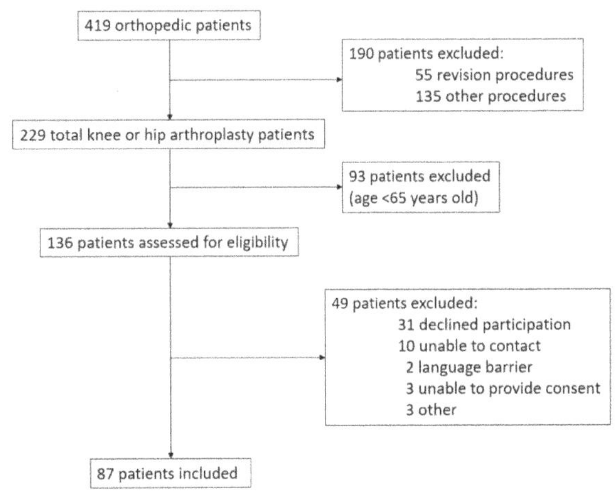

Fig. 1 Patient recruitment flow chart

to vulnerability [14]. Based on the current literature [9], the 2 most commonly-used frailty models in surgical settings are Rockwood's deficit accumulation model [15] and Fried's phenotypic model [16]. Rockwood's model was quantified with the Clinical Frailty Scale, and Fried's model was assessed with the FRAIL Scale. The Clinical Frailty Scale, derived from the Frailty Index, is an ordinal scale from 1 to 8, where 1 represents a state of robustness, and 8 indicates a very severe frailty state. Patients were asked to identify which level on the scale best corresponded to their perceived well-being. They can be further grouped as being robust (score 1 to 3), pre-frail (score 4), and frail (score 5 to 8), based on the initial study by Rockwood et al. [17]. It is well-validated in predicting adverse outcomes in community-dwelling elders [15].

The Clinical Frailty Scale was selected over the Frailty Index as being more feasible in clinical practice. The FRAIL Scale was created at a consensus meeting of the International Academy on Nutrition and Aging Task Force. Its conceptual underpinnings are heavily rooted in Fried's phenotypic model [18]. It is composed of 5 items (fatigue, resistance, ambulation, weight loss, illness) with the first 4 components taken from Fried's phenotypic model. Also, it is assessed subjectively, and each item is scored by a binary system. Summed scores range from 0 to 5, where 0 epitomizes robustness, 1 or 2 signifies pre-frail, and scores greater than 2 indicate frailty. Since its creation, it has been successfully applied in community-dwelling elders with excellent prognostic capabilities [19].

The Fried phenotypic model was discarded because our research team deemed gait speed measurements to be potentially difficult to perform and less feasible in a purely orthopedic population. As scaling systems differ, frailty prevalence with both screening instruments was estimated after reclassification as robust or not robust (pre-frail or frail). After obtaining consent, patients were asked to grade their perceived well-being on the

Clinical Frailty Scale and to answer all 5 questions of the FRAIL Scale.

Variables

Patient characteristics were collected before surgery (age, gender, co-morbidity, daily living activities, living status before admission, body mass index (BMI), baseline Hb level), and type of procedure, i.e., total hip or knee arthroplasty (THA or TKA). Hospital mortality, LOS and disposition at discharge were collected by chart review after discharge. Co-morbidity was defined as the co-existence of at least 2 separate chronic illnesses [20]. We quantified the burden of co-morbidity by calculating age-adjusted scores on the Charlson Comorbidity Index [21]. Disability was characterized as difficulty or inability to perform activities essential for independent living, including essential roles, self-care tasks, living independently in a home, and desired activities important to quality of life [19]. We quantified disability with the Katz Index of Independence [22].

Outcomes

Our primary outcomes were hospital LOS and disposition at discharge. Both have been consistently associated with greater burden and cost to the healthcare system in orthopedic surgery settings [3, 23]. We divided LOS into 3 categories: 1–2 days, 3–5 days, and > 5 days. Short-stay patients (≤2 days) incur the lowest care costs, even when compared to those with LOS of 3–5 days [23], and this can be considered an achievable goal with early, aggressive, in-patient rehabilitation of most of them [24]. LOS of 5 days is often reported as the median value in Canadian patients undergoing TJR [25], and patients with LOS exceeding 5 days incur the highest care costs [23]. Disposition at discharge was characterized by the need to transfer to a rehabilitation center. Secondary outcomes were robust and not robust patient proportions, as defined by both frailty instruments and their agreement.

Analysis

Frailty prevalence was reported as proportions on both scales. Continuous variables were assessed for normal distribution by the Shapiro-Wilk test, and continuous variables were compared by independent sample t-test (BMI) and the Mann-Whitney test (age, Charlson Comorbidity Index and Hb level). Categorical variables were compared by the Chi-square test or Fisher's exact test, if absolute patient count was ≤5 for any given category: gender distribution, disposition before surgery, categorized hospital LOS and disposition at discharge. Associations between hospital LOS, discharge to rehabilitation center and frailty were assessed by the Chi-square test or Fisher's exact test. Unfortunately, our small sample size prevented regression analysis with covariates. Finally, agreement between the 2 frailty scales was evaluated by Cohen's kappa test. All analyses were performed with SPSS 20.0.

Results

The baseline characteristics of study subjects are presented in Table 1. Median age of our cohort was 72.0 years (interquartile range (IQR) = 9.0), ranging from 65.0 to 88.0 years, and 65.5% were female patients. More than half of our cohort were living at home with their spouses (57.5%), while 5.6% were living in a residence. The median Charlson Comorbidity Index in our cohort was 4.0 (IQR = 1.0), and 87.4% were fully independent in their daily living activities. TKA represented 51.7% of all procedures, followed by THA and bilateral TJR (39.1% and 9.2%, respectively). The mean time period between pre-operative clinic visit and surgery was 74.3 ± 34.8 days.

The Clinical Frailty Scale classified 46.0% of our cohort as robust while the FRAIL Scale grouped 15.0% as robust. Baseline characteristics (gender, disposition before surgery and BMI) differed significantly between robust and not robust patients based on the Clinical Frailty Scale ($p < 0.05$), while fully independent status almost reached statistical significance ($p = 0.058$). Robust and not robust patients did not differ significantly on the FRAIL Scale, except in terms of gender, mean BMI and median baseline Hb level ($p < 0.05$).

Median hospital LOS of our cohort was 5 days (IQR = 3). Eight patients (9.1%) were discharged within 48 h after surgery, 49 patients (56.3%) were discharged between 3 and 5 days, and total LOS was over 5 days in 30 patients (34.4%) (Table 2). No patient died during hospital stay. Based on the Clinical Frailty Scale, 17.5% ($N = 7$) of robust patients had hospital LOS over 5 days compared to 48.9% ($N = 23$) of not robust patients. Hospital LOS distribution differed significantly between robust and not robust patients ($p = 0.005$). When classified according to the FRAIL Scale, hospital LOS distribution did not differ significantly between robust and not robust patients ($p = 0.700$).

A total of 17 patients (19.5%) were discharged to rehabilitation center after surgery. Based on the Clinical Frailty Scale, 10.0% ($N = 4$) of robust patients were transferred to rehabilitation center compared to 27.7% ($N = 13$) of not robust patients ($p = 0.038$). Robust ($N = 3$, 23.1%) and not robust ($N = 14$, 23.3%) patients did not differ significantly on the FRAIL Scale ($p = 0.727$).

Table 3 reports patient classification according to frailty status on the Clinical Frailty Scale and the FRAIL Scale. Since both instruments are not rated by the same scaling system, the results are presented after reclassification into robust, pre-frail and frail patients. The Clinical Frailty Scale classified 40 patients (45.9%) as robust, 43 patients (49.4%) as pre-frail, and 4 patients (4.5%) as frail, while the

Table 1 Baseline characteristics of patients stratified by frailty status according to the Clinical Frailty Scale and the FRAIL Scale

	Total patients (N = 87)	Clinical Frailty Scale			FRAIL Scale		
		Robust (n = 40)	Not robust (n = 47)	p-value	Robust (n = 13)	Not robust (n = 74)	p-value
Age (median (IQR))	72.0 (9.0	71.0 (8.0)	73.0 (11.0)	0.145	73.0 (6.0)	71.5 (9.0)	0.330
Gender (female) (%)	57 (65.5)	21 (52.5%)	36 (76.6%)	0.018	4 (30.8%)	53 (71.6%)	0.009
Disposition before surgery (%)							
- Home with loved ones	50 (57.5%)	30 (75.5%)	20 (42.6%)	0.02	8 (61.5%)	42 (56.8)	1.00
Charlson comorbidity index (median (IQR))	4.0 (1.0)	4.0 (1.0)	5.0 (1.0)	0.273	5.0 (1.0)	4.0 (1.0)	0.239
Fully independent (%)	76 (87.4)	38 (95%)	38 (82.6%)	0.058	0	11 (14.9%)	0.205
BMI (mean ±SD)	30.5 ± 6.4	28.3 ± 4.7	32.3 ± 7.0	0.002	28.1 ± 3.1	30.9 ± 6.7	0.02
Baseline Hb (median (IQR))	135.0 (16.0)	139.0 (20.0)	134.0 (12.0)	0.109	146.0 (19.0)	134.0 (16.0)	0.004

SD: standard deviation; BMI: body mass index; Hb: hemoglobin; IQR: interquartile range

FRAIL Scale categorized 12 patients (13.7%) as robust, 54 patients (62.0%) as pre-frail, and 20 patients (22.9%) as frail. Both scales agreed on 39 evaluations (38.0%) and disagreed on 48 evaluations (62.0%). Out of the 20 patients considered as frail by the FRAIL Scale, 5 were classified as robust with the Clinical Frailty Scale. Due to the small numbers of patients considered as frail by the latter, both scales were dichotomized into robust versus not robust (sum of pre-frail and frail) (Table 4). Cohen's kappa agreement was 0.245 (p = 0.002) between both scales after dichotomization.

Discussion

Frailty is progressively acknowledged as a marker of functional decline and a potentially modifiable risk factor for patient improvement. It is even more relevant in peri-operative patients where interventions can be applied before the surgical procedure. In our study, pre-frail and frail patients, as defined by the Clinical Frailty Scale and undergoing TKA or THA, had longer hospital LOS and higher percentage of discharge to rehabilitation center compared to robust patients. These results are consistent with current literature on the general surgical population. Most studies, using Rockwood's or Fried's model, have reported associations between increasing frailty and major post-operative outcomes (in-hospital mortality, hospital LOS, post-operative complications, etc.).

In orthopedic surgery, involving the Ontario Healthcare Database, McIsaac et al. [26] found an increase in hospital LOS among frail elderly undergoing THA or TKA based on Johns Hopkins Adjusted Clinical Groups frailty-defining diagnoses indicators (odds ratio: 1.78, confidence interval: 1.74–1.81). The latter model is based on another conceptual underpinning and is also difficult to apply in clinical practice as it relies on variables from multiple datasets. Cooper et al. [27] considered both Fried's phenotypic model and the Frailty Index in a cohort of 415 orthopedic patients. Both instruments predicted discharge to post-acute institutional care and hospital LOS > 5 days. This discrepancy between results can be explained by the higher prevalence of frailty (35% with Fried's phenotypic model and 41% with the Frailty Index) in older patients with greater functional decline. They included patients undergoing other types of surgery, such as lumbar and cervical laminectomy.

The FRAIL Scale was not associated with hospital LOS or discharge to rehabilitation center in our cohort. Both scales differed significantly in the percentage of patients classified as robust and not robust, with moderate agreement at best. Part of the difference in performance by both scales can be explained by the modest agreement between them. The 2 instruments are not conceptually identical in their definition of frailty. The Clinical Frailty Scale is derived from the Frailty Index developed by Rockwood and colleagues [17]. It is based on a mathematical model of deficit accumulation and the complex interplay between co-morbidities [15]. The FRAIL Scale is heavily rooted in Fried's phenotypic model, a

Table 2 Hospital LOS and discharge to rehabilitation home stratified by frailty status according to the Clinical Frailty Scale and the FRAIL Scale

		Hospital length of stay				Discharge to rehabilitation center		
Frailty scales (N)		1–2 days (8)	3–5 days (49)	> 5 days (30)	p-value	Yes (17)	No (70)	p-value
Clinical Frailty Scale	Robust	6	27	7	0.005	4	36	0.038
	Not robust	2	22	23		13	34	
FRAIL Scale	Robust	2	7	4	0.700	3	10	0.727
	Not robust	6	42	26		14	60	

Table 3 Comparison of the Clinical Frailty Scale and the FRAIL Scale

Clinical Frailty Scale	FRAIL Scale			
		Robust (0)	Prefrail (1–2)	Frail (3–5)
	Robust (1–3)	11	24	5
	Prefrail (4)	2	27	14
	Frail (5–7)	0	3	1

syndrome-based definition of weight loss, fatigue and diminished energy expenditure, all related to sarcopenia [28]. Cooper et al. [27] obtained similar results with the phenotypic and deficit accumulation models with moderate agreement (kappa = 0.42). Furthermore, our cohort of orthopedic patients awaiting TJR did not suffer from significant co-morbidities or disabilities, which are all related to frailty. By excluding urgent surgeries, such as hip fracture patients and those deemed too ill for surgery, we further selected a subgroup of healthier and more functional orthopedic patients. In a cohort with higher prevalence of frail patients, the FRAIL Scale may have been associated with clinical outcomes. Also, even with our small sample size, the power of our analyses with the FRAIL scale was 99% for both clinical outcomes. It is unlikely that our results were due to beta errors.

Our study has some limitations. First, it was conducted in a single center with a small sample size, and lacked power to assess other known risk factors and their interactions with frailty status. For example, Hb level was significantly higher in robust patients (with the FRAIL scale) compared to not robust patients, although a multi-centered interventional trial did not show improved outcome with a liberal transfusion strategy in hip surgery patients [29]. Hypoalbuminemia, another risk factor associated with sepsis after TJRs [30], was not captured due to a significant amount of missing data. It is not a mandatory test in our pre-operative clinic. Since it is not, validation is also needed across other cohorts of TJR patients. Second, these results cannot be applied to other surgical specialties, since frailty prevalence might differ from orthopedic patients, and it is still unclear which frailty instrument is better suited for a specific surgical subgroup. Third, as mentioned, we excluded urgent surgical procedures as the prevalence of frailty is usually higher in this group. In a previous study evaluating frailty with the Frailty Index in hip fracture patients, the prevalence of being very frail on admission was 36%. Therefore, our findings may not apply to them.

Table 4 Comparison of robustness between the clinical frailty scale and the FRAIL Scale

Clinical Frailty Scale	FRAIL Scale		
		Robust	Not robust
	Robust	11	29
	Not robust	2	45

Cohen's kappa: 0.245 ($p = 0.002$)

As for our study's strengths, the recruitment process did not delay surgery and usual care, and was easily implemented in routine assessment due to the simplicity of both selected scales. Our results agree with the existing literature and, to our knowledge, it is the first time that the Clinical Frailty Scale and the FRAIL Scale have been applied in a TJR population.

Conclusion

In conclusion, the Clinical Frailty Scale was, while the FRAIL scale was not, significantly associated with hospital LOS and discharge to rehabilitation center in our cohort of TJR patients. Whether either instrument can be generalized to other surgical patients and used to target vulnerable elderly patients for pre-operative intervention needs to be investigated.

Abbreviations

BMI: Body mass index; Hb: Hemoglobin; IQR: Interquartile range; LOS: Length of stay; THA: Total hip arthroplasty; TJR: Total joint replacement; TKA: Total knee arthroplasty

Acknowledgements

No acknowledgments.

Funding

Not applicable.

Authors' contributions

HTW, JF, SA, PAV and PH all contributed to study design and data interpretation. HTW analyzed the data and wrote the manuscript. All authors provided valuable comments on the manuscript and approved the final version for submission/publication.

Authors' information

See title page.

Consent for publication

Not applicable.

Competing interests

The authors declare that they have no competing interests.

Author details

[1]Department of Internal medicine and Critical Care Medicine, Centre Integre Universitaire de Sante et Services Sociaux (CIUSSS) de l'est de l'île de Montréal, Hopital Maisonneuve-Rosemont, 5415 boul. l'Assomption, H1T 2M4, Montreal, Quebec, Canada. [2]Department of Surgery, Centre Integre Universitaire de Sante et Services Sociaux (CIUSSS) de l'est de l'île de Montréal, Hôpital Maisonneuve-Rosemont, 5415 boul. l'Assomption, H1T 2M4, Montreal, Quebec, Canada. [3]Departments of Medicine and Critical Care Medicine and Centre de recherche, Centre hospitalier de l'Université de Montréal (CRCHUM), 900 St-Denis, H2X 0A9, Montréal, Québec, Canada.

A. References

1. Canadian Institute for Health Information. Hip and Knee Replacements in Canada: Canadian Joint Replacement Registry 2014 Annual Report. https://

secure.cihi.ca/estore/productFamily.htm?pf=PFC3391&lang=en&media=0 (2014). Accessed February 2, 2017.

2. Romero-Artuno R, Kenny RA. The frailty index in Europeans: association with age and mortality. Age Ageing. 2012;41(5):684–98.
3. Gobbens RJ, Luijkx KG, Wijnen-Sponselee MT, Schols JM. Toward a conceptual definition of frail community dwelling older people. Nurs Outlook. 2010;58(2):76–86.
4. De Lepeleire J, Lliffe S, Mann E, Degryse JM. Frailty: An emerging concept for general practice. Br J Gen Pract. 2009;59(562):e177–82.
5. Collard RM, Boter H, Schoevers RA, Oude Voshaar RC. Prevalence of frailty in community-dwelling older persons: a systematic review. J Am Geriatr Soc. 2012;60(8):1487–92.
6. Makary MA, Segev DL, Pronovost PJ, Syin D, Bandeen-Roche K, Patel P, et al. Frailty as a predictor of surgical outcomes in older patients. J Am Coll Surg. 2010;210(6):901–8.
7. Afilalo J, Mottillo S, Eisenberg MJ, Alexander KP, Noiseux N, Perrault LP, et al. Addition of frailty and disability to cardiac surgery risk scores identifies elderly patients at high risk of mortality or major morbidity. Circ Cardiovasc Qual Outcomes. 2012;5(2):222–8.
8. Ganapathi AM, Englum BR, Hanna JM, Schechter MA, Gaga JG, Hurwitz LM, et al. Frailty and risk in proximal aortic surgery. J Thorac Cardiovasc Surg. 2014;147(1):186–91.
9. Buigues C, Juarros-Folgado P, Fernande-Garrido J, Navarro-Martinez R, Cauli O. Frailty syndrome and risk of pre-operative evaluation: a systematic review. Arch Gerontol Geriatr. 2015;61(3):309–21.
10. Cigolle CT, Ofstedal MB, Tian Z, Blaum CS. Comparing models of frailty: the health and retirement study. J Am Geriatr Soc. 2009;57(5):830–9.
11. Ibrahim MS, Twaij H, Giebaly DE, Nizam I, Haddad FS. Enhanced recovery in total hip replacement: a clinical review. Bone Joint J. 2013;95-B(12):1587–94.
12. Snow R, Granata J, Ruhil AV, Vogel K, McShane M, Wasielewski R. Associations between preoperative physical therapy and post-acute care utilization patterns and cost in total joint replacement. J Bone Joint Surg Am. 2014;96(19):e165.
13. Kehlet H, Thienpont E. Fast-track Knee arthroplasty – status and future challenges. Knee. 2013;20(Suppl 1):S29–33.
14. Walston J, Hadley EC, Ferrucci L, Guralnik JM, Newman AB, Studenski SA, et al. Research agenda for frailty in older adults: toward a better understanding of physiology and etiology: summary from the American Geriatrics Society/National Institute on Aging research conference on frailty in older adults. J Am Geriatr Soc. 2006;54(6):991–1001.
15. Mitniski AB, Graham JE, Mogilner AJ, Rockwood K. Frailty, fitness and late-life mortality in relation to chronological and biological age. BMC Geriatr. 2002;27(2):1–8.
16. Fried LP, Tangen CM, Walston J, Newman AB, Hirsch C, Gottdiener J, et al. Frailty in older adults: evidence for a phenotype. J Gerontol A Biol Sci Med Sci. 2001;56(3):M146–56.
17. Rockwood K, Song X, MacKnight C, Bergman H, Hogan DB, McDowell I, et al. A global clinical measure of fitness and frailty in elderly people. CMAJ. 2005;173(5):489–95.
18. Abellan van Kan G, Rolland Y, Bergman H, Morley JE, Kritchevsky SB, Vellas B. The I.A.N.A task force on frailty assessment of older people in clinical practice. J Nutr Health Aging. 2008;12(1):29–37.
19. Morley JE, Malmstrom TK, Miller DK. A simple frailty questionnaire (FRAIL) predicts outcomes in middle aged African Americans. J Nutr Health Aging. 2012;16(7):601–8.
20. Fried LP, Ferrucci L, Darer J, Williamson JD, Anderson G. Untangling the concepts of disability, frailty, and comorbidity: implications for improved targeting and care. J Gerontol A Biol Sci Med Sci. 2004;59(3):255–63.
21. Charlson M, Szatrowski TP, Peterson J, Gold J. Validation of a combined comorbidity index. J Clin Epidemiol. 1994;47(11):1245–51.
22. Brorsson B, Asberg KH. Katz Index of independence in ADL. Reliability and validity in short-term care. Scand J Rehabil Med. 1984;16(3):125–32.
23. Lovald ST, Ong KL, Malkani AL, Lau EC, Schmier JK, Kurtz SM, et al. complications, mortality, and costs for outpatient and short-stay total knee arthroplasty patients in comparison to standard-stay patients. J Arthroplast. 2004;29(3):510–5.
24. Cook JR, Warren M, Ganley KJ, Prefontaine P, Wylie JW. A comprehensive joint replacement program for total knee arthroplasty: a descriptive study. BMC Musculoskelet Disord. 2008;9(154)
25. Hart A, Bergeron SG, Epure L, Huk O, Zukor D, Antoniou J. Comparison of US and Canadian perioperative outcomes and hospital efficiency after Total hip and knee arthroplasty. JAMA Surg. 2015;150(10):990–8.
26. McIsaac DI, Beaule PE, Bryson GL, Van Walraven C. The impact of frailty on outcomes and healthcare resource usage after total joint arthroplasty: a population-based cohort study. Bone Joint J. 2016;98-B(6):799–805.
27. Cooper Z, Rogers SO Jr, Ngo L, Guess J, Schmitt E, Jones RN, et al. Comparison of frailty measures as predictors of outcomes after orthopedic surgery. J Am Geriatr Soc. 2016;64(12):2464–71.
28. Afilalo J. Conceptual models of frailty: the sarcopenia phenotype. Can J Cardiol. 2016;32:1051–5.
29. Carson JL, Terrin ML, Noveck H, Sanders DW, Chaitman BR, Rhoads GG, et al. Liberal or restrictive transfusion in high-risk patients after hip surgery. N Engl J Med. 2011;365(26):2453–62.
30. Bohl DD, Shen MR, Kayupov E, Cvetanovich GL, Della Valle CJ. Is hypoalbuminemia associated with septic failure and acute infection after revision Total joint arthroplasty? A study of 4517 patients from the National Surgical Quality Improvement Program. J Arthroplast. 2016;31(5):963–7.

Supervised neuromuscular exercise prior to hip and knee replacement: 12-month clinical effect and cost-utility analysis alongside a randomised controlled trial

Linda Fernandes[1,2*], Ewa M. Roos[3], Søren Overgaard[1,4], Allan Villadsen[1] and Rikke Søgaard[5,6]

Abstract

Background: There are indications of beneficial short-term effect of pre-operative exercise in reducing pain and improving activity of daily living after total hip replacement (THR) and total knee replacement (TKR) surgery. Though, information from studies conducting longer follow-ups and economic evaluations of exercise prior to THR and TKR is needed. The aim of the study was to analyse 12-month clinical effect and cost-utility of supervised neuromuscular exercise prior to THR and TKR surgery.

Methods: The study was conducted alongside a randomised controlled trial including 165 patients scheduled for standard THR or TKR at a hospital located in a rural area of Denmark. The patients were randomised to replacement surgery with or without an 8-week preoperative supervised neuromuscular exercise program (Clinical Trials registration no.: NCT01003756). Clinical effect was measured with Hip disability and Osteoarthritis Outcome Score (HOOS) and Knee injury and Osteoarthritis Outcome Score (KOOS). Quality adjusted life years (QALYs) were based on EQ-5D-3L and Danish preference weights. Resource use was extracted from national registries and valued using standard tariffs (2012-EUR). Incremental net benefit was analysed to estimate the probability for the intervention being cost effective for a range of threshold values. A health care sector perspective was applied.

Results: HOOS/KOOS quality of life [8.25 (95% CI, 0.42 to 16.10)] and QALYs [0.04 (95% CI, 0.01 to 0.07)] were statistically significantly improved. Effect-sizes ranged between 0.09-0.59 for HOOS/KOOS subscales. Despite including an intervention cost of €326 per patient, there was no difference in total cost between groups [€132 (95% CI −3942 to 3679)]. At a threshold of €40,000, preoperative exercise was found to be cost effective at 84% probability.

Conclusion: Preoperative supervised neuromuscular exercise for 8 weeks was found to be cost-effective in patients scheduled for THR and TKR surgery at conventional thresholds for willingness to pay. One-year clinical effects were small to moderate and favoured the intervention group, but only statistically significant for quality of life measures.

Keywords: Osteoarthritis, Exercise, Cost-benefit analysis, Arthroplasty, Replacement

* Correspondence: linda.fernandes1@gmail.com
[1]Department of Orthopaedic Surgery and Traumatology, Odense University Hospital, Odense, Denmark
[2]Department of Rehabilitation, Odense University Hospital, Sdr. Boulevard 29, 5000 Odense C, Denmark
Full list of author information is available at the end of the article

Background

Total hip and knee replacement (THR and TKR) surgery are recognized treatments for pain relief in patients with severe symptoms from hip or knee osteoarthritis (OA) [1]. Nevertheless, one year after surgery up to 50% of patients undergoing THR and TKR may not experience clinically important improvements in pain and activities of daily living (ADL) [2, 3]. Supervised exercise has shown to be effective treatment for reducing pain and improving ADL in patients with OA [4–9]. It seems exercise at later stages of the disease, and prior to joint replacement surgery, also has beneficial results [10, 11].

However, before a new treatment strategy such as preoperative exercise is implemented, one key input into the decision-making process is the effect and cost-effectiveness of the strategy in question. Today, information on the post-operative effect of exercise prior to surgery is sparse and sufficiently powered studies with feasible interventions and longer follow-ups along with high-quality economic evaluations are warranted [11–15].

We previously conducted a randomised controlled trial (RCT) evaluating an 8-week supervised neuromuscular exercise prior to THR and TKR [10, 16]. The study showed overall improvements in favour of the exercise group in ADL prior to surgery and at 6 weeks postoperatively. At 3 months postoperatively the effects were diminished [16]. Although demonstrating short-term effects only, the addition of preoperative exercise may be clinically important in early mobilisation and returning to prior activities. Our aim with this study was to evaluate one-year clinical effect and cost-utility of the supervised neuromuscular exercise programme prior to THR and TKR. If supervised exercise prior to THR and TKR is shown to be cost-effective, health policy decision makers should consider changing the pre-operative care trajectory to include supervised exercise prior to THR and TKR.

Methods

Overview of study design and participants

165 patients were included between 4 January 2010 and 21 March 2011.[10, 16] Inclusion criteria were; ≥18 years of age and scheduled for THR or TKR due to symptomatic OA. Exclusion criteria were; scheduled for bilateral surgery, previous fractures in or adjacent to the joint, inflammatory arthritis and severe heart disease or neurologic deficits. Included patients were randomly allocated to the intervention group, i.e. supervised neuromuscular exercise and preoperative educational package (EP); or to the control group, i.e. EP alone (Fig. 1). The primary outcome was the ADL subscale of the Hip disability and Osteoarthritis Outcome Score (HOOS) and Knee injury and Osteoarthritis Outcome Score (KOOS) [17–19].

Clinical effect was measured with HOOS and KOOS at one year post-surgery. Assessments points were at baseline, 8 weeks (post-intervention), 15 weeks (6 weeks post-surgery), 21 weeks (3 months post-surgery) and 61 weeks (one year post-surgery). The economic evaluation was conducted alongside the RCT and applied the health care sector perspective, incorporating cost of health care services, including cost of the exercise program. It took form of a cost-utility analysis using Quality Adjusted Life Years (QALYs). The time horizon was 61 weeks within the start and end date of the study (4 January 2010 – 13 August 2012).

Intervention

The neuromuscular exercise programme was supervised by a physiotherapist and focused on lower extremity muscular control and quality of movement.[10, 16, 20, 21] It consisted of three parts: warm-up, circuit programme and cool-down. The majority of the exercises were weight-bearing exercises imitating functions of daily living and the patients learned how to control hip-knee-foot alignment in each exercise. Progression of exercise level was guided by neuromuscular control and quality of the performance (determined by the physiotherapist) and with acceptable exertion (determined by the patient). The programme was delivered in groups of 6–12 patients twice weekly lasting 1 h per session at the Department of Rehabilitation at Odense University Hospital, Svendborg, in a rural part of Southern Denmark. An attendance of 12 sessions or more was considered good compliance.

The EP was standard preoperative information on the operating procedure, expected postoperative progression and a leaflet on various exercises [16]. All patients were offered the EP.

Intervention cost

Valuation of formal care of the exercise program was based on tariff-based costs for physiotherapy in primary care (https://fysio.dk/globalassets/documents/raadgivning/overenskomster/praksisoverenskomster/takster-for-fysioterapi-oktober-2016.pdf). The fees reflect the physiotherapist's wage, capital cost and expenses, e.g. rental costs, use of equipment, dispensable material and electricity. Implementation cost of the exercise program was not included. Costs for the 3-h patient education package were not included as this was offered to all participants in the trial. All monetary units were reported in 2012-EUR with an exchange rate of DKK 7.45 to 1 EUR.

Health care utilisation and cost

Individual data was extracted from two national registers: The National Health Insurance Service Registry and The Danish National Patient Register [22, 23]. The former includes details about all services provided in primary care including national reimbursement fees [22].

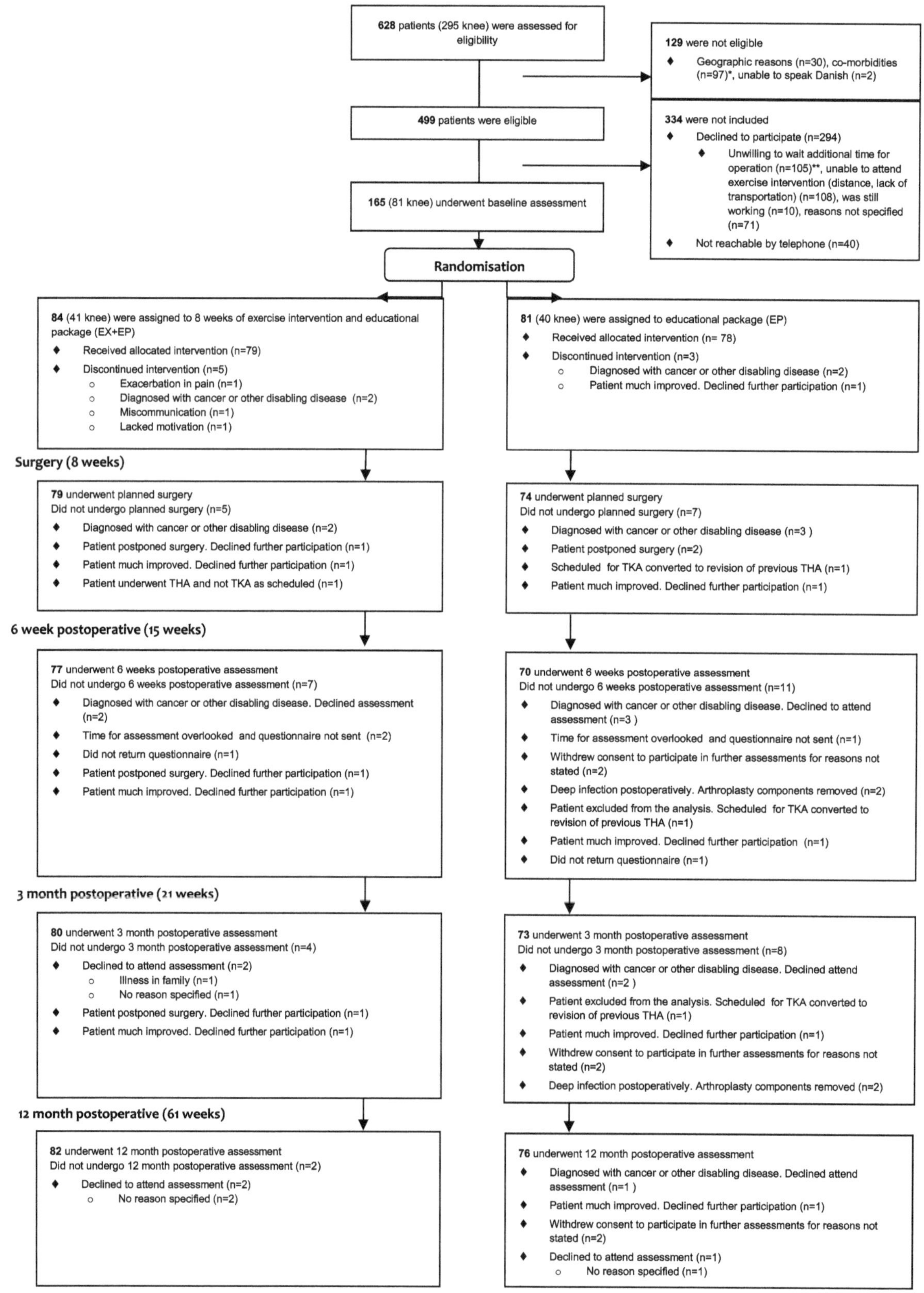

Fig. 1 (See legend on next page.)

(See figure on previous page.)
Fig. 1 Flow diagram of patients participating in this study. * Co-morbidities (n = 97). ◆ Previous fracture in or adjacent to the joint (*n* = 13) (1 knee). ◆ Inflammatory arthritis (*n* = 11) (5 knee). ◆ Revision arthroplasty (*n* = 7) (4 knee). ◆ Previously enrolled with another joint (*n* = 9) (7 knee). ◆ Unicompartemental replacement (knee) (*n* = 27). ◆ Bilateral procedure in same session or within 3 month (*n* = 16). ◆ Necrosis of the femoral head (hip) (*n* = 6). ◆ Neurological disorders (*n* = 6), Hemiparesis (*n* = 2), Parkinsons Disorder (*n* = 2), Dementia (n = 2). ◆ Dysplasia of the femoral head (*n* = 1). ◆ Possible cancer metastasis in proximal femur (*n* = 1). ** The Danish Healthcare System has a one month treatment guarantee. Entering this study meant all patients accepting an additional wait of up to 5 weeks in comparison to the treatment guarantee. After randomization, this additional wait applied only for patients randomized to the 8 week exercise intervention. The control group was operated on when originally scheduled

The latter includes details about all contacts to hospitals including diagnoses, procedures and diagnosis-related-grouping casemix tariffs [23].

Patient expenses

Valuation of patients' time and transport for attending the exercise classes were included in a sensitivity analysis. Valuation of informal time (i.e. time spent by patients attending the exercise regimen) was based on a human capital approach, for which the value of a person's time is reflected by wage rates (productivity loss). The wage rate was estimated by applying age- and gender matched national average gross income for year 2012 extracted from Statistics Denmark [24]. Informal time for one exercise session was set to a fixed value of 1.25 h. Patients' expenses for travelling to and from the gym were calculated by using the national fees for travel reimbursement for 2012 (DKK 3.80/km or €0.51/km) times the distance (km) between the exercise facility and patients' homes.

Patient reported outcome measures

The HOOS and KOOS assesses pain, symptoms, ADL, function in sport and recreation and knee related quality of life in five separate subscales scored on a 0–100 (worst to best) scale [18, 19, 25, 26].

Utility was expressed as QALYs measured with the generic outcome measure European Quality of Life 5-Dimension 3-Level Health Outcome (EQ-5D-3L) [27]. Health state valuations from the Danish general population were adopted [28].

Analysis

Baseline subject characteristics were summarised as number (%) or mean (SD). QALYs were produced by calculating the area under the curve of the EQ-5D-3L utility scores from baseline and all follow-ups assuming linear trend between observations. Visits and costing for primary care were categorised based on care provider. In hospital stay and costing for secondary care were categorised based on primary unit. All parameters were tested for normality and distribution. Because of skewed data all comparative analyses, including the net benefit, were based on bootstrapped standard errors. Non-parametric bootstrapping with 10,000 replications was applied [29].

Group comparisons were based on intention-to-treat analysis.[30] Since no interaction (group allocation joint involved) was seen in the original RCT,[16] the analyses did not adjust for hip or knee involvement. One-year clinical effect was expressed as the between-group mean difference [95% confidence interval (CI)] of change values (61 weeks – baseline) and effect-size (d = mean difference of change values/pooled baseline standard deviation) of the five subscale scores of the HOOS and KOOS. Analysis of linear regression was used for between-group comparisons of QALYs and costs and presented as between-group mean differences (95% CI) over the time horizon. An adjustment for baseline health utility was included in the analysis to account for baseline imbalances in the estimation of mean differential QALYs [31].

Handling of missing EQ-5D-3L utility scores was based on comparison of complete item response and two different imputation methods: last observation carried forward (LOCF), in which missing values are imputed based on existing values, and linear trend at point (LTAP), in which missing values are imputed by values based on a linear regression model using nonmissing observations in the series to fit the regression. Analysis comparing responders and non-responders was performed for QALYs. Since imputed data using the LTAP method showed the lowest mean difference estimate for QALYs (Table 2), and thereby the lowest risk of overestimating results, it was decided to be used in the analyses. A significance level of 0.05 was used.

Cost-utility

The cost-utility analysis adopted a health care sector perspective. We estimated the value for money of the intervention by calculating the incremental net monetary benefit using a range of hypothetical threshold values for decision-makers' willingness-to-pay for a unit of effect [32]. The threshold values ranged from €0 to €100,000. The net benefits were presented visually in cost-effectiveness acceptability curves (CEAC). These curves illustrate the probability that the intervention is cost-effective compared to the control at various threshold values of willingness-to-pay for a QALY gain. A willingness-to-pay of €40,000 per QALY gained was used as the threshold indicating good value for money [33, 34].

Sensitivity analyses

Four sensitivity analyses were performed to assess robustness of results for cost-utility and presented in the CEAC.

1. Complete item response analysis leaving out patients not filling in the EQ-5D-3L one or more times during the follow-up period.
2. Per-protocol analysis including only patients who complied to exercise.
3. Not adjusting analysis for the potentially skewed baseline EQ-5D-3 L.
4. Including patients' travel and time costs associated with attending exercise.

Results

Overall, 92.1% of the observations of the HOOS or KOOS and the EQ-5D-3L at the five assessment points were complete. There were 122 (74%) complete item responses for QALYs. There was no significant difference between number of patients with missing QALY in the intervention ($n = 21$) and control group ($n = 22$) ($p = 0.75$). Cost data had no missing values. Except for the EQ-5D-3L, there were no differences at baseline. Baseline characteristics are presented in Table 1. Five patients did not go through THR or TKR surgery during the 61 weeks. Reasons for declining surgery were: intervention group, much improved after exercise ($n = 1$) and no reason specified ($n = 1$); and control group, cancer ($n = 1$), started to exercise on her own ($n = 1$) and anxious about surgical procedure ($n = 1$).

Table 1 Baseline subject characteristics

	Intervention group	Control group	Mean difference (95%CI)
n	84	81	
Female sex	47 (56%)	45 (56%)	
Age–years	67.9 (8.6)	66.9 (8.3)	1.08 (−1.52 to 3.67)
BMI–kg/m^2	29.6 (4.5)	31.1 (6.1)	−1.41 (−3.05 to 0.24)
Waiting list THA	43 (51%)	41 (51%)	
Waiting list TKA	41 (49%)	40 (49%)	
EQ-5D-3L	0.63 (0.15)	0.57 (0.19)	0.06 (0.01 to 0.12)
HOOS/KOOS			
ADL	50.5 (15.1)	45.6 (16.9)	4.9 (−0.02 to 9.83)
Pain	46.8 (14.3)	42.7 (14.4)	4.0 (−0.39 to 8.46)
Symptoms	49.4 (19.7)	44.6 (18.6)	4.8 (−0.98 to 10.55)
Sport & Recreation	24.6 (17.2)	19.9 (18.2)	4.6 (−0.80 to 10.09)
Quality of life	31.2 (12.1)	28.9 (15.9)	2.3 (−2.01 to 6.60)

Continuous variables are expressed as the mean (SD); non-continuous variables are expressed as the number of patients (%); *THA*, Total hip arthroplasy; *TKA*, Total knee arthroplasty; *EQ5D-3L*, European Quality of Life 5 Dimension 3 Level Health Outcome; *HOOS*, Hip disability and Osteoarthritis Outcome Score; *KOOS*, Knee injury and Osteoarthritis Outcome Score; *ADL*, function in daily living

Patient reported outcomes

The intervention was associated with a statistically significant QALY gain of 0.04 (95% CI, 0.01 to 0.07). The QALYs showed similar results for complete item response, different imputation methods and unadjusted analyses (Table 2). Mean differences at 61 weeks favoured the exercise group for all HOOS/KOOS subscales, however only significantly so for the quality of life subscale [mean difference 8.25 points (95% CI, 0.42 to 16.10)] (Table 2). Effect-sizes for HOOS/KOOS subscales ranged from 0.09 – 0.59 (Table 2).

Resource use

All patients in both groups attended the preoperative education package prior to surgery. In total, 144 exercise sessions were provided during the intervention period with a mean of 7.7 patients per session. On average, patients in the intervention group had attended the exercise programme 13.1 times (Table 3). Sixty-two of the 84 patients in the intervention group (74%) displayed good compliance.

The average number of health care visits in primary and secondary care, including the number of inhospital days was not significantly different between groups, with the exception of visits with a chiropractor (Table 3). In total, 4 and 36 visits with chiropractor were registered in the intervention and control groups, respectively. 95% of the visits in the subgroup "other" had visited the dentist. None of the participants had visited psychologist funded by the national health care system during the follow-up period. Summarizing all inhospital days, 75% were to orthopaedic units.

Cost

Participating in the supervised neuromuscular exercise program cost on average (SE) €326 (12.9) per patient (Table 4). A mean of 7.7 patients attended each session. Hence, the tariff to the physiotherapist was based on groups of eight equivalent to a cost of €186/session (https://fysio.dk/praksis/Overenskomst-og-takster/Almen-fysioterapi1/Almen-fysioterapi/). No differences between groups (€-132; 95% CI −3668 to 3405) were found for costs in primary or secondary health care sector (Table 4). The largest cost was, as expected, found for inpatient hospital stay.

Table 2 Mean differences of QALYs and HOOS or KOOS for the 61-week follow-up period

	Intervention ($n = 84$)		Control ($n = 81$)			
	n	Mean (SE)	n	Mean (SE)	Mean difference (95% CI)	ES
QALY, LTAP[a]	84	0.66 (0.04)	81	0.61 (0.04)	0.04 (0.01 to 0.07)	
QALY, LTAP[b]	84	0.80 (0.01)	81	0.74 (0.01)	0.06 (0.02 to 0.09)	
QALY, LOCF[a]	82	0.64 (0.05)	79	0.58 (0.05)	0.05 (0.02 to 0.09)	
QALY, complete[a]	63	0.68 (0.05)	59	0.63 (0.05)	0.05 (0.02 to 0.09)	
QALY, per-protocol[a]	62	0.63 (0.04)	81	0.59 (0.05)	0.04 (0.01 to 0.07)	
HOOS/KOOS						
ADL	84	35.9 (2.1)	81	32.1 (2.4)	3.80 (−2.45 to 10.07)	0.24
Pain	84	41.2 (2.2)	81	37.1 (2.4)	4.13 (−2.33 to 10.60)	0.29
Symptoms	84	33.9 (2.7)	81	32.2 (2.6)	1.69 (−5.79 to 9.17)	0.09
Sport and Recreation	84	33.1 (3.6)	81	26.3 (2.8)	6.79 (−2.10 to 15.69)	0.39
Quality of Life	84	43.4 (2.6)	81	35.2 (3.0)	8.25 (0.42 to 16.10)	0.59

Mean (bootstrap SE) and mean differences (95% confidence interval). ES, effect-size (mean difference/pooled standard deviation)
QALY, quality-adjusted life-years; complete, complete item response analysis; *LTAP*, linear trend at point; *LCOF*, last observation carried forward; per-protocol, per-protocol analysis equals attending ≥12 exercise sessions. *HOOS*, Hip disability and Osteoarthritis Outcome Score; *KOOS*, Knee injury and Osteoarthritis Outcome Score; *ADL*, function in daily living
[a]Adjusted for baseline EQ-5D-3 L scores
[b]Unadjusted analysis

Patients attending exercise travelled on average 21.5 km (range 0.5–78.3 km) to the exercise facility and had a mean (SE) transportation cost of €137 (12.2). The mean (SE) informal time valuation was €302 (15.3) for the intervention period. When including patients' expenses, the cost for the intervention increased to a mean (SE) of €765 (33.5) per patient during the intervention period.

Cost-utility

At conventional thresholds, decision-makers willingness to pay around €40,000 the probability for the intervention being cost-utile was estimated at 84%. Sensitivity analyses showed that the cost-utility result was robust (Fig. 2).

Discussion

The present analysis demonstrates that a pre-operative 8-week supervised exercise intervention was cost-effective, showing a probability of 84% for decision-makers willingness to pay around €40,000 for a QALY gained. This is comparable to the typical threshold between £20,000 and £30,000 per QALY gained used by the British National Health Service when instituting new treatments.[34] Compared to care as usual, we found no overall additional health care cost during the first post-operative year despite adding 8 weeks of physiotherapist-supervised exercise prior to TKR and THR surgery. In return one can expect QALY gain over the following year.

This study is one of few RCTs that estimates costs and cost-effectiveness of exercise as treatment in patients with hip and knee OA, and, to our knowledge, the first to analyse cost-utility of exercise prior to THR and TKR. Previous cost-effectiveness analyses evaluating exercise, as the only intervention and not prior to surgery, in patients with knee OA found better health outcomes at lower costs, i.e. exercise was cost saving [13]. One RCT found that water-based exercise saved £123-175 per patient per year despite a relatively high intervention cost (£830 per patient) [35]. A second RCT found that both aerobic and resistance training were cost saving, $114 and $117, respectively, along with improvements in self-reported functioning [36]. A third RCT found QALY gains of 0.023 (SE 0.04) from class-based exercise compared to home-based exercise and a probability of 70% of being cost-effective at a willingness to pay of £30.000 [37]. Further, two RCTs have shown less total costs for patients with hip OA and chronic knee pain, respectively, following patient education and exercise programs compared to usual care [38, 39]. Comparing our study of exercise prior to OA surgery to studies evaluating exercise interventions in other patient groups, the results are quite similar. A Cochrane review of exercise for patients with heart failure reported a QALY gain of 0.03 and a probability of 90% for willingness to pay around 50.000 USD [40], group-based exercise for the prevention of falling showed an incremental cost per QALY gain of 72.700 AUD [41], and pelvic-floor muscle training showed cost-effectiveness with a probability of >70% for the willingness to pay around £50.000 [42].

We found that patients allocated to exercise had a lower total length of hospital stay and total cost during the follow-up period. The results were not statistically significant. However, should these findings not be due to

Table 3 Health care utilization during 61 weeks

	Intervention group ($n = 84$)	Control group ($n = 81$)	Mean difference (95% CI)
Intervention			
Exercise sessions, mean (range)	13.1 (0–24)	0	13.1 (12.2 to 14.0)
Primary health care, visits			
General practice	18.2 (1.3)	19.5 (1.7)	−1.36 (−5.46 to 2.74)
Physiotherapist	0.3 (0.1)	0.5 (0.2)	−0.27 (−0.81 to 0.27)
Medical specialist	0.9 (0.2)	1.0 (0.2)	−0.05 (−0.57 to 0.48)
Chiropractor	0	0.4 (0.03)	−0.40 (−0.77 to −0.03)
Other[a]	2.0 (0.1)	2.2 (0.2)	−0.28 (−0.72 to 0.16)
Subtotal	21.4 (1.3)	23.7 (1.7)	−2.36 (−6.61 to 1.90)
Secondary health care, visits			
Outpatient	8.4 (0.9)	8.5 (1.0)	−0.13 (−2.80 to 2.55)
Emergency	0.2 (0.1)	0.5 (0.1)	−0.24 (−0.52 to 0.03)
Subtotal	8.6 (0.9)	9.0 (1.1)	−0.37 (−3.16 to 2.43)
Secondary health care, inhospital days			
Orthopeadic	3.6 (0.4)	4.6 (1.1)	−0.95 (−3.32 to 1.42)
Surgery[b]	0.3 (0.1)	1.2 (0.7)	−0.91 (−2.28 to 0.45)
Medicine[c]	0.7 (0.3)	0.8 (0.3)	−0.12 (−0.92 to 0.68)
Oncology[d]	0	0.4 (0.3)	−0.37 (−0.95 to 0.22)
Other	0.3 (0.2)	0.3 (0.3)	−0.01 (−0.72 to 0.70)
Subtotal	4.8 (0.7)	7.2 (1.8)	−2.36 (−6.11 to 1.38)

Variables are expressed as the mean (bootstrap SE) number of outpatient visits or in-hospital days per patient during the 61 week follow-up period and the mean difference (95% confidence interval) between groups
[a]Other, includes visits at the dentistry, laboratory or foot care clinic
[b]Surgery, gastrointestinal, urology, plastic, thoracic
[c]Medicine, internal medicine, cardiology, medical gastroenterology, neurology, geriatrics, general practice
[d]Other, includes inhospital stay at oftamology, odontology or physiotherapy units

Table 4 Costs of the intervention, outpatient and emergency visits and inpatient hospital stay during 61 weeks

	Intervention group ($n = 84$)	Control group ($n = 81$)	Mean difference (95% CI)
Intervention			
Physiotherapy	326 (13)	0	326 (301 to 351)
Primary health care sector			
General Practice	331 (28)	345 (29)	−14 (−92 to 64)
Physiotherapist	22 (10)	98 (61)	−76 (−197 to 45)
Specialists	99 (21)	97 (29)	2 (−68 to 72)
Chiropractor	2 (1)	6 (2)	−4 (−9 to 0)
Other[a]	75 (7)	83 (8)	−7 (−28 to 14)
Subtotal	530 (35)	629 (74)	−99 (−258 to 60)
Secondary health care sector			
Outpatient	2240 (560)	1917 (317)	323 (−933 to 1579)
Emergency	12 (4)	32 (11)	−20 (−43 to 4)
Subtotal	2252 (557)	1949 (316)	303 (−949 to 1555)
Secondary health care sector			
Orthopaedics	11760 (572)	11695 (1038)	66 (−2250 to 2382)
Surgery[b]	280 (180)	773 (363)	−493 (−1285 to 300)
Medicine[c]	883 (322)	865 (350)	18 (−919 to 955)
Oncology	0	213 (170)	−213 (−547 to 120)
Other[d]	150 (149)	189 (169)	−40 (−494 to 415)
Subtotal	13074 (706)	13735 (1249)	−662 (−3478 to 2154)
TOTAL	16181 (1174)	16313 (1374)	−132 (−3668 to 3405)

Variables are expressed as the mean (bootstrap SE) per patient during the 61 week follow-up period and the mean difference (95% confidence interval) between groups. The monetary units are presented in EUR2012
[a]Other, includes visits at the dentistry, laboratory or foot care clinic
[b]Surgery, gastrointestinal, urology, plastic, thoracic
[c]Medicine, internal medicine, cardiology, medical gastroenterology, neurology, geriatrics, general practice
[d]Other, includes inhospital stay at oftamology, odontology or physiotherapy units

random variation, a reduction of 2.4 days in hospital per patient and year is a relevant difference for the health care system. In 2012, a total of 8787 and 8008 patients underwent THR and TKR, respectively, at Danish hospitals [43, 44]. Extrapolating the resource use to the Danish THR and TKR population in 2012, exercise prior to surgery could potentially save 39.500 days in hospital per year. Seventy-five percent of all in hospital days during the 61 week period were at orthopaedic units, leaving 25% at other units. We did not ask the patients about comorbidities, but the data show that at least some had concurrent diseases. The second largest cost, after admission to orthopaedic units, was admission to internal medicine and cardiology units (Table 4). Over half of the population with hip and knee OA have been found to have concomitant cardiovascular disease and 86% of patients going through THR or TKR have one or more comorbidities [45, 46]. There have also been found significant associations between number and type of comorbidity and lower ADL, pain and HRQoL scores, with largest impact on ADL in THR patients, suggesting that functional limitations due to other diseases have to be taken into account to optimize outcome after THR and TKR [45, 46]. A national database study from Taiwan found a reverse dose-relationship of having coronary artery disease and dyslipidemia in patients attending physiotherapy due to symptoms from their OA, i.e. patients receiving a higher dose of physiotherapy showed a lowered risk of coronary artery disease and dyslipidemia [47]. Since comorbidities are common in OA and possibly can be influenced by the intervention given in our study, we find the inclusion of the total cost and resource use important for this study (Table 3 and 4).

The sensitivity analyses showed that the health care sector perspective using LTAP imputed data was robust

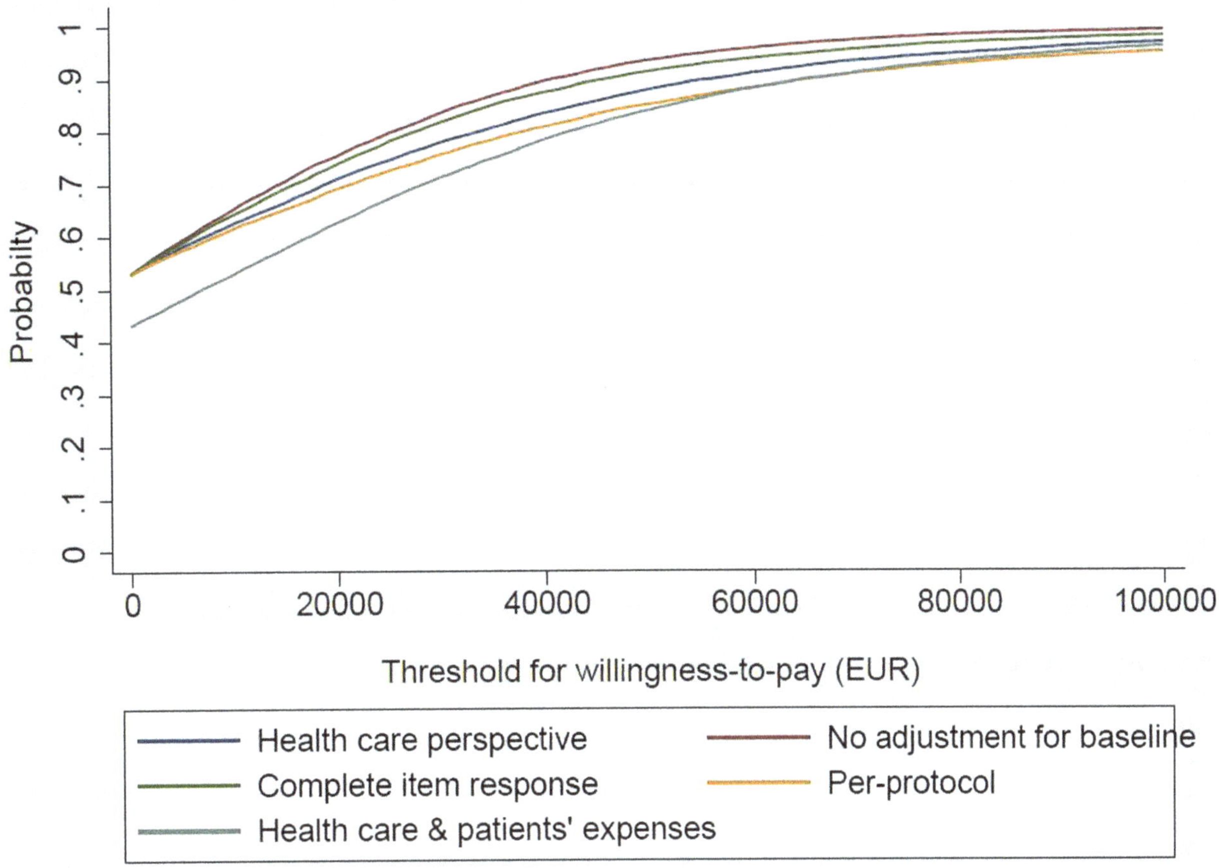

Fig. 2 Cost effectiveness acceptability curves for incremental net monetary benefit to estimate the probability for the intervention being cost effective at conventional thresholds for willingness to pay. Health care perspective, Health Care Sector perspective (base-case analysis); Complete item response, only complete item response of the EQ-5D-3L included in the analysis; Health care & patients' expenses, Health Care Sector and patients' own expenses perspective; No adjustment for baseline, adjustments for baseline EQ-5D-3L scores were not included; Per-protocol, only patients attending 12 or more exercise sessions were included in the analysis

as compared to complete item response, unadjusted and per-protocol analyses. The analysis using the health care sector plus patients' expenses differed slightly from the base-case analysis showing a slightly lower probability for willingness to pay thresholds. This was expected since adding patients' average expenses by €439 to the average cost of the intervention (€326) would result in higher costs for the intervention group, i.e. €765 versus €326 for the intervention per patient calculated with or without patient expenses, respectively. This study had a follow-up period of 61 week. We did not find it necessary to discount for costs or consequences as the study only passed one year by 9 weeks. Implementation cost of the intervention was not included in the analysis as the intervention today is available at 377 private and public physiotherapy clinics nationwide in Denmark [48]. Hence, the exercise program is already on the market in Denmark and could be implemented as standard care for patients undergoing THR or TKR without extra costs for education and training of care providers.

With regards to generalisability of the cost-utility results there are challenges in interpretation due to the vast differences in health care structure worldwide. In Denmark, all health care utilization and cost for different services and procedures performed in primary and secondary care are registered in national registers [22, 23]. To enable comparison to other health care structures, the overall average unit costs in this study can be found by dividing the cost estimates in table 4 with the resource use in table 3 or by viewing the tariff catalogues [49]. However, the efficacy of the intervention is well documented and it is of general interest to optimise the pre- as well as postoperative period with increased activities of daily living and through this a possible reduction in postoperative complications (e.g. joint stiffness, thrombosis/emboli) and a faster return to work for the younger part of this patient group.

Strength and limitations

Some strengths of this RCT were a rigorous design by applying the CONSORT recommendations [30], evaluating a time horizon of one year, in which changes in ADL and HRQoL are expected to appear [50, 51], and using a common generic HRQoL measurement (EQ-5D-3L) to calculate QALYs [52]. Our sample size of 165 allowed us however to detect moderate, as opposed to small, effect sizes. We found a significant effect size of 0.59 favouring the exercise group in HOOS/KOOS quality of life, but the effect size of 0.39 in HOOS/KOOS sport and recreation function remained non-significant (Table 2). One limitation of this RCT was that the Danish national registers do not include costs for care delivered directly by the municipality. In Denmark, the municipality is responsible for post-operative care after hospital discharge, e.g. standard post-operative exercise and home-care. Although group allocation was stratified on municipality, differences in resource use and costs between the groups during the follow-up period may exist. Another limitation was that we had no data on patients' work status (sick-leave, disability pension, retired or in the workforce) or OA-related medicine. The majority of participants in this study were assumed to be retired, as the retirement age in Denmark is 65 years and the average age in the study was 67.5 years at baseline. Even though the majority was assumed to be retired, a recent study has shown that the year after THR and TKR patients cost €6000 more compared to a reference population due to loss of employment income, use of medication and need for home care [53]. A broader societal perspective including also work status, medication and municipality-based services would therefore have been optimal. If this intervention would be implemented in routine clinical practice, the intervention could be provided in the primary care setting usually located within 15 km from peoples' homes. The private pocket cost of transportation would then be reduced whereas program administration costs might increase and gains from economies of scale could be lost. This should be considered and balanced with the potential benefit of extra participation and/or compliance by patients sensitive to provider and/or transportation distance. Finally, of those meeting eligibility criteria for this study only 30% were included which may impact external validity.

Conclusion

Preoperative supervised neuromuscular exercise for 8 weeks was found to be cost-effective in patients scheduled for THR and TKR surgery at conventional thresholds for willingness to pay. One-year clinical effects were small to moderate and favoured the intervention group, but only statistically significantly so for quality of life measures.

Abbreviations

ADL: Activities of Daily Living; CEAC: Cost-Effectiveness Acceptability Curves; CI: Confidence Interval; CONSORT: Consolidated Standards of Reporting Trials; DKK: Danish Krona; EQ-5D-3L: European Quality of Life 5-Dimension 3-Level Health Outcome; HOOS: Hip disability and Osteoarthritis Outcome Score; HRQoL: Health Related Quality of Life; KOOS: Knee injury and Osteoarthritis Outcome Score; LOCF: Last Observation Carried Forward; LTAP: Linear Trend At Point; OA: Osteoarthritis; QALY: Quality Adjusted Life Year; RCT: Randomised Controlled Trial; SD: Standard Deviation; SE: Standard Error; THR: Total Hip Replacement; TKR: Total Knee Replacement; USD: US Dollar

Funding

This study was financed by research grants from OUH Svendborg Hospital (nr. 12/9062) and the Association of Danish Physiotherapists' Foundation for research, CPD and professional development. The funders had no role in the study design, data collection and analysis, decision to publish or preparation of the manuscript.

Authors contribution

All authors were responsible for concept and design. LF and AV were responsible of collection of data. LF was responsible for assembly of data and drafting of the article. LF and RS were responsible for the analysis of data. RS was responsible for statistical expertise. LF, RS, ER, AV and SO were responsible for interpretation of data, critical revision of the article for important intellectual content and for final approval of the article. LF and RS take responsibility for the integrity of the work as a whole from inception to finished article.

Competing interests

LF is co-owner of Ther-ex Ltd, Denmark . AV is co-owner of Ther-ex Ltd., Denmark. Ther-ex Ltd distribute (free of charge and commercial free) the mobile application Ther-ex which offers functional and neuromuscular exercise, exercise diary and pain monitoring for people with hip and knee osteoarthritis. ER is developer of the Good Life with Osteoarthritis in Denmark (GLA:D) program. GLA:D is a not-for-profit initiative to implement clinical guidelines for osteoarthritis, hosted at the University of the Southern Denmark. All other authors declare no competing interests.

Consent for publication

Not applicable.

Author details

[1]Department of Orthopaedic Surgery and Traumatology, Odense University Hospital, Odense, Denmark. [2]Department of Rehabilitation, Odense University Hospital, Sdr. Boulevard 29, 5000 Odense C, Denmark. [3]Research Unit for Musculoskeletal Function and Physiotherapy, Institute of Sports Science and Clinical Biomechanics, University of Southern Denmark, Odense, Denmark. [4]Department of Clinical Research, University of Southern Denmark, Odense, Denmark. [5]Department of Public Health, Aarhus University, Aarhus, Denmark. [6]Department of Clinical Medicine, Aarhus University, Aarhus, Denmark.

References

1. Felson DT, Lawrence RC, Hochberg MC, McAlindon T, Dieppe PA, Minor MA, Blair SN, Berman BM, Fries JF, Weinberger M, et al. Osteoarthritis: New insights. Part 2: treatment approaches. Ann Intern Med. 2000;133(9):726–37.
2. Hawker GA, Badley EM, Borkhoff CM, Croxford R, Davis AM, Dunn S, Gignac MA, Jaglal SB, Kreder HJ, Sale JE. Which patients are most likely to benefit from total joint arthroplasty? Arthritis Rheum. 2013;65(5):1243–52.
3. Paulsen A, Roos EM, Pedersen AB, Overgaard S. Minimal clinically important improvement (MCII) and patient-acceptable symptom state (PASS) in total hip arthroplasty (THA) patients 1 year postoperatively. Acta Orthop. 2014;85(1):39–48.
4. Fransen M, McConnell S. Exercise for osteoarthritis of the knee. Cochrane Database Syst Rev. 2008;4:CD004376.

5. Fransen M, McConnell S, Hernandez-Molina G, Reichenbach S. Exercise for osteoarthritis of the hip. Cochrane Database Syst Rev. 2009;3:CD007912.
6. Lange AK, Vanwanseele B, Fiatarone Singh MA. Strength training for treatment of osteoarthritis of the knee: a systematic review. Arthritis Care Res. 2008;59(10):1488–94.
7. Fernandes L, Hagen KB, Bijlsma JW, Andreassen O, Christensen P, Conaghan PG, Doherty M, Geenen R, Hammond A, Kjeken I, et al. EULAR recommendations for the non-pharmacological core management of hip and knee osteoarthritis. Ann Rheum Dis. 2013;72(7):1125–35.
8. Hernandez-Molina G, Reichenbach S, Bin Z, Lavalley M, Felson DT. Effect of therapeutic exercise for hip osteoarthritis pain: results of a meta-analysis. Arthritis Care Res. 2008;59(9):1221–8.
9. Juhl C, Christensen R, Roos EM, Zhang W, Lund H. Impact of exercise type and dose on pain and disability in knee osteoarthritis: a systematic review and meta-regression analysis of randomized controlled trials. Arthritis Rheumatol. 2014;66(3):622–36.
10. Villadsen A, Overgaard S, Holsgaard-Larsen A, Christensen R, Roos EM. Immediate efficacy of neuromuscular exercise in patients with severe osteoarthritis of the hip or knee: a secondary analysis from a randomized controlled trial. J Rheumatol. 2014;41(7):1385–94.
11. Wallis JA, Taylor NF. Pre-operative interventions (non-surgical and non-pharmacological) for patients with hip or knee osteoarthritis awaiting joint replacement surgery - a systematic review and meta-analysis. Osteoarthritis Cartilage. 2011;19(12):1381–95.
12. Hoogeboom TJ, Oosting E, Vriezekolk JE, Veenhof C, Siemonsma PC, de Bie RA, van den Ende CHM, van Meeteren NLU. Therapeutic validity and effectiveness of preoperative exercise on functional recovery after joint replacement: a systematic review and meta-analysis. PLoS ONE. 2012;7(5):e38031.
13. Pinto D, Robertson MC, Hansen P, Abbott JH. Cost-effectiveness of Nonpharmacologic, nonsurgical interventions for Hip and/or knee osteoarthritis: systematic review. Value Health. 2012;15(1):1–12.
14. Puig-Junoy J, Ruiz Zamora A. Socio-economic costs of osteoarthritis: a systematic review of cost-of-illness studies. Semin Arthritis Rheum. 2015;44(5):531–41.
15. Kwok IH, Paton B, Haddad FS. Does Pre-operative physiotherapy improve outcomes in primary total knee arthroplasty? - a systematic review. J Arthroplasty. 2015;30(9):1657–63.
16. Villadsen A, Overgaard S, Holsgaard-Larsen A, Christensen R, Roos EM. Postoperative effects of neuromuscular exercise prior to hip or knee arthroplasty: a randomised controlled trial. Ann Rheum Dis. 2014;73(6):1130–7.
17. Roos EM, Roos HP, Lohmander LS, Ekdahl C, Beynnon BD. Knee injury and osteoarthritis outcome score (KOOS)–development of a self-administered outcome measure. J Orthop Sports Phys Ther. 1998;28(2):88–96.
18. Roos EM, Toksvig-Larsen S. Knee injury and osteoarthritis outcome score (KOOS) - validation and comparison to the WOMAC in total knee replacement. Health Qual Life Outcomes. 2003;1:17.
19. Nilsdotter AK, Lohmander LS, Klassbo M, Roos EM. Hip disability and osteoarthritis outcome score (HOOS)–validity and responsiveness in total hip replacement. BMC Musculoskelet Disord. 2003;4:10.
20. Ageberg E, Link A, Roos EM. Feasibility of neuromuscular training in patients with severe hip or knee OA: the individualized goal-based NEMEX-TJR training program. BMC Musculoskelet Disord. 2010;11:126.
21. Ageberg E, Nilsdotter A, Kosek E, Roos EM. Effects of neuromuscular training (NEMEX-TJR) on patient-reported outcomes and physical function in severe primary hip or knee osteoarthritis: a controlled before-and-after study. BMC Musculoskelet Disord. 2013;14:232.
22. Sahl Andersen J, De Fine ON, Krasnik A. The Danish national health service register. Scand J Public Health. 2011;39(7 suppl):34–7.
23. Lynge E, Sandegaard JL, Rebolj M. The Danish national patient register. Scand J Public Health. 2011;39(7 suppl):30–3.
24. Gross and Disposable income by region, gender and age range, Table INDKP5. http://www.statistikbanken.dk/statbank5a/default.asp?w=1920.
25. Roos EM, Lohmander LS. The knee injury and osteoarthritis outcome score (KOOS): from joint injury to osteoarthritis. Health Qual Life Outcomes. 2003;1:64.
26. Peer MA, Lane J. The knee injury and osteoarthritis outcome score (KOOS): a review of its psychometric properties in people undergoing total knee arthroplasty. J Orthop Sports Phys Ther. 2013;43(1):20–8.
27. EuroQol Group; Oemar MO, M.: EQ-5D-3 L User Guide. Basic information on how to use the EQ-5D-3 L instrument. . In. http://www.euroqol.org/; 2013.
28. Wittrup-Jensen KU, Lauridsen J, Gudex C, Pedersen KM. Generation of a Danish TTO value set for EQ-5D health states. Scand J Public Health. 2009;37(5):459–66.
29. Efron BT, Tibshirani R. Bootstrap methods for standard errors, confidence intervals and other measures of statistical accuracy. Stat Sci. 1986;1(1):54–77.
30. Schulz KF, Altman DG, Moher D, Group C. CONSORT 2010 statement: updated guidelines for reporting parallel group randomised trials. BMJ. 2010;340:c332.
31. Manca A, Hawkins N, Sculpher MJ. Estimating mean QALYs in trial-based cost-effectiveness analysis: the importance of controlling for baseline utility. Health Econ. 2005;14(5):487–96.
32. Hernández MAN, Vázquez-Polo FJ, González-Torre FJG, Bas EM. Complementing the net benefit approach: a new framework for Bayesian cost-effectiveness analysis. Int J Technol Assess Health Care. 2009;25(04):537–45.
33. Eichler H-G, Kong SX, Gerth WC, Mavros P, Jönsson B. Use of cost-effectiveness analysis in health-care resource allocation decision-making: How Are cost-effectiveness thresholds expected to emerge? Value Health. 2004;7(5):518–28.
34. The National Institute for Health and Care Excellence. How NICE measures value for money in relation to public health interventions. 2013. https://www.nice.org.uk/Media/Default/guidance/LGB10-Briefing-20150126.pdf.
35. Cochrane T, Davey R, Matthes Edwards S. Randomised controlled trial of the cost-effectiveness of water-based therapy for lower limb osteoarthritis. Health Technol Assess. 2005;9(31):130.
36. Sevick MA, Bradham DD, Muender M, Chen GJ, Enarson C, Dailey M, Ettinger WH. Cost-effectiveness of aerobic and resistance exercise in seniors with knee osteoarthritis. Med Sci Sports Exerc. 2000;32(9):1534–40.
37. Richardson G, Hawkins N, McCarthy CJ, Mills PM, Pullen R, Roberts C, Silman A, Oldham JA. Cost-effectiveness of a supplementary class-based exercise program in the treatment of knee osteoarthritis. Int J Technol Assess Health Care. 2006;22(1):84–9.
38. Juhakoski R, Tenhonen S, Malmivaara A, Kiviniemi V, Anttonen T, Arokoski JP. A pragmatic randomized controlled study of the effectiveness and cost consequences of exercise therapy in hip osteoarthritis. Clin rehabil. 2011;25(4):370–83.
39. Hurley MV, Walsh NE, Mitchell H, Nicholas J, Patel A. Long-term outcomes and costs of an integrated rehabilitation program for chronic knee pain: a pragmatic, cluster randomized, controlled trial. Arthritis Care Res. 2012;64(2):238–47.
40. Rees K, Taylor RS, Singh S, Coats AJ, Ebrahim S. Exercise based rehabilitation for heart failure. Cochrane Database Syst Rev. 2004;3:CD003331.
41. Church J, Goodall S, Norman R, Haas M. An economic evaluation of community and residential aged care falls prevention strategies in NSW. N S W Public Health Bull. 2011;22(3–4):60–8.
42. Imamura M, Abrams P, Bain C, Buckley B, Cardozo L, Cody J, Cook J, Eustice S, Glazener C, Grant A, et al. Systematic review and economic modelling of the effectiveness and cost-effectiveness of non-surgical treatments for women with stress urinary incontinence. Health Technol Assess (Winch Eng). 2010;14(40):1–188. iii-iv.
43. Dansk Hoftealloplastik Register. Årsrapport 2013. . In: Dækker fra 1 januar til 31december 2012 Opgørelseperiode fra 1 januar 2012 til 31 December 2012 Edited by Overgaard SP, A.B. www.dhr.dk; 2013.
44. Dansk Knæalloplastikregister. Årsrapport 2013. Administrativt ekstrakt. . In: Kvalitetsindikatorer for operationer foretaget i perioden 2008–2012 Den fulde rapport dækker perioden 01011997 – 31122012 Edited by Pedersen A, B.; Haagen Hjelm, A.; Odgaard, A. www.dkar.dk; 2013.
45. Peter WF, Dekker J, Tilbury C, Tordoir RL, Verdegaal SHM, Onstenk R, Bénard MR, Vehmeijer SB, Fiocco M, Vermeulen HM, et al. The association between comorbidities and pain, physical function and quality of life following hip and knee arthroplasty. Rheumatol Int. 2015;1–9.
46. Kirkness CS, Yu J, Asche CV. The effect on comorbidity and pain in patients with osteoarthritis. J Pain Palliat Care Pharmacother. 2008;22(4):336–48.
47. Yeh HJ, Chou YJ, Yang NP, Cheng CC, Huang N. Physical therapy reduces coronary artery disease and dyslipidemia among osteoarthritis patients: a nationwide database study. Arch Phys Med Rehabil. 2015;97:8–16.
48. Skou ST, Odgaard A, Rasmussen JO, Roos EM. Group education and exercise is feasible in knee and hip osteoarthritis. DanMed J. 2012;59(12):A4554.

49. Ministeriet for sundhed og forebyggelse. Takstsystem 2012. http://sundhedsdatastyrelsen.dk/-/media/sds/filer/finansiering-og-afregning/takster/2012/takstsystem2012.pdf. In.; 2012.
50. Vissers MM, Bussmann JB, Verhaar JAN, Arends LR, Furlan AD, Reijman M. Recovery of physical functioning after total Hip arthroplasty: systematic review and meta-analysis of the literature. Phys Ther. 2011;91(5):615–29.
51. Hopley CDJ, Crossett LS, Chen AF. Long-term clinical outcomes and survivorship after total knee arthroplasty using a rotating platform knee prosthesis: a meta-analysis. J Arthroplast. 2013;28(1):68–77. e63.
52. The National Institute for Health and Clinical Excellence. Methods for the development of NICE public health guidance (third edition). In., 3rd edn. https://www.nice.org.uk/process/pmg4/chapter/introduction; 2012.
53. Kjellberg J, Kehlet H: A nationwide analysis of socioeconomic outcomes after hip and knee replacement. Dan Med J 2016, 63 (8).

Permissions

All chapters in this book were first published in MD, by BioMed Central; hereby published with permission under the Creative Commons Attribution License or equivalent. Every chapter published in this book has been scrutinized by our experts. Their significance has been extensively debated. The topics covered herein carry significant findings which will fuel the growth of the discipline. They may even be implemented as practical applications or may be referred to as a beginning point for another development.

The contributors of this book come from diverse backgrounds, making this book a truly international effort. This book will bring forth new frontiers with its revolutionizing research information and detailed analysis of the nascent developments around the world.

We would like to thank all the contributing authors for lending their expertise to make the book truly unique. They have played a crucial role in the development of this book. Without their invaluable contributions this book wouldn't have been possible. They have made vital efforts to compile up to date information on the varied aspects of this subject to make this book a valuable addition to the collection of many professionals and students.

This book was conceptualized with the vision of imparting up-to-date information and advanced data in this field. To ensure the same, a matchless editorial board was set up. Every individual on the board went through rigorous rounds of assessment to prove their worth. After which they invested a large part of their time researching and compiling the most relevant data for our readers.

The editorial board has been involved in producing this book since its inception. They have spent rigorous hours researching and exploring the diverse topics which have resulted in the successful publishing of this book. They have passed on their knowledge of decades through this book. To expedite this challenging task, the publisher supported the team at every step. A small team of assistant editors was also appointed to further simplify the editing procedure and attain best results for the readers.

Apart from the editorial board, the designing team has also invested a significant amount of their time in understanding the subject and creating the most relevant covers. They scrutinized every image to scout for the most suitable representation of the subject and create an appropriate cover for the book.

The publishing team has been an ardent support to the editorial, designing and production team. Their endless efforts to recruit the best for this project, has resulted in the accomplishment of this book. They are a veteran in the field of academics and their pool of knowledge is as vast as their experience in printing. Their expertise and guidance has proved useful at every step. Their uncompromising quality standards have made this book an exceptional effort. Their encouragement from time to time has been an inspiration for everyone.

The publisher and the editorial board hope that this book will prove to be a valuable piece of knowledge for researchers, students, practitioners and scholars across the globe.

List of Contributors

Liang-Tseng Kuo
Division of Sports Medicine, Department of Orthopedic Surgery, Chang Gung Memorial Hospital, Chiayi, Taiwan
Centre for Evidence-Based Medicine, Chang Gung Memorial Hospital, Chiayi, Taiwan
Chang Gung University of Science and Technology, Chiayi, Taiwan

Wei-Hsiu Hsu
Division of Sports Medicine, Department of Orthopedic Surgery, Chang
Gung Memorial Hospital, Chiayi, Taiwan
College of Medicine, Chang Gung University, Taoyuan, Taiwan

Ching-Chi Chi
Centre for Evidence-Based Medicine, Chang Gung Memorial Hospital, Chiayi, Taiwan
College of Medicine, Chang Gung University, Taoyuan, Taiwan
Department of Dermatology, Chang Gung Memorial Hospital, Linkou, 5, Fuxing St, Guishan Dist, Taoyuan 33305, Taiwan

Jae Chul Yoo
Department of Orthopedic Surgery, College of Medicine, Samsung Medical Center, Sungkyunkwan University School of Medicine, 81 Irwon-ro, Gangnam-gu, Seoul 135-710, Republic of Korea

Han Ting Wang, Josée Fafard and Stéphane Ahern
Department of Internal medicine and Critical Care Medicine, Centre Integre Universitaire de Sante et Services Sociaux (CIUSSS) de l'est de l'île de Montréal, Hopital Maisonneuve-Rosemont, 5415 boul. l'Assomption, H1T 2M4, Montreal, Quebec, Canada

Pascal-André Vendittoli
Department of Surgery, Centre Integre Universitaire de Sante et Services Sociaux (CIUSSS) de l'est de l'île de Montréal, Hôpital Maisonneuve-Rosemont, 5415 boul. l'Assomption, H1T 2M4, Montreal, Quebec, Canada

Paul Hebert
Departments of Medicine and Critical Care Medicine and Centre de recherche, Centre hospitalier de l'Université de Montréal (CRCHUM), 900 St-Denis, H2X 0A9, Montréal, Québec, Canada

Sophie Moerman, Nina M. C. Mathijssen, Dieu D. Niesten and Tim L. Molenaar
Department of Orthopaedics, Reinier de Graaf Group, Reinier de Graafweg 5, 2625 AD Delft, The Netherlands

Roeland Riedijk
Tergooi hospital, Hilversum, The Netherlands

Willard J. Rijnberg
Rijnstate Hospital, Arnhem, The Netherlands

Sander Koëter and Keetie Kremers van de Hei
Canisius Wilhelmina Hospital, Nijmegen, The Netherlands

Wim E. Tuinebreijer
Department of Surgery/ Traumatology, Erasmus MC, Rotterdam, The Netherlands

Rob G. H. H. Nelissen
Leiden University Medical Center, Leiden, The Netherlands

Anne J. H. Vochteloo
Centre for Orthopedic Surgery OCON, Hengelo, The Netherlands

Weiping Ji, Qiuping Fan and Bo Wang
Department of Orthopaedic Surgery, Lishui City People's Hospital, the Sixth Affiliated Hospital of Wenzhou Medical University, Lishui, China

Xianfeng Lin, Ruoxia Zhang, Pan Tang, Jian Mo, Xinyi Teng, Shunwu Fan, Jianfeng Zhang, Shuai Chen and Kangmao Huang
Department of Orthopaedic Surgery, Sir Run Run Shaw Hospital, Medical College of Zhejiang University, Hangzhou, China

Deborah Kennedy
Sunnybrook Holland Orthopaedic and Arthritic Centre, 43 Wellesley Street East, Toronto, ON M4Y 1H1, Canada
School of Rehabilitation Science, McMaster University, 1400 Main St. W, Hamilton, ON L8S 1C7, Canada
Department of Physical Therapy, University of Toronto, 500 University Avenue, Toronto, ON M5G 1V7, Canada

Amy Wainwright
Sunnybrook Holland Orthopaedic and Arthritic Centre, 43 Wellesley Street East, Toronto, ON M4Y 1H1, Canada
Department of Physical Therapy, University of Toronto, 500 University Avenue, Toronto, ON M5G 1V7, Canada

Lucy Pereira and Susan Robarts
Sunnybrook Holland Orthopaedic and Arthritic Centre, 43 Wellesley Street East, Toronto, ON M4Y 1H1, Canada

Patricia Dickson
Sunnybrook Holland Orthopaedic and Arthritic Centre, 43 Wellesley Street East, Toronto, ON M4Y 1H1, Canada
Department of Occupational Science and Occupational Therapy, University of Toronto, 500 University Avenue, Toronto, ON M5G 1V7, Canada

Jennifer Christian
Centre for Addiction and Mental Health, 33 Russell Street, Toronto, ON M5S 2S1, Canada

Fiona Webster
Institute of Health Policy Management and Evaluation, Dalla Lana School of Public Health, University of Toronto, 155 College Street, Toronto, ON M5T 3M7, Canada

Jasvinder A. Singh
University of Alabama at Birmingham, Birmingham, AL, USA
Birmingham Veterans Affairs Medical Center, Birmingham, AL, USA

Michael Dohm
Department of Orthopaedic Surgery, University of Arizona, Tucson, AZ, USA

Chen Wang, Chen Zhang, De-Lin Liu, Wen-Wen Tong, Chong-Ru He, Xuan Huang and Wei-Dong Xu
Department of Orthopedics, Changhai Hospital, Second Military Medical University, No. 168, Changhai Road, Shanghai 200433, China

Xiaozhen Han and Guiqing Gong
Department of Orthopedics, Jinan Zhangqiu District Hospital of Traditional Chinese Medicine, No. 1463 Xiushui Street, Mingshui subdistrict office, Zhangqiu district, Jinan 250200, Shandong, China

Naili Han
Clinical Laboratory, Jinan Zhangqiu District Hospital of Traditional Chinese Medicine, No. 1463 Xiushui Street, Mingshui subdistrict office, Zhangqiu district, Jinan 250200, Shandong, China

Mei Liu
Department of Intensive Care Unit, Wuhan No.1 Hospital, No.215 Zhongshan Ave, Wuhan 430022, Hubei, China

Akihiko Takeuchi, Norio Yamamoto, Katsuhiro Hayashi, Hidenori Matsubara, Hiroaki Kimura, Shinji Miwa, Takashi Higuchi, Kensaku Abe, Yuta Taniguchi and Hiroyuki Tsuchiya
Department of Orthopaedic Surgery, Kanazawa University Graduate School of Medical Sciences, 13-1 Takara-machi, Kanazawa 920-8641, Japan

Dirk Zajonz and Christoph Josten
Department of Orthopaedic Surgery, Trauma Surgery and Plastic Surgery, University Hospital Leipzig, Liebigstrasse 20, D-04103 Leipzig, Germany
ZESBO –Zentrum zur Erforschung der Stuetz- und Bewegungsorgane, Semmelweisstrasse 14, D-04103 Leipzig, Germany

Undine Birke, Mohamed Ghanem, Andreas Roth and Johannes K. M. Fakler
Department of Orthopaedic Surgery, Trauma Surgery and Plastic Surgery, University Hospital Leipzig, Liebigstrasse 20, D-04103 Leipzig, Germany

Torsten Prietzel
Department of Orthopaedics and Trauma Surgery, HELIOS Clinic Blankenhain, Wirthstrasse 5, D-99444 Blankenhain, Germany
ZESBO - Zentrum zur Erforschung der Stuetz- und Bewegungsorgane, Semmelweisstrasse 14, D-04103 Leipzig, Germany

Christoph Ihle, Christoph Weiß, Ulrich Stöckle, Christian Bahrs, Andreas Nüssler and Anna Janine Schreiner
Siegfried Weller Institute for Trauma Research, BG Trauma Center Tübingen, Eberhard Karls University Tübingen, Schnarrenbergstrasse 95, 72076 Tübingen, Germany

Gunnar Blumenstock
Department of Clinical Epidemiology and Applied Biometry, Eberhard Karls University Tübingen, Silcherstrasse 5, 72076 Tubingen, Germany

Björn Gunnar Ochs
Department of Orthopedics and Trauma Surgery, Medical Center, Albert-Ludwigs-University of Freiburg, Faculty of Medicine, Freiburg, Germany

Alf Inge Hellevik
The HUNT Research Centre, Department of Public Health and Nursing, Faculty of Medicine and Health Sciences, Norwegian University of Science and Technology (NTNU), Levanger, Norway
Division of Orthopaedic Surgery, Oslo University Hospital, Oslo, Norway

Marianne Bakke Johnsen, Kjersti Storheim and John Anker Zwart
Division of Orthopaedic Surgery, Oslo University Hospital, Oslo, Norway
Research and Communication Unit for Musculoskeletal Health, Division of Clinical Neuroscience, Oslo University Hospital, Oslo, Norway
Faculty of Medicine, University of Oslo, Oslo, Norway

Arnulf Langhammer
The HUNT Research Centre, Department of Public Health and Nursing, Faculty of Medicine and Health Sciences, Norwegian University of Science and Technology (NTNU), Levanger, Norway

Anne Marie Fenstad
The Norwegian Arthroplasty Register, Department of Orthopedic Surgery, Haukeland University Hospital, Bergen, Norway

Ove Furnes
The Norwegian Arthroplasty Register, Department of Orthopedic Surgery, Haukeland University Hospital, Bergen, Norway
Department of Clinical Medicine, Institute of Medicine and Dentistry, University of Bergen, Bergen, Norway

Gunnar Flugsrud
Division of Orthopaedic Surgery, Oslo University Hospital, Oslo, Norway

Lars Nordsletten
Division of Orthopaedic Surgery, Oslo University Hospital, Oslo, Norway
Faculty of Medicine, University of Oslo, Oslo, Norway

Sandra Mathews, Nakita Frater and Frank-Jakobus Rühli
Institute of Evolutionary Medicine (IEM), University of Zurich, Winterthurerstrasse 190, CH-8057 Zurich, Switzerland

Marco Burkhard, Ingeborg Franke, Helena Bischofberger and Oliver Ullrich
Division of Gross Anatomy, Institute of Anatomy, University of Zurich, Zurich, Switzerland

Nabil Serrano, Karl Link and Martin Häusler
Institute of Evolutionary Medicine (IEM), University of Zurich, Winterthurerstrasse 190, CH-8057 Zurich, Switzerland
Division of Gross Anatomy, Institute of Anatomy, University of Zurich, Zurich, Switzerland

Florian M. Buck
Medical Radiology Institute, Schulthess Clinic, Zurich, Switzerland
Medical Faculty, University of Zurich, Zurich, Switzerland

Dominic Gascho and Michael Thali
Institute of Forensic Medicine, University of Zurich, Zurich, Switzerland

Steffen Serowy
Institute of Neuroradiology, University Hospital Magdeburg, Magdeburg, Germany

Magdalena Müller-Gerbl
Musculoskeletal Research Unit, Department of Biomedicine, University of Basel, Basel, Switzerland

Gareth Harper
Shoulder Unit, Queen Alexandra Hospital, Portsmouth, UK

Ford Qureshi
Shoulder Unit, Doncaster Royal Infirmary, Doncaster, UK

Thomas Böni
Institute of Evolutionary Medicine (IEM), University of Zurich, Winterthurerstrasse 190, CH-8057 Zurich, Switzerland
Technical Orthopedics Unit, University Hospital Balgrist, Zurich, Switzerland

Hans-Rudolf Bloch
Shoulder Surgery Unit, Ospedale Civico, Lugano, Switzerland

Elisabeth Eppler
Division of Gross Anatomy, Institute of Anatomy, University of Zurich, Zurich, Switzerland
Institute of Neuroradiology, University Hospital Magdeburg, Magdeburg, Germany
Musculoskeletal Research Unit, Department of Biomedicine, University of Basel, Basel, Switzerland

Bill Reynolds and Peter Schoch
Physiotherapy Department, Barwon Health, Geelong, VIC 3220, Australia

Nick Maister, Shaun Waring and Andrew Thomson
Orthopaedic Department, Barwon Health, Geelong, Victoria 3220, Australia

Sally Beattie
Barwon Centre for Orthopaedic Research and Education (B-CORE), St John of God Hospital and Barwon Health, Geelong, VIC 3220, Australia

Stephen D. Gill
Physiotherapy Department, Barwon Health, Geelong, VIC 3220, Australia
Barwon Centre for Orthopaedic Research and Education (B-CORE), St John of God Hospital and Barwon Health, Geelong, VIC 3220, Australia
School of Medicine, Deakin University, Waurn Ponds, VIC 3220, Australia

Richard S. Page
Orthopaedic Department, Barwon Health, Geelong, Victoria 3220, Australia
Barwon Centre for Orthopaedic Research and Education (B-CORE), St John of God Hospital and Barwon Health, Geelong, VIC 3220, Australia
School of Medicine, Deakin University, Waurn Ponds, VIC 3220, Australia

Perla J. Marang-van de Mheen
Department of Medical Decision Making, Leiden University Medical Center, J10-S, 2300 RC Leiden, The Netherlands

Ellie Bragan Turner
Dr Foster Ltd, London, UK

Susan Liew
Department of Orthopaedic Surgery, Alfred Hospital, Melbourne, Australia

Ton Tran
Department of Orthopaedic Surgery, Monash Health, Dandenong, Australia

Nora Mutalima
Department of Orthopaedic Surgery, Monash Health, Dandenong, Australia
Department of Surgery, Monash University, Dandenong, Australia

Sten Rasmussen
Orthopaedic Surgery Research Unit, Aalborg University Hospital, Aalborg, Denmark
Department of Clinical Medicine, Aalborg University, Aalborg, Denmark

Rob G. H. H. Nelissen
Department of Orthopaedic Surgery, Leiden University Medical Center, Leiden, The Netherlands

Andrew Gordon
Department of Orthopaedic Surgery, Sheffield Teaching Hospitals NHS trust, Sheffield, UK

Yuan Zhu and Xiang-yang Xu
Department of Orthopedics, Shanghai Ruijin Hospital, Shanghai Jiaotong University School of Medicine, Shanghai 200025, China

Yang Xu
Department of Orthopedics, Shanghai Ruijin Hospital, Shanghai Jiaotong University School of Medicine, Shanghai 200025, China
Shanghai Institute of Traumatology and Orthopedics, Shanghai, China

Juan Shiguetomi-Medina, Jorgen Baas, Kjeld Soballe and Ole Rahbek
Orthopaedic Research Laboratory, Department of Orthopaedics, Aarhus
University Hospital, Norrebrogade 44, Building 1A, DK-8000 Aarhus, Denmark

Thomas Jakobsen and Søren Kold
Orthopaedic Research Laboratory, Department of Orthopaedics, Aarhus
University Hospital, Norrebrogade 44, Building 1A, DK-8000 Aarhus, Denmark
Department of Orthopaedics, Aalborg University Hospital, Aalborg, Denmark

Jasvinder A. Singh
University of Alabama at Birmingham, 510 20th Street S, Faculty Office Tower 805B, Birmingham, AL 35294, USA
Birmingham Veterans Affairs Medical Center, 700 19th St S, Birmingham, AL 35233, USA

Michelle Dowsey and Peter F. Choong
Department of Surgery, University of Melbourne, St. Vincent's Hospital, Melbourne, Australia

Lin-nan Wang, Bo-wen Hu, Lei Wang, Yue-ming Song, Xi Yang, Li-min Liu and Hao Liu
Department of Orthopedics, West China Hospital, Sichuan University, 37 Guoxue Rd, Chengdu 610041, China
Jenni N. E. Harjula and Ville Äärimaa Department of Orthopedics and Traumatology, Turku University Hospital, University of Turku, Turku, Finland

Juha Paloneva
Department of Surgery, Central Finland Hospital, Jyväskylä, Finland

Jaason Haapakoski
National Institute for Health and Welfare, Helsinki, Finland

Juha Kukkonen
Department of Surgery, Division of Orthopaedic and Trauma Surgery, Satakunta Central Hospital and University of Turku, Turku, Finland

U. Plenge and B. M. Biccard
Department of Anaesthesia and Perioperative Medicine, Groote Schuur
Hospital and Faculty of Health Sciences, University of Cape Town, Cape Town, South Africa

M. B. Nortje
Department of Orthopaedic Surgery, Groote Schuur Hospital and Faculty of Health Sciences, University of Cape Town, Cape Town, South Africa

L. C. Marais
Department of Orthopaedic surgery, School of Clinical Medicine, University of KwaZulu-Natal, Pietermaritzburg, South Africa

J. D. Jordaan
Department of Orthopaedic Surgery, Tygerberg Medical School, University of Stellenbosch, Cape Town, South Africa

P. Rowe
Department of Orthopaedic surgery, Victoria Hospital, Cape Town, South Africa

J. G. van der Walt
Department of Anaesthesia, Victoria Hospital, Cape Town, South Africa

R. Isaacs Noordien
Department of Physiotherapy, Victoria Hospital, Cape Town, South Africa

A. Theron
Department of Anaesthesiology and Critical Care, Tygerberg Academic Hospital, University of Stellenbosch, Cape Town, South Africa

Samantha Bay and Neil McLean
M304, School of Psychological Science, The University of Western Australia, 35 Stirling Highway, Perth, Western Australia 6009, Australia

Lukas Kuster
Sir Charles Gairdner Hospital, Hospital Ave, Perth, Western Australia 6009, Australia

Michelle Byrnes
Perron Institute for Neurological and Translational Science, The University of Western Australia, RR Block, QEII Medical Centre, 8 Verdun Street, Perth, Western Australia 6009, Australia

Markus Stefan Kuster
Sir Charles Gairdner Hospital, Hospital Ave, Perth, Western Australia 6009, Australia
Medical School, The University of Western Australia, 35 Stirling Hwy, Perth, Western Australia 6009, Australia

Mirko Brandes
Department of Prevention and Evaluation, Unit Applied Health Intervention
Research, Leibniz Institute for Prevention Research and Epidemiology - BIPS GmbH, Achterstraße 30, 28359 Bremen, Germany

Norman Wirsik
Department of Biometry and Data Management, Unit Statistical Modelling of Primary Data, Leibniz Institute for Prevention Research and Epidemiology - BIPS GmbH, Bremen, Germany

Peter F. Choong
Department of Surgery, University of Melbourne, Melbourne, Australia
Department of Surgery, St. Vincent's Hospital, Melbourne, Australia

Jörg Heimsoth and Bernd Möhring
Orthopaedic Department, Rehabilitation Centre Oldenburg, Oldenburg, Germany

Marion Lindner, Anett Keller-Pliessnig, Per Teigelack, Martin Teufel and Sefik Tagay
Department of Psychosomatic Medicine and Psychotherapy, University of Duisburg-Essen, Virchowstraße 174, 45147 Essen, Germany

Olaf Nosseir
Department of General, Orthopedic and Accident Surgery, Sankt Josef-Hospital GmbH, In der Hees 4, 46509 Xanten, Germany

Anne Jacobsen, Frank Seehaus, Yutong Hong, Han Cao and Raimund Forst
Department of Orthopaedic Surgery, Friedrich-Alexander-Universität Erlangen-Nürnberg (FAU), Rathsberger Str. 57, 91054 Erlangen, Germany

Alexander Schuh
Muskuloskelettales Zentrum, Klinikum Neumarkt, Nürnberger Str. 12, 92318 Neumarkt i. d. OPf, Germany

Stefan Sesselmann
Department of Orthopaedic Surgery, Friedrich-Alexander-Universität Erlangen-Nürnberg (FAU), Rathsberger Str. 57, 91054 Erlangen, Germany
Institute for Medical Technology, Ostbayerische Technische Hochschule Amberg-Weiden, Hetzenrichter Weg 15, 92637 Weiden, Germany

Hanna Niehoff
Institute of Sports Science, Oldenburg University, Oldenburg, Germany

Linda Fernandes
Department of Orthopaedic Surgery and Traumatology, Odense University Hospital, Odense, Denmark
Department of Rehabilitation, Odense University Hospital, Sdr. Boulevard 29, 5000 Odense C, Denmark

Ewa M. Roos
Research Unit for Musculoskeletal Function and Physiotherapy, Institute of Sports Science and Clinical Biomechanics, University of Southern Denmark, Odense, Denmark

Søren Overgaard
Department of Orthopaedic Surgery and Traumatology, Odense University Hospital, Odense, Denmark
Department of Clinical Research, University of Southern Denmark, Odense, Denmark

Allan Villadsen
Department of Orthopaedic Surgery and Traumatology, Odense University Hospital, Odense, Denmark

Rikke Søgaard
Department of Public Health, Aarhus University, Aarhus, Denmark
Department of Clinical Medicine, Aarhus University, Aarhus, Denmark

Index

www.ingramcontent.com/pod-product-compliance
Lightning Source LLC
LaVergne TN
LVHW080708210926
848485LV00003B/435